T5-BBO-902

PENICILLIN

ITS PRACTICAL APPLICATION

Under the General Editorship of

PROFESSOR SIR ALEXANDER FLEMING
M.B., B.S., F.R.C.P., F.R.C.S., F.R.S.

PROFESSOR OF BACTERIOLOGY IN THE UNIVERSITY OF LONDON,
ST. MARY'S HOSPITAL, LONDON

THE BLAKISTON COMPANY
Philadelphia
1946

Published July 1946

PRINTED IN GREAT BRITAIN
CHAPEL RIVER PRESS, ANDOVER, HANTS
6.46

PREFACE

THE publishers approached me to write a book for them on penicillin. This request I had to refuse for two very good reasons: first I had too many commitments to spare the time to do justice to such a book, and secondly it would have been impossible for me, a laboratory worker, to place penicillin therapy in its proper perspective relative to other forms of medical and surgical treatment in a great variety of conditions.

It was agreed, therefore, that a number of authorities should be invited to contribute articles on different aspects of penicillin therapy, and almost without exception they consented. This book, therefore, is not a continuous textbook but a series of independent contributions giving each author's view on the use of penicillin therapy in a disease or in infections of some region of the body. This being so there is inevitably a certain amount of overlapping, but that is not a disadvantage. There are some slight differences of opinion between different authors, but that may be a distinct advantage. Penicillin therapy is very young and is rapidly evolving and has not as yet crystallized sufficiently for complete agreement as to dosage and methods of administration.

It is likely that in a year or two such further advances will have been made and fresh developments taken place that there will have to be some reconsideration of a number of the statements put forward by the various authors. This series of articles gives a fair presentation of penicillin therapy as it exists today.

The authors were instructed that this book was not intended to be merely a *résumé* of all the work which had been done on penicillin but that its object was to tell the practitioner how to use penicillin to best advantage when it should become readily available to the whole medical profession.

In addition to the more purely medical sections there are chapters on the use of penicillin in dental and veterinary surgery. These chapters should be of interest to medical practitioners whose mental outlook is not confined within too narrow limits.

Penicillin therapy to some extent has been influenced by the fact that the drug has hitherto been in short supply and many of the methods used have been designed to economize in its use.

There is ample proof, however, that it is to all intents and purposes a non-toxic substance and when there is a plentiful supply the dosage can be increased in many cases with advantage. It is almost impossible to give an overdose in the ordinary sense of the word. It is certainly possible to give much more than is necessary but in days of plenty that will not be a serious crime. The guiding rule should be always to give enough; it is much better to give more than enough than too little. It may be that gonorrhoea can be cured in almost every case with 100,000 units or even less if the doses are spaced out in such a way as to be inconvenient for the ordinary civilian sufferer but, by an increase in the amount of penicillin used, the same result can be achieved without inconvenience. It will surely be wrong to persist in a system irksome to the patient merely to economize in penicillin when there is plenty. Such a system, especially in gonorrhoea, leads to default in treatment, incomplete cure and to further spread of the disease.

The development of penicillin on a large scale has been a wonderful story. Governments, manufacturers, scientists and everyone down to the most humble workmen have played their part. There was the stimulus of war and a large proportion of the workers in every grade had near relatives in the Fighting Forces. Penicillin had been shown to increase considerably a wounded man's chance of recovery and to lessen his suffering materially. The workers felt that they were doing something for their own kith and kin and in this they were assisted by the authorities. A reproduction is given of one of the many posters displayed on the sites where factories were being erected to manufacture penicillin.

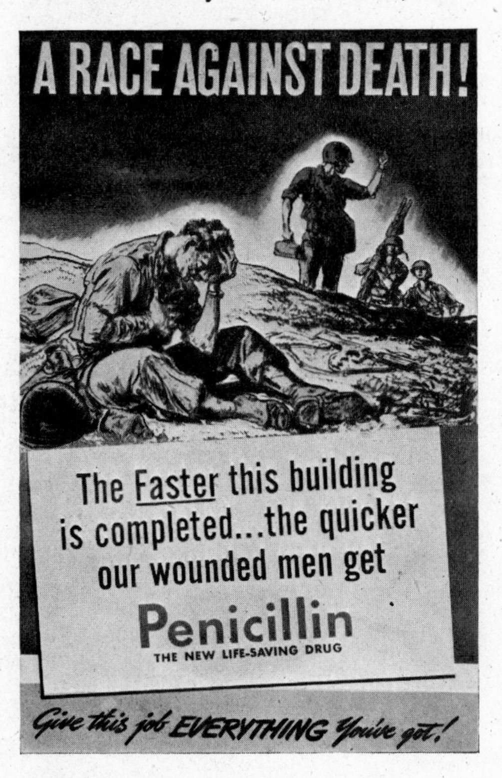

There is also reproduced the small pamphlet with which the workers in penicillin factories in England received their pay packets. All this helped to give an extra spur without which there would not have been sufficient penicillin for the wounded when D-day arrived. It was largely due to the American factories that this happy state of affairs was reached so soon and we in Great Britain have to thank them. Without their help our wounded during the invasion of Europe would have been woefully short of penicillin, but we can look back with a certain amount of satisfaction to the earlier work in England without which there would have been no penicillin for anyone.

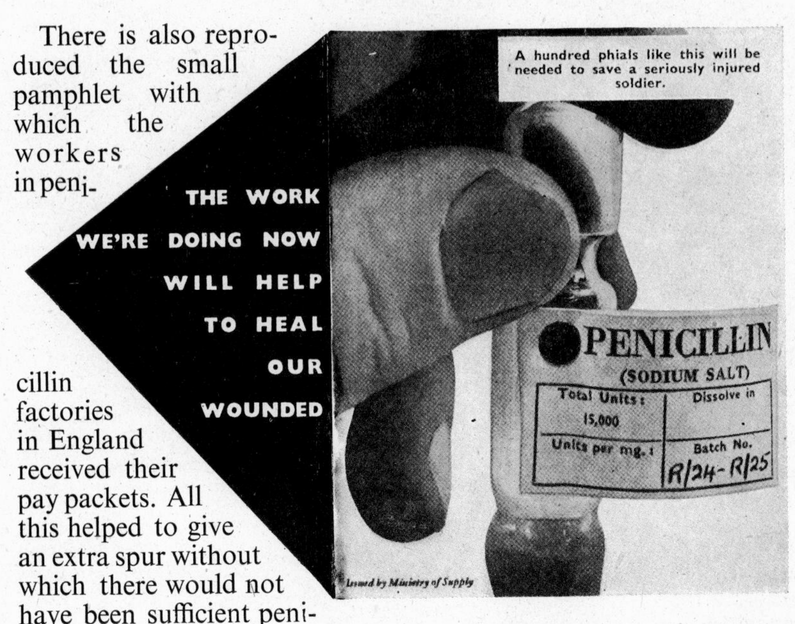

Press publicity in the last few years has given many people the idea that penicillin is a panacea, but throughout the book it is emphasized that penicillin is not a "cure-all". There are many of our most common ailments on which it has no effect. When the supply of penicillin is plentiful many patients will demand it from their doctor for degenerative nerve conditions and the like for which there is not any possibility of its doing good. Perhaps this volume will help the doctor to resist the pressure.

The remarkable success of penicillin has stimulated research into substances produced by moulds and bacteria in the hope that something even better may be found. Many antibacterial agents have been discovered and some of them will some day be used in medical practice. The time has not yet arrived, however, when any of these antibiotics should be included in a book such as this.

My own contribution to this book is small but the whole

volume gives the views of many experienced and eminent men who have worked with penicillin here in Great Britain, and I think we may say that it fairly represents the present state of our knowledge. It is a general guide to the potentialities of the drug and it should be of use to the senior student and the hospital resident medical and surgical officers as well as to the more experienced practitioner. The specialist who wants more detailed information must necessarily refer to the literature pertaining to his speciality. I hope this book will be useful—I think it will.

July, 1946 ALEXANDER FLEMING

CONTENTS

PAGE

Preface - iii
List of Illustrations - ix
Acknowledgements - xi

GENERAL

HISTORY AND DEVELOPMENT OF PENICILLIN - 1
Sir Alexander Fleming, M.B., B.S., F.R.C.P., F.R.C.S., F.R.S.

CHEMISTRY AND MANUFACTURE OF PENICILLIN - 24
A. L. Bacharach, M.A., F.R.I.C.
B. A. Hems, Ph.D., F.R.I.C.

PHARMACY OF PENICILLIN - 46
H. Berry, B.Sc., Ph.C., Dip. Bact. Lond., F.R.I.C.

PHARMACOLOGY OF PENICILLIN - 59
L. P. Garrod, M.D., F.R.C.P.

BACTERIOLOGICAL CONTROL OF PENICILLIN THERAPY - 76
Sir Alexander Fleming, M.B., B.S., F.R.C.P., F.R.C.S., F.R.S.

METHODS OF ADMINISTRATION - 93
W. Howard Hughes, M.D., B.S.

CLINICAL

PROPHYLACTIC USE OF PENICILLIN - 105
A. E. Porritt, C.B.E., M.Ch., F.R.C.S.
G. A. G. Mitchell, O.B.E., M.B., Ch.M.

GENERALIZED INFECTIONS - 116
R. Vaughan Hudson, F.R.C.S.

BACTERIAL ENDOCARDITIS - 134
Ronald V. Christie, M.D., D.Sc., F.R.C.P.

CHEST INFECTIONS - 141
A. Hope Gosse, M.D., F.R.C.P.

CHEST SURGERY - 150
T. Holmes Sellors, D.M., M.Ch., F.R.C.S.

WOUNDS AND GAS GANGRENE - 162
A. E. Porritt, C.B.E., M.Ch., F.R.C.S.
G. A. G. Mitchell, O.B.E., M.B., Ch.M.

BURNS AND PLASTIC SURGERY - 180
Rainsford Mowlem, F.R.C.S.

ORTHOPAEDIC SURGERY AND FRACTURES - 189
V. H. Ellis, F.R.C.S.

OSTEOMYELITIS - 200
Ian Aird, Ch.M., F.R.C.S.Ed.

PAGE

HAND INFECTIONS - - - - - - - - - - 211
E. C. B. Butler, F.R.C.S.

ABDOMINAL INFECTIONS - - - - - - - - - 229
R. M. Handfield-Jones, M.S., F.R.C.S.

OBSTETRICS AND GYNAECOLOGY - - - - - - - 241
Leslie Williams, M.D., M.S., F.R.C.S., F.R.C.O.G.

SEPSIS NEONATORUM - - - - - - - - - - 252
Donald Paterson, M.D., F.R.C.P.
Martin Bodian, M.D. Vienna, L.R.C.P. & S. Ed.

BRAIN AND MENINGEAL INFECTIONS - - - - - 265
A. Dickson Wright, M.S., F.R.C.S.

VENEREAL DISEASES - - - - - - - - - 278
G. L. M. McElligott, M.R.C.S., L.R.C.P.

OPHTHALMOLOGY - - - - - - - - - - 291
Arnold Sorsby, M.D., F.R.C.S.

OTORHINOLARYNGOLOGY - - - - - - - - - 301
John F. Simpson, F.R.C.S.

DERMATOLOGY - - - - - - - - - - 317
A. C. Roxburgh, M.D., F.R.C.P.

DENTAL AND ORAL INFECTIONS - - - - - - - 324
E. Wilfred Fish, M.D., D.D.Sc., D.Sc.

PENICILLIN IN ANIMAL DISEASES - - - - - - - 337
Reginald Lovell, M.Sc., Ph.D., M.R.C.V.S., D.V.S.M.

PENICILLIN AND THE GENERAL PRACTITIONER - - - 350
G. B. Mitchell-Heggs, O.B.E., M.D., F.R.C.P.

INDEX

LIST OF ILLUSTRATIONS

FIG.		PAGE
1.	Germinated spore of *Penicillium notatum*	1
2.	Colonies of *P. notatum* 2, 3, 4, 5, 6 and 10 days old	2
3.	Typical penicillus of *P. notatum*—	
	(a) Westling's original strain	3
	(b) Fleming's strain	4
4.	Original culture plate on which action of penicillin was observed	5
5.	Inhibited action of *P. notatum* on different bacteria	6
6.	Comparison of diffusibility of penicillin and some other antiseptics	7
7.	Gutter method of demonstrating selective inhibition	8
8.	Lysis of staphylococci under the influence of penicillin	9
9.	The selective action of penicillin	10
10.	Effect of phenol on bacteria and leucocytes	11
11.	Effects of penicillin on *B. welchii*	12
12.	Effect of penicillin on gonococcus	13
13.	Penicillin flask	34
14.	Sterilization	35
15.	Cooling sterilized penicillin flasks	36
16.	Inoculation	37
17.	Inoculation room	38
18.	Incubation	39
19.	Deep fermentation—lower section of large vertical fermentation vats for deep culture	40
20.	Deep fermentation—middle section of large vertical fermentation vats for deep culture	41
21.	Concentration	42
22.	Extraction	43
23.	Freeze-drying	44
24.	Bacteriostatic power of serum following injection of 15,000 units of penicillin intravenously, intramuscularly and subcutaneously	60
25.	Bacteriostatic power of serum following intramuscular injection of 50,000 and 100,000 units of penicillin	61
26.	Average results of bacteriostatic estimations of serum after single intramuscular injections	62
27.	Result of rapidly repeated intravenous injections of penicillin	63
28.	Result of rapidly repeated intramuscular injections of penicillin	64
29.	Assay plate. Test organism staphylococcus	77
30.	Typical curve relating diameter zone of inhibition with concentration of penicillin solution causing it	78

FIG. PAGE

31. Estimation of penicillin in serum by slide cell method – – – 81
32. Titrations in capillary tubes using streptococcus as test organism and human blood as indicator – – – – – – – – – 82
33. Assay of penicillin in sputum 12 hours after inhalation – – – 85
34. Test of sensitivity to penicillin in the primary culture – – – 86
35. Simple method of discovering penicillinase producing bacteria – – 88
36. Demonstration of the action of penicillinase on agar plate – – 89
37. Demonstration of the action of penicillinase on agar plate – – 90
38. Bacteriostatic effect of penicillin contained in pus collected 24 hours after injection into an axillary abscess – – – – – – – – 91
39. Eudrip No. 1. A modification of the standard transfusion apparatus for continuous intravenous or intramuscular administration – – 94
40. Eudrip No. 3. A continuous drip apparatus giving simpler control than earlier models – – – – – – – – – 94
41. A clock drip for continuous administration of small volumes of penicillin 96
42. The Collinson apparatus for administration of atomized penicillin – 99
43. Hand atomizer with mask suitable for either systemic administration or for the treatment of lung conditions – – – – – – 101
44. Catheter in antero-posterior and lateral views traversing the wound in front of the finger and passing the whole length of the tendon sheath 219
45. Case of suppurative tenosynovitis showing range of movement of the fingers after treatment – – – – – – – – 221
46. Case of suppurative tenosynovitis showing almost full movement of the fingers after treatment – – – – – – – – 222
47. Osteomyelitis of the head of the fifth metacarpal with necrosis of a portion of the bone – – – – – – – – – 224
48. Reformation of the head of the fifth metacarpal bone – – – 225
49. Congenital syphilis. X-ray photograph before treatment – – – 260
50. Congenital syphilis. X-ray photograph after treatment – – – 261
51. Osteomyelitis of skull. Before treatment – – – – – – 266
52. Osteomyelitis of skull. After treatment – – – – – – 267
53. Extradural abscess tracking over the base of the skull – – – 268
54. Spreading osteomyelitis of the skull illustrating spread of infection – 269
55. In aural cases abscesses may be present both above and below the tentorium – – – – – – – – – – – – 270
56. Illustrating how an infection in the frontal sinus may cause single or multiple abscesses in the brain – – – – – – – 271
57. Multiple abscesses of the brain secondary to thoracic suppuration – 272
58. Introduction of penicillin in pneumococcal meningitis by means of catheter passed over surface of brain after aspirating the ventricle – 274
59. Sites for introduction of penicillin in cases of meningitis – – – 275

ACKNOWLEDGEMENTS

We wish to express our thanks for permission to reproduce the following illustrations: to the Editors of the *British Journal of Surgery* (Fig. 29), the *Journal of the Royal Institute of Public Health and Hygiene* (Figs. 1, 5, 6, 8, 11 and 12), the *Lancet* (Fig. 32), the *Proceedings of the Royal Society of Medicine* (Figs. 38 and 44); Glaxo Laboratories, Ltd. (Figs. 13 to 16, 18 to 20, 22 and 23); Dr. Bernard Schlesinger (Figs. 49 and 50); Wellcome Foundation, Ltd. (Figs. 17 and 21).

THE BLAKISTON COMPANY.

HISTORY AND DEVELOPMENT OF PENICILLIN

By Sir Alexander Fleming, M.B., B.S., F.R.C.P., F.R.C.S., F.R.S.
Professor of Bacteriology, St. Mary's Hospital, London

INTRODUCTION

The name "penicillin" was given by me in 1929 to an antibacterial substance produced by a mould of the genus *Penicillium*. The nomenclature therefore follows old established custom, for example, digitalin from digitalis, aloin from aloes.

Penicillin belongs to a class of antibacterial substances produced by living organisms which as far back as 1889 were termed antibiotics. This word, although introduced so long ago, fell into

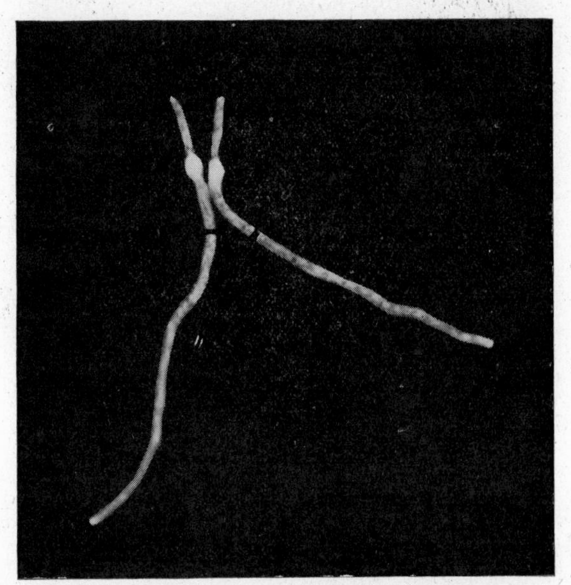

Fig. 1.—Germinated spore of *Penicillium notatum*
(*J. R. Inst. publ. Hlth. Hyg.*)

disuse but has been revived in recent years and serves a useful purpose.

Many instances of micro-organisms producing antibiotic substances have been described since the time of Pasteur but it will serve no useful purpose to detail these. A review of this literature has been given by Florey[1] but none of the older work had any influence on the birth of penicillin.

Before going on to describe the beginnings of penicillin it

would be well to say something of *Penicillium*. Its life history commences as a spore which, when it germinates, produces septate hyphae which grow and branch forming a thick felted colony (see Figs. 1 and 2). Meantime many special reproductive hyphae are produced. Each of these subdivides in a peculiar fashion forming a body (penicillus) resembling a brush or pencil—hence the name. From the terminal branches of these reproductive hyphae spores are budded off (see Figs. 3 (a) and 3 (b)) so that each penicillium colony may liberate millions of spores. These spores are disseminated by air currents or otherwise and, when they fall on a suitable culture medium, they grow out into a

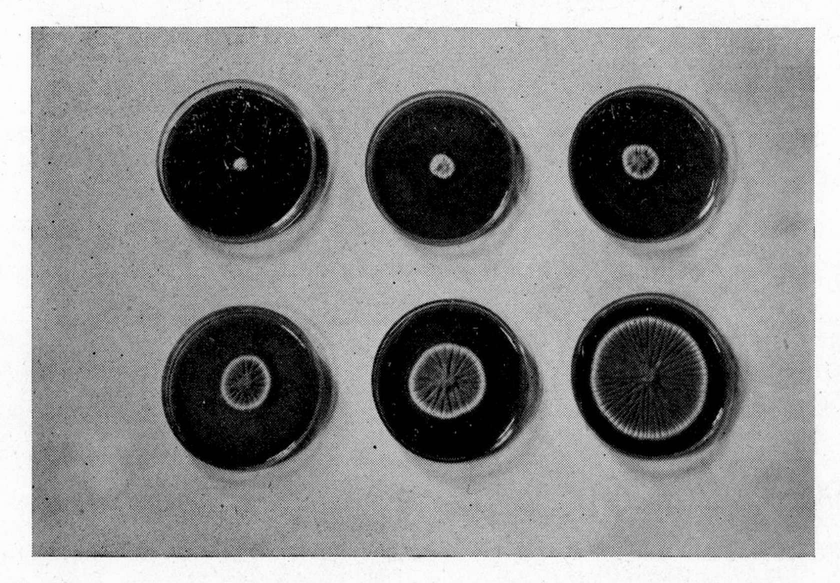

FIG. 2.—Colonies of *P. notatum* 2, 3, 4, 5, 6 and 10 days old

mould colony such as is seen on jam, bread or other organic matter which is sufficiently moist.

The contamination in 1928 of a culture plate by spores of a species of *Penicillium* was the beginning of the study of penicillin. Such contamination is not uncommon in a bacteriological laboratory and is usually regarded as a reflection on the technique of the bacteriologist. Sometimes, however, it is unavoidable, as in this particular instance when the culture plate had to be opened for examination under a dissecting microscope and then left for future examination. When next observed, mould spores which had gained access had developed into a large colony. This in itself did not call for comment but what was very surprising was that the staphylococcal colonies in the neighbourhood of the mould, which had been well developed, were observed now to be showing signs of dissolution (see Fig. 4). This was an extraordinary and unexpected appearance and seemed to demand investigation.*

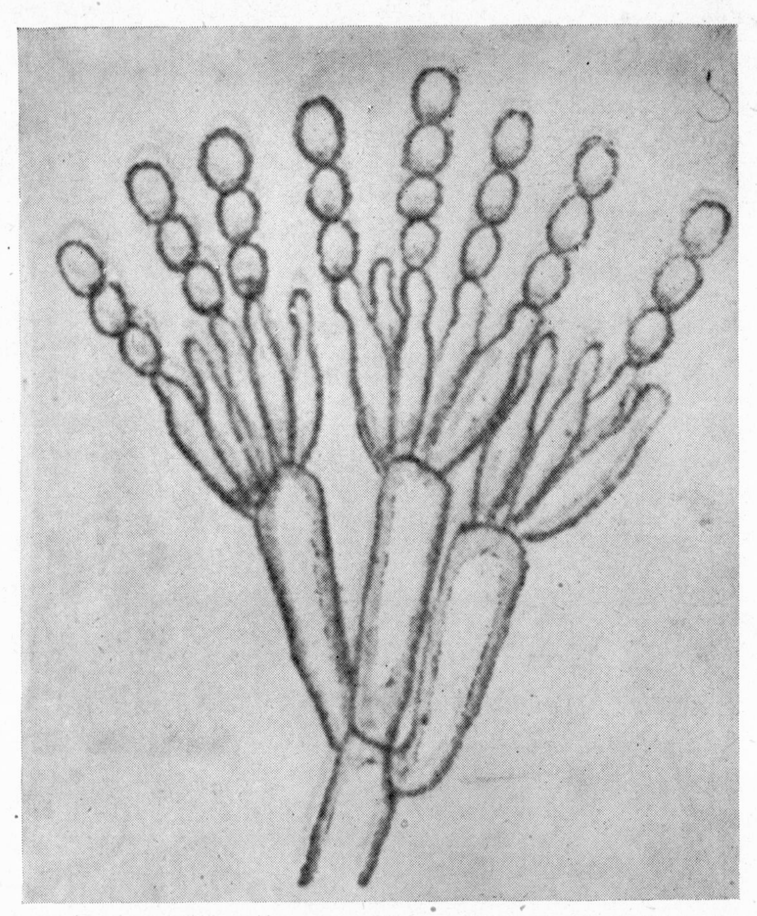

FIG. 3a.—Typical Penicillus of *P. notatum*. Copy of Westling's illustration of original strain isolated in 1911

The mould was therefore isolated in pure culture for further examination. It was found to belong to the genus *Penicillium* but it was not so easy to identify the species. There are some hundreds of species of *Penicillium* and the mycologist attached to St. Mary's Hospital classed it as *P. rubrum*, and in the first publication on penicillin this name appeared. Later work, however, by Raistrick

* This culture plate has been preserved in the author's laboratory at St. Mary's Hospital, London.

and Thom showed that it really was *P. notatum*, a species closely allied to *P. chrysogenum* (Thom). *P. notatum* was first described in 1911 by Westling[2] who discovered it in decaying hyssop in Scandinavia.

Preliminary experiments with the contaminating mould

Some spores were transferred to a spot on an agar plate and were allowed to grow at room temperature for 4 or 5 days. Then

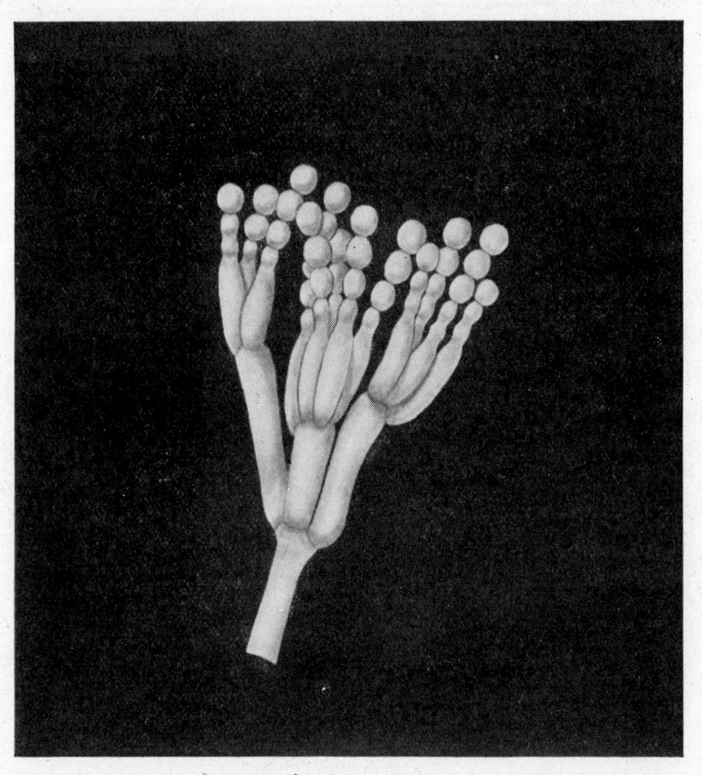

FIG. 3b.—Typical Penicillus of *P. notatum*. Fleming's strain (from Raper and Alexander, 1945)

different bacteria were planted in streaks radially to the mould culture. Some of these bacteria grew right up to the mould colony while others were completely inhibited for a considerable distance (see Fig. 5). This showed that the mould produced a selective antibacterial substance which was freely diffusible in agar. This diffusibility is an important property in antiseptics. Penicillin is extremely diffusible, but the older antiseptics which had been used for the treatment of established infections in the human body, without great success, were deficient in this respect. This is brought out in Fig. 6.

Then the mould was grown on a fluid medium: ordinary nutrient broth. Here it grew as a thick corrugated felted mass on the surface and after a few days an intense yellow colour developed in the underlying clear fluid.

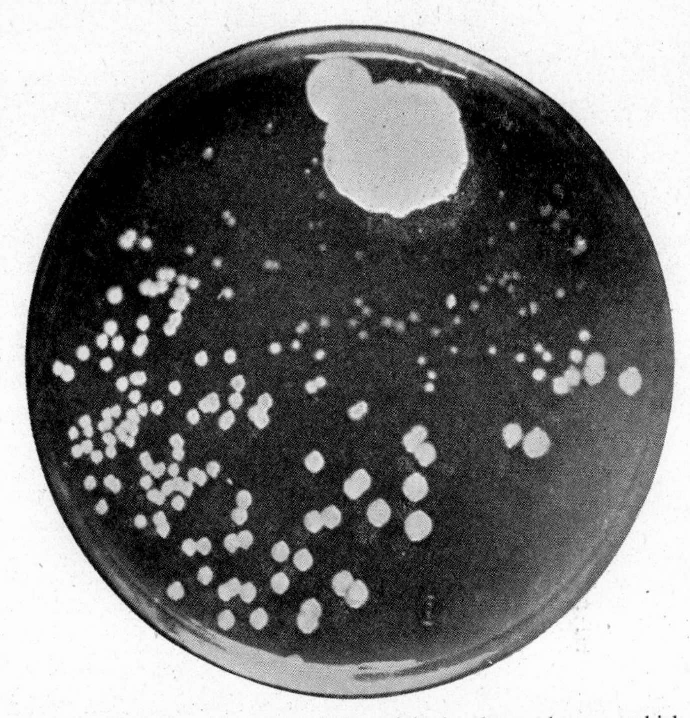

FIG. 4.—Photographic print of the original culture plate on which the action of penicillin was observed, showing contaminating colony of *P. notatum*; staphylococci undergoing lysis; normal staphylococcal colony

The antibacterial power was tested by making serial dilutions of the culture fluid in broth which had been infected with the staphylococcus, a microbe which had already been seen to be sensitive to the action of penicillin. It was found that the culture fluid could be diluted several hundred times before it lost its power of completely inhibiting the growth of the staphylococci. Table 1, reproduced from the first article published on penicillin, shows the rate of development of the antibacterial substance in nutrient broth.

2

TABLE 1

DEVELOPMENT OF PENICILLIN AT ROOM TEMPERATURE IN NUTRIENT BROTH

Test organism = Staphylococcus

After	days				
After 5	days complete inhibition in a	1 in 20 dilution
,, 6	,, ,, ,, ,,	1 in 40 ,,
,, 7	,, ,, ,, ,,	1 in 200 ,,
,, 8	,, ,, ,, ,,	1 in 500 ,,

The antibacterial power of the culture fluid was also assayed in another way, by measuring the rate of diffusion into agar.

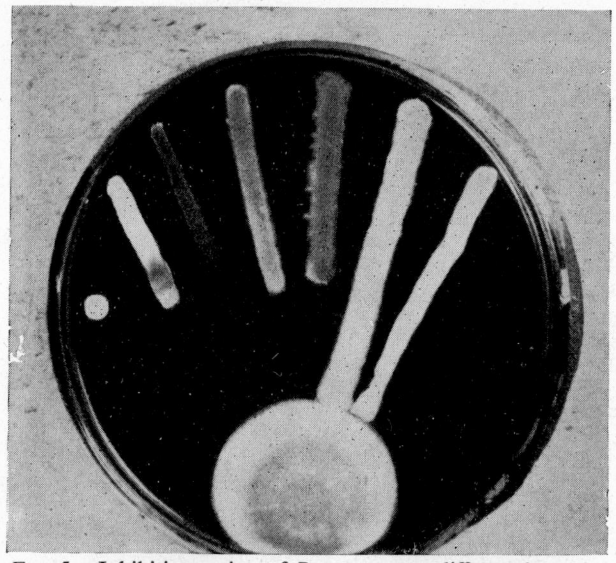

FIG. 5.—Inhibiting action of *P. notatum* on different bacteria.
1. Staphylococcus
2. Streptococcus
3. Diphtheria bacillus
4. Anthrax bacillus
5. *Esch. coli*
6. Typhoid bacillus

(*J. R. Inst. publ. Hlth. Hyg.*)

This method was similar to that used by Fleming and Allison[3] in connexion with Lysozyme. With a knife a gutter was cut out of the agar in a Petri dish and was filled with agar containing the fluid from the mould culture. Different microbes were then planted in streaks from the edge of the plate to the gutter. After incubation some of these were found to grow right up to the gutter while others were inhibited for a considerable distance. This showed that the mould produced in the culture fluid a substance which had a powerful inhibitory action on some bacteria but not on others, and that among the sensitive bacteria were some of the commonest agents of infection in man. Herein penicillin differed from lysozyme (see Fig. 7). Penicillin suppressed the growth of many of the common pathogens of man whereas the bacteria most susceptible to the action of lysozyme were non-pathogenic.

It had now been shown that the mould produced an anti-bacterial substance which inhibited the growth of many pathogenic

TABLE 2. BACTERICIDAL POWER OF CRUDE PENICILLIN: NUMBER OF COLONIES DEVELOPING AFTER SOJOURN IN PENICILLIN

Time in hours	Control	Concentration of penicillin			
		1 in 80	1 in 40	1 in 20	1 in 10
At beginning	27	27	27	27	27
After 2 hours	116	73	51	48	23
After 4½ hours	116	13	1	2	5
After 8 hours	116	0	0	0	0
After 12 hours	116	0	0	0	0

bacteria. It did more, however, than merely inhibit growth. It also had bactericidal properties (see Table 2) and the very first

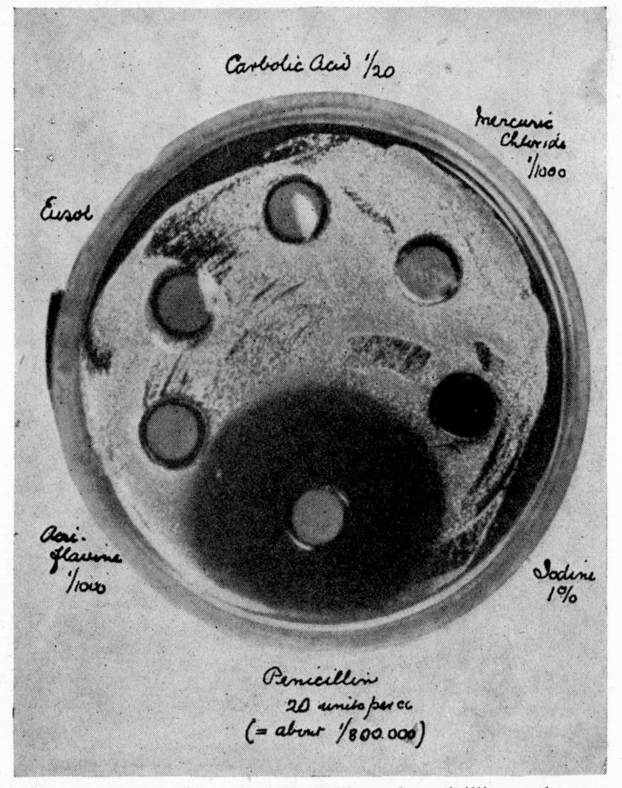

FIG. 6.—Comparison of diffusibility of penicillin and some other antiseptics. Discs of blotting paper soaked in antiseptic imbedded in agar plate inoculated with staphylococcus

(*J. R. Inst. publ. Hlth. Hyg.*

observation (see Fig. 4) showed that it was capable of inducing lysis of the bacteria. The lytic effect was brought out in a further experiment.

The surface of an agar plate was thickly inoculated with staphylococci. Discs were cut out with a cork-borer and the holes so made were filled with fluid from a number of cultures of *P. notatum* to find out whether or not they were active. It will be seen that each hole is surrounded by a zone of complete inhibition of growth (see Fig. 8, I), but there are areas where the staphylococci have grown profusely. Fig. 8, II, shows the same plate after it had lain for one week at room temperature. In each of the holes the unfiltered fluid from the mould cultures had grown out into

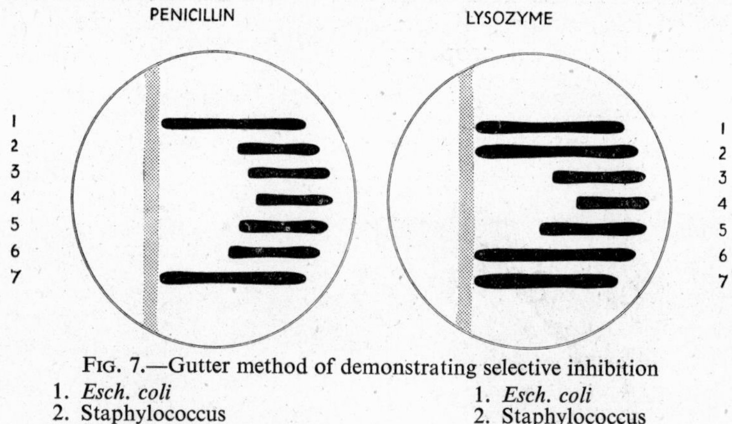

FIG. 7.—Gutter method of demonstrating selective inhibition

Penicillin	Lysozyme
1. *Esch. coli*	1. *Esch. coli*
2. Staphylococcus	2. Staphylococcus
3. Haemolytic streptococcus	3. Sarcina
4. Gonococcus	4. *M. lysodiekticus*
5. *B. diphtheriae*	5. *B. subtilis*
6. *B. anthracis*	6. Streptococcus
7. *B. typhosus*	7. *B. typhosus*

fresh mould colonies, these had produced more penicillin, and the staphylococcal growth had practically disappeared.

From the results of the agar diffusion and serial dilution methods a list was made of the common microbes which were sensitive or insensitive to penicillin. This list brought up to date is to be found on page 19. A consideration of the list led to the first practical use to which penicillin was put. This was to render easier the isolation of penicillin-insensitive organisms from amongst a mass of penicillin-sensitive ones. In the respiratory tract Pfeiffer's influenza bacillus (*H. influenzae*) and the whooping cough bacillus (*H. pertussis*) are found often with large numbers of pneumococci or streptococci. The pneumococci and streptococci are sensitive to penicillin so that when there is penicillin in the culture medium they do not develop, while the growth of *H. influenzae* or *H.*

pertussis is not hindered. For practical purposes when there is an enormous difference in the sensitivity of the different microbes it is sufficient to plate out the material in the ordinary way and then to spread over half of the plate 4 or 5 drops of the crude penicillin, or of purified penicillin of a strength of 5 units per millilitre. On one half of the plate, therefore, is an ordinary culture and on the other half only the penicillin-insensitive microbes grow (see Fig. 9). By a careful gradation of the strength of the penicillin in the medium it was found that, even when the difference between the sensitivity of the microbes was relatively small, the more sensitive ones could be suppressed while the less sensitive ones grew freely. Thus Craddock[5] was able consistently

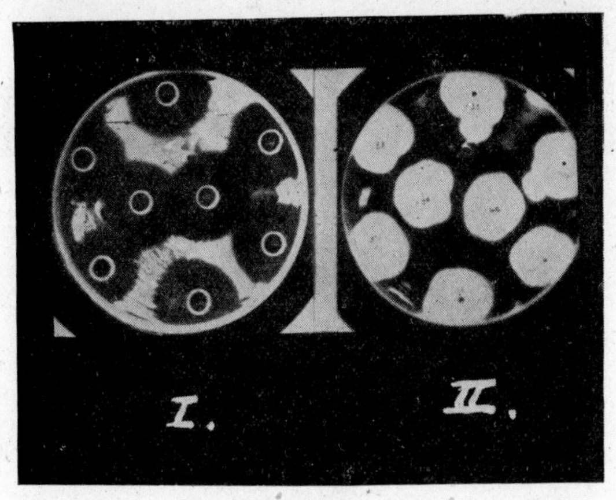

FIG. 8.—Lysis of staphylococci under the influence of penicillin

(*J. R. Inst. publ. Hlth. Hyg.*)

to obtain pure cultures of the acne bacillus (*C. acnes*) from lesions, many of which were infected with staphylococci, by incorporating in the medium just sufficient penicillin to inhibit the staphylococci.

Penicillin was an unstable substance. A culture might have reached its maximum potency in 10 days, but in another 7–10 days it might become inert. Even if it were filtered and the *p*H adjusted to about 6·8, its potency rapidly disappeared although, if it were kept at a temperature of about 4° C. in the refrigerator, it might retain its potency for one or two months. Heating momentarily to 100° C. had little effect but after boiling for one hour penicillin lost almost all its potency. Autoclaving destroyed it. Heating to 65° C. for half an hour did not reduce the potency and this is useful when titrating the potency of penicillin in materials infected with bacteria which are killed at this temperature.

The toxicity of penicillin was tested by injection into animals and it was found to be not more toxic than the same quantity of the broth used for growing the mould. It had no irritant effect when applied to the human cornea or to large infected surfaces. Its toxicity to human leucocytes was tested by the method

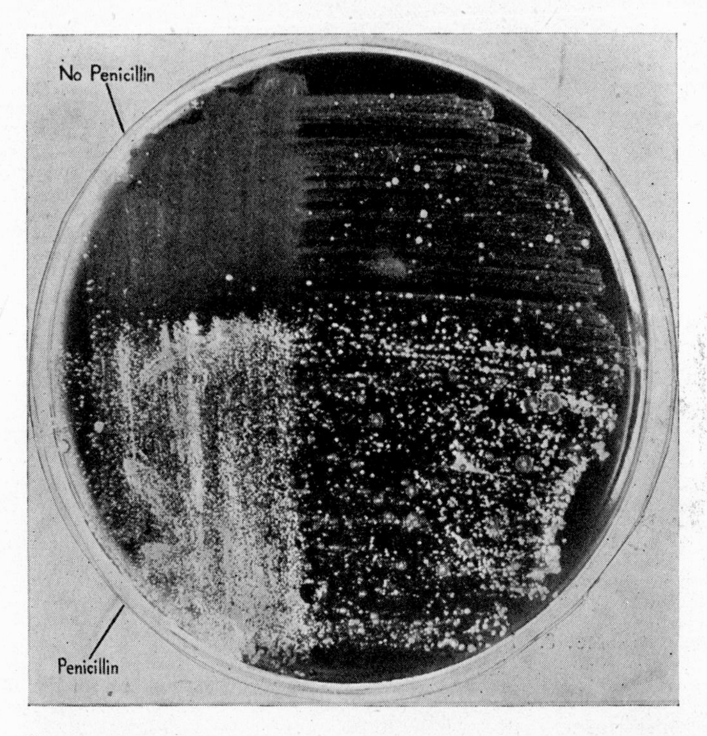

FIG. 9.—Illustrating the Selective Action of Penicillin. Culture from a tooth socket on boiled blood agar. An infected swab was rubbed over the left half of the plate. The rest of the plate was then more thinly planted by streaking a wire from the infected to the uninfected part. The lower half was treated with penicillin after planting. The thickly planted portion untreated with penicillin gave an almost pure culture of streptococci. The less thinly planted portion of the upper half shows many streptococci with a few other colonies. The lower portion (treated with penicillin) shows a very copious growth of Gram negative cocci and haemophilic bacteria

previously used by me for other antiseptics. Infected human defibrinated blood is mixed with serial dilutions of the antiseptic and incubated in slide cells. In the control cell where the antiseptic was replaced by physiological saline solution, the blood—by virtue of its leucocytes—killed off about 95 per cent of the infecting microbes. With the older antiseptics there was invariably a range of concentration which destroyed the leucocytes and allowed the bacteria to grow out (see Fig. 10).

Penicillin was the first substance ever encountered which did

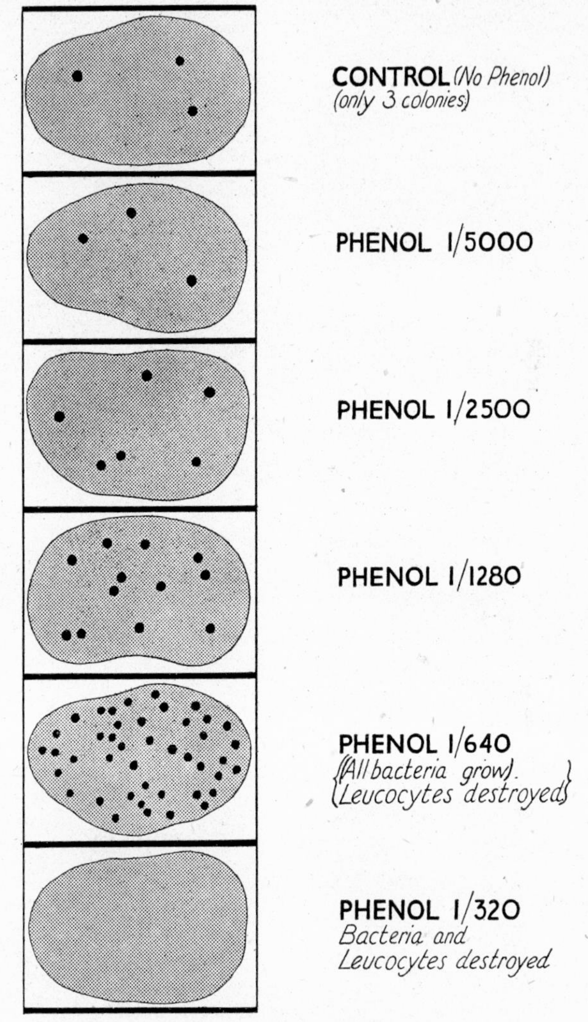

FIG. 10.—Effect of phenol on bacteria and leucocytes

not show this effect and which destroyed the bacteria without any apparent destructive action on the leucocytes. It was this observation more than any other which stimulated me in my first paper on penicillin to say : "It may be an efficient antiseptic for application to, or injection into, areas infected with penicillin-sensitive microbes."

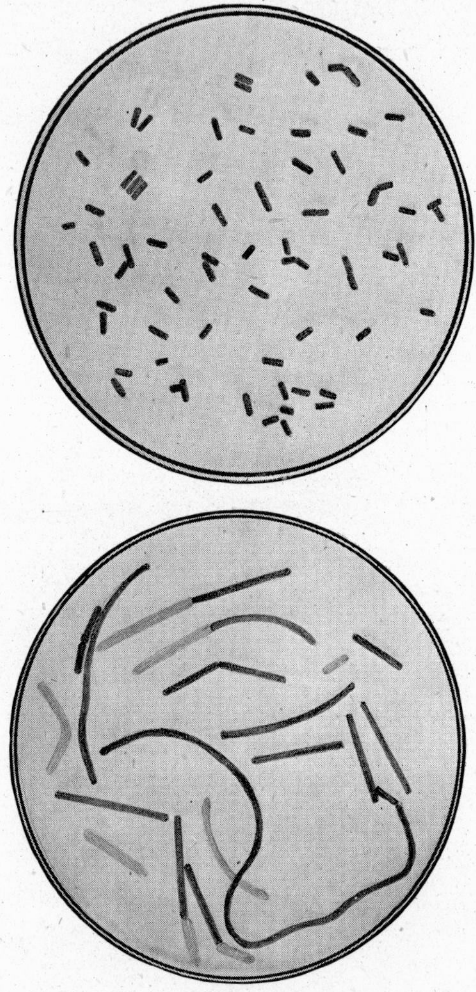

FIG. 11
Effect of penicillin on *B. welchii*. Upper plate shows normal *B. welchii* culture on blood agar. Lower plate shows *B. welchii* culture on blood agar containing a very small amount of penicillin
(*J. R. Inst. publ. Hlth. Hyg.*)

In 1929 the position was that a mould—a *Penicillium*—produced in culture a remarkable antibacterial substance (penicillin). This acted on many of the common bacteria pathogenic to man. The strength of a broth culture of this mould was such that it could be diluted to nearly 1 in 1,000 before it lost its bacteriostatic power against staphylococci. This is about 3 times the dilution at which phenol ceases to be bacteriostatic. In contrast to all the older

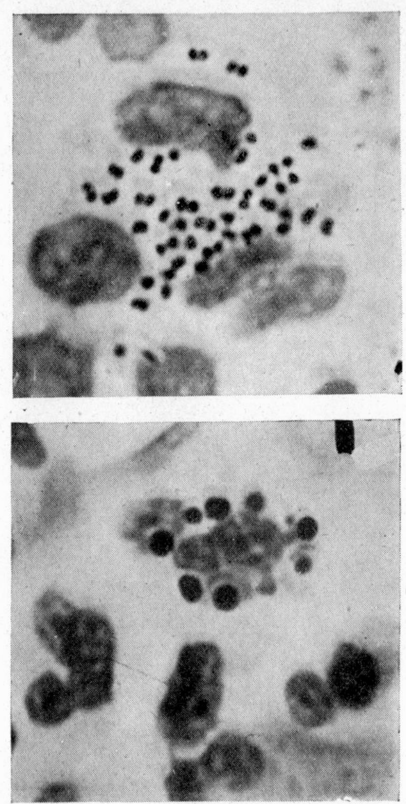

FIG. 12
Effect of penicillin on gonococcus. Upper plate shows gonococci in urethral pus before treatment. Lower plate shows effect between 2 and 3 hours after first intramuscular injection of 15,000 units of penicillin
(J. R. Inst. publ. Hlth. Hyg.

antiseptics it was apparently without toxicity to human leucocytes, but it was unstable and easily destroyed. The earliest attempts at concentration failed, but the crude fluid continued to be used for selective culture in the bacteriological laboratory.

In 1930 Raistrick and his colleagues obtained a culture of the mould and showed that it produced penicillin on Czapex-Dox medium—a simple synthetic medium containing some salts and glucose. They showed that the yellow colour was due to a pigment chrysogenin which was not related to penicillin. They demonstrated that it could be extracted from the culture fluid by ether in acid solution, but in their process a large part of the penicillin was destroyed. Difficulties arose, however, over bacteriological cooperation, which was absolutely necessary, as there was, and still is, no satisfactory method other than a bacteriological one for testing the potency of the extracts. In 1932[8] they published their results and transferred their attention to other problems.

I had failed to advance further for the want of adequate chemical help. Raistrick and his associates had lacked bacteriological cooperation, so the problem of the effective concentration of penicillin remained unsolved.

Nothing further of importance occurred in connexion with penicillin for 7 years. During that time a remarkable change had happened in medical thought in regard to the chemotherapy of bacterial infections. In 1930 there had not been any real advance in this direction since Ehrlich had introduced Salvarsan 20 years before. There was an idea that the common pyogenic cocci, after they invaded the body, were beyond the reach of all chemicals. Then in the middle thirties the sulphonamides appeared. Sulphanilamide was shown to have a remarkable antibacterial effect on streptococci and some other organisms, and later sulphapyridine to a large extent conquered the pneumococcus. The medical profession became chemotherapeutically minded and there was the urge to treat all manner of infections with these newer chemicals. Dubos, also, had shown that a certain bacillus could be induced to make in culture a substance which had an extraordinary effect on some pneumococci and that *B. brevis* produced a powerful antibacterial substance which affected most of the Gram positive organisms.

It was in this atmosphere that Florey and Chain at Oxford, having brought to a successful conclusion their work on lysozyme, decided to engage on a systematic investigation of antibiotic substances. After studying the literature they considered that it would be worth while attempting to concentrate penicillin. They obtained my culture and grew it on the modified Czapek-Dox medium used by Clutterbuck, Lovell and Raistrick, and eventually the successful extraction of penicillin was accomplished by acid ether rapidly at a very low temperature. It is unnecessary here to go into detail but they concentrated the penicillin 1,000 times or more and dried it. When dry it was relatively stable. Even now with much purer preparations it is only when penicillin is dry that it is stable.

The Oxford workers tested its action on various bacteria and obtained almost the same results as those obtained with the crude penicillin except that the bacteriostatic dilution was as much as 1 in 1,000,000 instead of the something less than 1 in 1,000 which it was with the crude preparation. Its power was not interfered with by the presence of blood as was that of many of the older antiseptics and, unlike the sulphonamides, its action was maintained in pus.

Even this concentrated material had little toxicity for animals or for leucocytes. Next, its chemotherapeutic properties were tested on experimentally infected animals. Mice were infected with streptococci, staphylococci and *V. septique* (*Cl. septicum*). Some of these were treated with a few milligrams of the concentrated penicillin while others were left as controls. All the controls were dead in 17 hours and the mice treated with all but the smallest doses survived. These experiments showed that penicillin thus concentrated was by far the most powerful chemotherapeutic agent which we possessed against these infections.

The results were published by Chain and his colleagues in 1940[9], and were the starting point of the more recent work on penicillin. The Oxford workers investigated the pharmacology of penicillin and showed especially that it could not be administered satisfactorily by the mouth and that when injected it was rapidly excreted by the kidney, so that to maintain a supply in the body, injections had to be repeated frequently. Then it was tried on man and although in the first series the patients were far from being ideal ones on which to test a drug, the results were sufficient to show that penicillin had remarkable curative properties. The first clinical results, together with the method of extraction, were published in 1941 by Abraham and his co-workers[10].

The real problem now was production of penicillin in quantity. In the pathological laboratory at Oxford University a miniature factory was set up which produced a small amount of concentrated penicillin for further clinical observation and chemical experiment. At that time World War II had taken a serious turn and the pharmaceutical industry was too hard pressed to undertake new ventures. Florey and Heatley went to the United States, who were still at peace, and laid all their information before the authorities there with the object of having large-scale production started. Some tentative work and one or two dramatic clinical results convinced Dr. A. N. Richards of the National Research Council and other American authorities of the value of penicillin, with the result that they gave every facility and help to the manufacturers and the production of "therapeutic" penicillin went on apace. This was not the first time that the penicillin-producing strain of *P. notatum* had reached the mycologists in America. In 1930 Raistrick had sent a culture of the strain, which he had received from me, to Thom to confirm his suspicion that the name first applied to it (*P. rubrum*) was wrong. It was distributed by Thom and Raper[11] to all who asked for it from 1930 onward, but apart from the identification of the mould nothing was done except some laboratory work by Reid[12] who confirmed and to some extent extended my findings.

At first the work on production was on entirely orthodox lines but, as was to be expected in the production of something new, improvements were introduced in several directions.

The culture medium.—At first the mould was grown on the same medium that was used by Raistrick in 1932 and later by the Oxford workers, namely, Czapek-Dox medium, with or without the addition of yeast extract. Much of the early laboratory work in America was done under the direction of Robert Coghill in the fermentation division of the Northern Regional Research Laboratory at Peoria, Illinois. This was in the midst of the "corn" country and this laboratory had a special interest in corn products. There was a by-product of a section of the corn industry, called corn steep liquor, for which it was desirable to find new uses. This was added to the culture medium and it increased the yield of penicillin about 10-fold. Corn steep liquor is now in general use in penicillin manufacture but it is not yet quite clear what its essential components are which favour a high yield of penicillin.

Method of culture.—At first all penicillin was made by a method similar to that originally used in 1928–1929, namely, by growing the mould on the surface of a shallow layer of culture medium in some type of bottle. In large-scale production this involved much labour in the handling of thousands of bottles a day, but in some factories the method is still in use. It was found, however, that good yields of penicillin could be produced if the mould were grown in submerged culture in large tanks and provided that the medium was sufficiently aerated and agitated. This method is now being generally adopted.

Nature of the mould.—At first all penicillin was made from direct descendants of the original spores which contaminated my culture plate in 1928. This had survived during the interval in various laboratories, grown on different culture media and subcultured at varying intervals, so it was not surprising that different cultures varied considerably in their penicillin production. One culture (1249) was found to give especially high yields and from this, by the cultivation of single spores, another culture (1249 B.21) was found to give even higher.

An intensive search, however, was made for better strains. Large numbers of strains from different natural sources were examined as well as museum cultures of *P. notatum*, but for surface growth nothing was found much better than the original strain, although another strain (1950) isolated in Peoria from a piece of Swiss cheese gave high yields, as did a mutant of this culture induced by exposure to ultra-violet light. From the museum cultures one (832) was found to give exceptional yields in submerged culture, very much higher than did the original strain.

In 1943 a *P. chrysogenum* was isolated in Peoria from a mouldy patch on a cantaloup and this was found to be an even better producer in submerged culture. This strain has been improved by selection and other methods and is now largely used in the mass production of penicillin.

During this time penicillin research and production in England had not been neglected. At Oxford a certain amount of penicillin was produced which enabled Sir Howard Florey and Lady Florey to treat another series of patients with extraordinarily good results.

My first experience of treating a patient with concentrated penicillin was in the summer of 1942. A middle-aged man with streptococcal meningitis appeared to be dying in spite of sulphonamide treatment. The streptococcus was sensitive to penicillin and Florey was good enough to give me his whole stock of penicillin to try on this, the first case of meningitis to be treated. After a few days' treatment with intramuscular and intrathecal injections the patient was out of danger and he made an uneventful recovery. The result was so dramatic that penicillin was brought to the notice of the Minister of Supply, who immediately called a meeting of everyone interested—academic and industrial. This became the Penicillin Committee under the Presidency of Sir Henry Dale which furthered the production of penicillin in Great Britain and which exchanged information freely with the American authorities. The close cooperation between the laboratories and factories on both sides of the Atlantic was a prime factor in furthering the large-scale production which was soon recognized as being a major war effort.

In England, production was hampered by shortage of labour and of some essential materials ; nevertheless, it progressed although at a slower rate than in the United States.

Meantime the chemists were busy with investigations regarding the purification and structure of penicillin, but this aspect of the question is dealt with elsewhere.

Extension of the use of penicillin in treatment

As the drug became more plentiful its use was extended. The earliest cases treated had been chiefly septic infections due to staphylococci and streptococci. Soon, however, pneumonia and other pneumococcal infections were treated successfully, and then penicillin was shown to have an almost miraculous effect on gonorrhoea. Later it was found that syphilis also could be successfully treated, as well as a large number of less common infections.

Morphological changes in bacteria exposed to penicillin

Penicillin apparently acts on bacteria only in the growing phase and fails to have a bactericidal action when conditions are such that the organism cannot grow. Gardner[13] was the first to point out that under the influence of sublethal concentrations of penicillin the bacteria lose their regular form. What is normally a short bacillus may become a long thread and cocci may take on a swollen and bloated appearance. These changes are illustrated in Figs. 11 and 12. In Fig. 11 *Cl. welchii* has been grown in very weak penicillin and in Fig. 12 the gonococci in pus taken from a patient after a single intramuscular injection of 15,000 units, are swollen and quite unlike the normal gonococcus.

The unit of penicillin

In the early days when penicillin was not yet concentrated there was no need for a unit. The strength could easily be expressed by the dilution which was necessary to inhibit the growth of a test organism. When, however, it was concentrated so that the inhibitory dilution ran into 7 figures, it became desirable to establish a unit for the more simple expression of the potency of the concentrates.

The Oxford workers established a unit which became known as the "Oxford unit". This unit was a purely arbitrary one corresponding to the potency of a certain sample of concentrated penicillin, but it roughly corresponded to the amount of penicillin which, when dissolved in 50 millilitres of broth, would just inhibit the growth of the test staphylococcus. More recently pure penicillin has been obtained and an international conference established the Oxford unit as an International unit and laid it down that the unit contained 0·0006 milligram of pure crystalline sodium salt of penicillin II which was to be maintained as a standard at the National Institute of Medical Research.

Thus 5,000 units of penicillin II weighs 3 milligrams, and it is probable that when pure or approximately pure penicillin is available for therapeutic purposes the doses will be indicated in milligrams instead of in units.

Purity of penicillin

The first crude penicillin contained not more than 20 units per millilitre. With better methods of culture the crude culture fluid, before concentration, may contain over 100 units per millilitre. The concentrated penicillin first used by the Oxford workers for therapeutic purposes was from 1 to 5 per cent pure. The purity has been steadily increasing with improvements in the extraction process and we may look forward to having, in the not too distant future, pure penicillin for the treatment of patients.

GENERAL RULES FOR PENICILLIN TREATMENT

There are a few simple rules for the use of penicillin in the treatment of bacterial infections. These may seem too simple—even childish—but experience in watching penicillin being used has made it quite clear that these rules are often broken with resulting disappointment.

(1) It should be used only when there is an infection by a

penicillin-sensitive microbe. The following list shows the sensitivity of the commoner microbes.

Sensitive	**Insensitive**
Staphylococcus	Enterococcus (*Streptococcus faecalis*)
Streptococcus pyogenes	Non-pathogenic Gram-negative cocci
Streptococcus viridans	Typhoid-coli-dysentery group
Some anaerobic streptococci	*Vibrio cholerae*
Pneumococcus	*Proteus*
Gonococcus	Pseudomonas group (*Ps. aeruginosa*, *B. fluorescens*)
Meningococcus	Haemophilus group (*H. influenzae*, *H. pertussis*)
Neisseria catarrhalis	Acid-fast group (tubercle, smegma etc.)
Micrococcus	Pasteurella group (*P. pestis* etc.)
Sarcina	Brucella
Actinomyces	Friedländer's bacillus (*Klebsiella pneumoniae*)
B. anthracis	Most of the viruses
Hay bacillus (*B. subtilis*)	Yeasts
Diphtheria group	Monilia
Clostridia (*tetani*, *welchii*, *septique*, *botulinum etc.*)	Moulds
Streptobacillus moniliformis	
Erysipelothrix rhusiopathiae (erysipeloid; swine erysipelas)	
Spirillum minus (rat-bite fever)	
Spirochaetes of relapsing fever	
syphilis	
yaws	
Vincent's angina	
Weil's disease	
Larger viruses (psittacosis, ornithosis)—partly	
Rickettsia —partly	

This list merely gives the general division but it must be recognized that among the sensitive microbes, for example, staphylococci, there are occasional strains which are relatively much less sensitive than the normal strains. There are, too, classed as insensitive bacteria some which, although insensitive to penicillin in concentrations which by systemic administration can be reached in the blood, are yet sensitive to the higher concentrations with which they may come in contact when penicillin is applied locally.

In most cases, however, there is a broad line of distinction between the sensitive and insensitive microbes and while success can be looked for in the treatment of infections by those listed as sensitive, failure is more than probable when the microbe is in the insensitive list.

The method of testing the sensitivity of a microbe is described elsewhere (p. 87) and whenever possible this test should be done. In the past it has often been the custom for patients to be treated without any bacteriological examination; bronchitis for instance was treated as bronchitis whatever the nature of the infection. The introduction, however, of highly selective antibacterial agents such as penicillin makes it very desirable that the nature of the infection should be known, not only for the prognosis but also for the adjustment of the dose of penicillin. It is obvious that a very sensitive microbe will be destroyed with smaller doses than will one which, although still in the "sensitive" list, is yet much less susceptible.

In acute conditions, however, it is not suggested that penicillin treatment should be delayed until a bacteriological diagnosis is established any more than that in suspected diphtheria, antitoxin should be withheld until a bacteriological diagnosis has been made. In such cases treatment should be instituted immediately and specimens taken. When the bacteriological report has been received the continuance of treatment can be further considered. A rigid adherence to the rule that the nature of the infection must be established before treatment can be commenced may jeopardize the patient's life.

Press publicity has given many people the idea that penicillin is a panacea. This idea must be dispelled, for however effective it is in many infections it is quite useless in many others.

(2) Penicillin must be administered in such a way that it comes in contact with the infecting microbe. This seems obvious but sometimes one sees a deep carbuncle having so-called penicillin treatment by the application of a little penicillin cream to the surface.

The methods of administration are described elsewhere, but there are two general methods of treatment. In the systemic method it is administered so that it gets into the blood and reaches the infecting microbe through the circulation, while with local treatment the penicillin is given in such a way that it reaches the microbes directly. The systemic method is technically not difficult but it is expensive in penicillin; the local method is very economical in the drug but it may be technically very difficult and, of course, in some cases it is impossible. In most cases if there is an ample supply of penicillin the systemic route will suffice, but there are exceptions ; these are emphasized in different chapters of this book. Especially, it must not be forgotten that penicillin does not readily pass from the blood to the cerebrospinal fluid. It is easy, however, to introduce it directly into the spinal canal, or into an empyema or other infected cavity, in far greater concentration than can possibly diffuse from the blood.

(3) The dose should be such that in the infected area the concentration of penicillin is sufficient to destroy the bacteria. In systemic treatment the dosage can be controlled by estimations of the blood concentration. After an injection there is a rapid rise in the concentration of penicillin in the blood ; some is excreted and some diffused into the tissues; then as the blood concentration falls below that of the tissues it will return from the tissues to the blood. This process will follow every injection. The method of estimating the concentration of penicillin in the blood and the amounts present after different doses, is described in other chapters.

Penicillin is the only chemotherapeutic substance which is almost completely non-toxic, so there is no fear of an overdose. While from 100,000 to 200,000 units daily is the normal dosage, one hundred times as much has been given to a patient, without toxic symptoms. The only reason for limiting the dose is an economic one and when there is any doubt it is wise to overdose rather than underdose.

It is fortunately not so easy to make organisms resistant to penicillin as it is with the sulphonamides and it has been shown that in the case of some microbes at least this fastness is only temporary[14]. Thus when there is not fear of toxic symptoms it seems a pity to underdose the patient and so run the risk of inducing a drug resistance (even temporary) in the infecting microbe.

(4) The treatment should be persisted in until the infection is defeated. It is difficult to give general directions regarding the time to stop penicillin treatment. It has been said that it should be continued until the infection has been completely eliminated. This is perhaps true for local treatment but in acute conditions treated systemically it is not so easy to know when the infection has disappeared. This is especially true in bacterial endocarditis in which the blood rapidly becomes sterile but the number of relapses is enormous unless the treatment is continued for some weeks. Here again, assuming that supplies are ample it is wise to prolong the treatment a little rather than to cut it short and favour relapses which may not be quite so easy to deal with.

These simple rules are elaborated in the various clinical chapters and if they are obeyed some remarkable results will be seen, but however effective penicillin can be it requires a certain amount of care and attention in its application.

Combination of penicillin with the sulphonamides

In infections with streptococci, pneumococci, gonococci and some other organisms the sulphonamides were extensively used before the advent of purified penicillin. The question is often asked, "Can one of the sulphonamides be used in conjunction with penicillin?". The answer is easy : there is not incompatibility. As will be seen in the section on the pharmacy of penicillin, dusting powders are used consisting of penicillin diluted in sulphathiazole or sulphanilamide. Indeed it has been suggested by various workers[15,16] that there is a definite synergism exercised by the combination. The combination of a sulphonamide with penicillin has been extensively used in practice and, apart from the possible toxic effects of the sulphonamide, there does not seem to be any satisfactory reason why they should not be combined in infections which are susceptible to both. Apparently they act on the microbe in a quite different manner. *p*-Aminobenzoic acid, which neutralizes sulphonamide action, has no such effect on penicillin, and microbes which have been rendered sulphonamide-fast are still fully sensitive to penicillin and *vice versa*.

Limitations of penicillin treatment

Infections with insensitive microbes.—The substance of rule (1) (see p. 19) may here be repeated. Infections like typhoid fever, dysentery, cholera, plague and undulant fever do not benefit from penicillin therapy. The same may be said of ulcerative colitis except in unusual cases. Some of the other common conditions which do not respond are cancer, tuberculosis, rheumatoid arthritis, nervous degenerations—for example, disseminated sclerosis and Parkinson's disease—psoriasis and almost all the virus diseases such as smallpox, measles, influenza and the common cold, although in this last class penicillin may be successfully used in the bacterial complications and sequelae. These are merely some of the diseases of many sufferers who, in the past 2 years, have, as a result of press reports, written to me for relief.

Sequestered infections.—Sometimes the infecting bacteria existed in situations sequestered from the blood stream as in sequestra in chronic osteomyelitis. The surrounding blood and tissues may be saturated with penicillin and theoretically, if this is maintained for a sufficient length of time, the penicillin might diffuse in and destroy the infection. This is often impracticable, however, and surgery must be combined with penicillin treatment.

Inconvenience.—The present methods of administration are inconvenient to both patient and doctor, but newer methods are remedying this so that a patient can have penicillin treatment and still carry on his work. Large doses morning and evening or a single daily dose in the oil-wax mixture suffice in many cases. Inhalation can be carried out by the intelligent patient and there are a number of methods of oral administration, which is, of course, the easiest of all, but none of these oral methods is quite satisfactory and all are extravagant in penicillin.

Instability.—The instability of penicillin in the presence of water is a very definite practical drawback. At present preparations containing water retain their potency for a comparatively short time—a matter of days or a few weeks—even if stored in a refrigerator, but there is hope that chemists will evolve a penicillin which is stable. This will be a great practical advance.

Penicillinase.—A considerable number of bacteria produce in their growth a substance, penicillinase, which destroys penicillin. Some of these, especially coliform bacilli, are found in infections in association with penicillin-sensitive organisms. In such cases the penicillinase produced may definitely militate against the success of penicillin treatment which otherwise would be effective.

SUMMARY

In penicillin we have a remarkable chemotherapeutic agent which affects many of the common infections of the human body. Other equally powerful antibacterial agents have been discovered but so far penicillin stands alone in combining this property with an almost complete lack of toxicity. The intensive research which it has stimulated may bring forth others as good, or even better, or the chemists may be able to modify the penicillin molecule so that its power is increased or its limitations are removed. There is still plenty of scope for further advance.

REFERENCES

[1] Florey, H. W. (1945) *Brit. med. J.*, **2**, 635.
[2] Westling, R. (1911) *Ueber die grünen spezces der gattung penicillium*, p. 96. Upsala.
[3] Raper, K. B., and Alexander, D. F. (1945) *J. Elisha Mitchell sci. Soc.*, **61**, 74.
[4] Fleming, A., and Allison, V. D. (1922) *Proc. roy. Soc.* Ser. B., **94**, 142.
[5] Craddock, S. (1942) *Lancet*, **1**, 558.
[6] Fleming, A. (1924) *Proc. roy. Soc.* Ser. B., **96**, 171.
[7] Fleming, A. (1929) *Brit. J. exp. Path.*, **10**, 226.
[8] Clutterbuck, P. W., Lovell, R., and Raistrick, H. (1932) *Bio-chem. J.*, **26**, 1907.
[9] Chain, E., Florey, H. W., Gardner, A. D., Heatley, N. G., Jennings, M. A., Orr-Ewing, J., and Sanders, A. G. (1940) *Lancet*, **2**, 226.
[10] Abraham, E. P., Chain, E., Fletcher, C. M., Florey, H. W., Gardner, A. D., Heatley, N. G., and Jennings, M. A. (1941) *Lancet*, **2**, 177.
[11] Thom, C. (1945) *Mycologia*, **37**, 460.
[12] Reid, R. D. (1935) *J. Bact.*, **29**, 215.
[13] Gardner, A. D. (1940) *Nature*, **146**, 837.
[14] Todd, E. W., Turner, G. S., and Drew, L. G. W. (1945) *Brit. med. J.*, **2**, 603.
[15] Ungar, J. (1943) *Nature*, **152**, 245.
[16] Bigger, J. W. (1944) *Lancet*, **2**, 142.

CHEMISTRY AND MANUFACTURE OF PENICILLIN

BY A. L. BACHARACH, M.A., F.R.I.C.

AND

B. A. HEMS, PH.D., F.R.I.C.

EARLY INVESTIGATIONS

THE first information, other than some incidental observations in Fleming's original paper, published about the chemical properties of penicillin, came from the London School of Hygiene, where Raistrick and his colleagues[1] demonstrated that penicillin is an organic acid lacking basic groups and readily extracted from aqueous solutions into various organic solvents, that it is fairly labile and that its activity is destroyed on mild acidification or on heating its aqueous solution.

Although there was nothing sensational about these discoveries it must be remembered that the properties described by Raistrick and his colleagues are fundamental to the methods adopted later for the concentration and purification of penicillin and, indeed, still remain the basis of manufacturing processes. Although the workers at the London School of Hygiene made no further attack on the problem because, as Coghill[2] writes of Raistrick, "his medical colleagues would not listen to his pleadings and he could get no clinical tests made", Raistrick himself has been prominently associated with subsequent developments of penicillin production.

The chemical properties of penicillin, described by Fleming and Raistrick and confirmed and further clarified by later workers, made it clear that penicillin is a compound of comparatively small molecular weight and is neither protein nor carbohydrate in nature. In 1941, however, when it had become certain that penicillin would be a valuable clinical agent, all the information available was at best scanty. It appeared to merit much more attention than it had received.

Several problems faced chemists concerned with the extraction and purification of penicillin and they had to be solved before its chemistry could be studied. These were due to the smallness of the yields obtainable from the metabolism solution, the instability of the active substance and the necessity of finding methods for separating a highly unstable compound from the inert materials accompanying it.

The extraordinary activity of penicillin was not at first appreciated nor, consequently, the fact that the yield obtained from the original metabolite solutions could not be any higher than 3–5 milligrams per litre. Although this yield has been very much increased since by improving strains, media and methods of extraction, the chemist has always had to contend with the difficulties of handling very small quantities of the substance.

At an early stage, in order to indicate what methods of isolation could be employed, studies of the stability of penicillin were undertaken. It was found that at a *p*H below 3 or above 9 penicillin was rapidly inactivated in aqueous solution even at low temperatures. It was, moreover, found thermolabile in aqueous solution at any *p*H. Since it was only with difficulty that it was extracted from aqueous solutions above *p*H 4, the conditions under which extraction could be successfully carried out, without at the same time causing too great destruction, were rather critical. For this reason attempts were made to find whether it could be adsorbed from aqueous solution on to a solid adsorbent and then eluted. This was successfully done with charcoal as the adsorbent and various mixtures of water with organic solvents as eluants; the method has been used in several penicillin production units. Many different solvents were tried for eluting the active principle from charcoal, partly to find convenient methods giving large yields and partly in attempts to achieve the highest possible degree of purity. It was also necessary to study the stability of penicillin in various solvents. It was found to be stable in most, although fairly rapidly destroyed by dry alcohols; on the other hand, aqueous solutions of alcohols have been used successfully for elution. It was also found to be unstable in the presence of primary and secondary organic bases, but is not destroyed by tertiary bases.

A study of the inactivation of penicillin in the presence of various metals was also undertaken for two reasons. First it was desired to find, if possible, a metallic salt of penicillin that was sparingly soluble in water and could therefore be used to help in its isolation; secondly it was necessary to know what metals were safe to use in plant required for its production and isolation. In very early attempts to isolate the zinc salt it was found that the antibacterial activity rapidly disappeared and that this could only be due to the zinc ions. Further investigation showed that penicillin was rapidly destroyed by ions of copper, mercury, lead or zinc, and less rapidly by iron ions. These metals were excluded as far as possible from production plant, although experience has shown that some of the precautions taken in the early days were unnecessary. A sparingly soluble metallic salt of penicillin was in fact not found.

Crude penicillin, usually about 40–150 units per milligram, having been isolated, the next step was to find suitable methods of purification, again bearing in mind all the diverse agents having a destructive action. Numerous procedures were tried, including precipitation and co-precipitation, adsorption and elution, fractional extraction, chromatography of various kinds and attempts to find sparingly soluble salts with organic bases.

The most successful methods, later universally adopted for investigation work, were those of chromatography. In this technique a solution of a mixture of substances is poured through a column of an adsorbent, commonly alumina, upon the top of which the substances are adsorbed. When further quantities of the solvent are allowed to flow through the column the various substances are washed down the column at different rates, the least strongly adsorbed travelling most and the most strongly adsorbed least, rapidly. In this way, under ideal conditions all the substances present in the original mixture become separated from one another and can be collected, either by cutting the column into bands, each containing an individual substance, or by washing them out of the column separately. The successful use of this method depends upon careful selection of the correct adsorbent and solvent or solvents to be used; many unsuccessful attempts were made to purify penicillin in this way before the problem was finally solved. A modification of this method, recently introduced, was particularly valuable in the purification of penicillin. This was the method known as partition chromatography and depends not on differential adsorption as described above, but on differential extraction. In this method the column consists of a watery phase—for penicillin a mildly acid strongly buffered solution—adsorbed into a porous solid, usually silicia gel. A solution of the mixture of substances to be separated, in a solvent not miscible with water, is poured on to the column and followed by further quantities of the solvent. The materials in the mixture are distributed unequally between the aqueous phase and the solvent phase, depending upon their relative solubility in the two liquids; as fresh solvent flows down the column continuous redistribution between the two phases takes place with the result that the substances less soluble in the aqueous phase travel down the column more rapidly than those that are more soluble. Separation is thus effected.

Before any of the penicillins had been crystallized, and while it was still believed that there was only one, some apparent anomalies had arisen between results obtained in studying materials prepared in Great Britain and in the United States of America, although it was not quite clear whether the variations were due to penicillin or to accompanying impurities. One of the early triumphs of the method of partition chromatography was the proof that there were at least two penicillins. This was achieved by mixing materials of British and American origin and showing that two separate bands with penicillin activity were got when the mixture was chromatographed. Since then several different penicillins have been produced, partly by using different strains of *Penicillium notatum* and partly by the addition to the culture media of certain organic compounds which are incorporated into the "penicillin" structure to produce a number of different substances with penicillin activity. Thus the original conception of penicillin as a unique compound has now been superseded by that of a class of penicillins having a similar general structure with minor modifications. These penicillins differ somewhat in their stabilities and in their antagonisms towards micro-organisms; although none of them has yet shown particular clinical advantages over others, future work may indicate the use of different penicillins for different purposes.

CHEMISTRY OF PENICILLIN

In discussing the chemistry of penicillin it is perhaps simplest to give the constitutional formula at present receiving the greatest measure of support, although it is not yet considered to be finally proved, and to relate the properties of penicillin to it. Of various formulae discussed from time to time, the most likely one seems to be that known as the β-lactam formula, which is as follows.

```
CH3
   \
    C — CH.COOH
CH3/ |    |
     S    N
      \  / \
       CH   \
       |     CO
       |    /
       CH  /
       |
     NH.CO.R
```

The different penicillins so far examined seem to have the same general structure and to vary only in the nature of the side chain R. There is a difference in the nomenclature of the substances in Great Britain and in the United States of America, as follows.

R	*British name*	*American name*
$-CH_2CH{=}CHCH_2CH_3$	Penicillin I	Penicillin F
$-CH_2C_6H_5$ 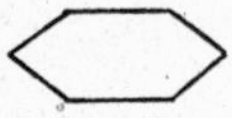	Penicillin II	Penicillin G
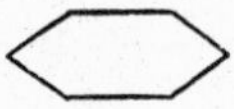 $-CH_2C_6H_4OH$	Penicillin III	Penicillin X
$-CH_2CH_2CH_2CH_2CH_2CH_2CH_3$	Penicillin K	Penicillin K

Penicillin I, with a Δ^2 pentenyl side chain, is the one produced by the original surface culture fermentation strains in England, whereas penicillin II is the one produced in largest amount by more recent surface culture strains and by the submerged culture strain used in the United States of America. Penicillin K is a later addition to the series and is produced by a recently isolated strain of *P. notatum.* These are the penicillins mainly produced by the present manufacturing methods. It will be seen from the formulae that they are monocarboxylic acids. Since the free acids are unstable in aqueous solution the usual derivative used for clinical purposes is the sodium salt, which is freely soluble in water and gives a neutral solution much more stable than that of the free acid. The carboxyl group can be esterified and several esters have been prepared. The esters are almost inactive *in vitro*, but *in vivo* they may be slowly rehydrolyzed to penicillin, presumably by esterases, and produce against a lethal dose of organisms a protective effect very similar to that of sodium penicillin itself. There are, however, pronounced species differences in the capacity of various animals to hydrolyze penicillin esters and their place in clinical practice is not yet clear.

Penicillin is completely broken down by hydrolysis with dilute acids, with the production of an amino-acid, ββ-dimethyl cysteine, known as penicillamine. It is interesting to note that the form of

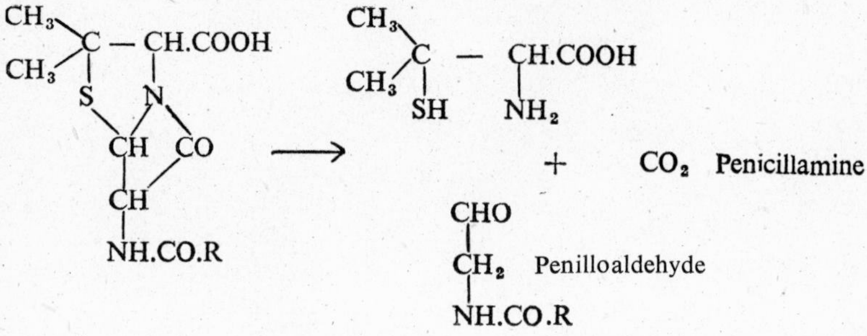

$(CH_3)_2C(-S-)-CH(COOH)-N<$; $S-CH(-N)-CH(NH.CO.R)-CO-N$ (β-lactam–thiazolidine structure) $\longrightarrow$ $(CH_3)_2C(SH)-CH(NH_2).COOH$ (Penicillamine) $+ CO_2 +$ $CHO-CH_2-NH.CO.R$ (Penilloaldehyde)

CH3 C — CH.COOH / CH3 / S N / CH CO / CH / NH.CO.R

⟶

CH3 C — CH.COOH / CH3 SH NH2 + CO2 Penicillamine

CHO / CH2 Penilloaldehyde / NH.CO.R

penicillamine obtained corresponds to the *d* or "unnatural" series of amino-acids; all those isolated from normal proteins belong to the *l* series. Carbon dioxide is also produced during hydrolysis and at the same time an acylated amino-acetaldehyde known as penilloaldehyde I, II or III, depending upon the penicillin from which it is derived.

Various intermediate breakdown products can be derived from penicillin by using milder conditions. A number of them have been satisfactorily identified by degradative work and the proposed constitutions have been confirmed by synthesis.

The instability of penicillin in alkaline or alcoholic solutions is due, for instance, to opening of the β-lactam ring with the formation of penicilloic acid derivatives,—salts by alkalis and esters by alcohols.

```
CH3                              CH3
   \                                \
    C—CH.COOH                        C—CH.COOH
   /  |  |                          /  |  |
CH3   |  |                       CH3   S  NH
      S  N                              \/
      \ /                               CH        Sodium penicilloate
      CH                                |
      |   \        +NaOH    ——→         CH.COONa (or Et)
      |    CO                           |
      |   /        or EtOH              NH.CO.R
      CH
      |
      NH.CO.R
```

A similar change takes place with organic bases, which react with penicillin to form amides of penicilloic acid.

The reactions taking place in acid solutions are quite different. In very mildly acid conditions penicillin undergoes rearrangement to a substance called penillic acid

```
CH3                              CH3
   \                                \
    C—CH.COOH                        C — CH.COOH
   /  |  |                          /  |    |
CH3   S  N                       CH3   S    N
      \ / \                             \  / \
      CH   \                            CH    CR    Penillic acid
      |     CO        ——→               |     ||
      |    /                            CH————N
      CH                                |
      |                                 COOH
      NH.CO.R
```

and this, on further treatment with acids, breaks down to penicillamine, penilloaldehyde and carbon dioxide as described above.

The action of various metallic ions is not entirely understood; different products are obtained under different conditions. Mercury ions are known to attack the sulphur-containing thiazolidine ring, but other metallic ions may have different actions.

The enzymatic breakdown of penicillin caused by penicillinase of bacterial origin leads to the production of acid; this similarity with the hydrolysis occurring under alkaline conditions suggests that the process is also hydrolytic. Enzyme systems catalyzing hydrolysis are, of course, well known, although a system that catalyzes the hydrolysis of a β-lactam ring is at least as unusual to find in nature as the β-lactam ring itself.

Thus it will be seen that explanations based on the known reactions of penicillin and on the constitutions of various breakdown products have been found for most of the actions of reagents shown to be destructive of penicillin.

MANUFACTURE OF PENICILLIN

The problems occurring in the large-scale production of penicillin arise from the biological properties of the mould and from the chemical properties of the antibiotic. The former are most characteristic of the stages up to incubation and the latter of the subsequent steps involved in preparing a concentrated dry preparation for therapeutic use. Both groups of properties have to be continually borne in mind during the planning and conduct of penicillin manufacture on the industrial scale.

The processes of this manufacture are conveniently considered under the following heads.

(1) Preparation of medium
(2) Sterilization and cooling of medium
(3) Preparation of spore suspensions and inoculation
(4) Incubation
(5) Harvesting
(6) Concentration
(7) Drying
(8) Packing

It will be clear that stages (1), (6), (7) and (8) are likely to be largely independent of the strain of mould used; they will be the same for surface culture and for deep fermentation. But the nature of stages (2), (3), (4) and (5) must be predominantly determined by the cultural characteristics of the organism.

In the stages up to harvesting two main principles form the basis of all modifications. First, the maximum production of penicillin per unit of culture medium is to be obtained; in other words, maximum "titre" (in units) of the metabolite fluid. Secondly, there must not at any stage be a risk of contamination with penicillinase-producing organisms; that is, all these stages must be conducted under aseptic conditions. Indeed, this is only a special and peculiarly problem-raising example of the first principle, for the presence of penicillinase at any stage up to harvesting will reduce and may even completely eliminate the "titre".

In the subsequent stages, which are in fact procedures not differing in fundamental nature from many of those undertaken in the fine chemical and pharmaceutical industries, the necessary special precautions arise mainly from the characteristic liability of penicillin to undergo an irreversible, easily catalyzed, hydrolysis to inactive substances, as described above, and other types of irreversible changes caused by certain amines and heavy metals. The risks of bacterial contamination during stages (5), (6) and (7) are slight, because most of the operations are conducted in closed vessels, organic solvents, themselves having some considerable antiseptic action, are present and all processes are pushed through at maximum speed. In the final drying stage, however, the possibility of contamination has to be remembered and avoided, but it is still more necessary to ensure that the final product is, and will remain, really dry with well under one per cent of moisture in the powder.

The scale of manufacturing operations is determined by four considerations. First, the "titre"; secondly, the losses during processing; thirdly, the size of dose required per patient; fourthly, the number of patients to be treated. The last two factors are variable, and therefore cannot be forecast. We have taken, just as example, the scale of operations necessary to produce 1,000 mega-units *per diem*, which would give 100,000 units for 10,000 patients or 1,000,000 units for 1,000 patients. The Table gives the relevant figures at different stages in the rapidly moving history of penicillin manufacture.

It will be seen that, even with the latest improvements in conditions of cultivating the mould and in the methods of handling the metabolism fluid and its concentrates, the volume of liquid involved is of the order of 2,000 gallons; until recently it was much greater. It must be emphasized that penicillin manufacture consists primarily in handling and subsequently in getting rid of large quantities of water, first under sterile conditions and later with minimum recourse to heat, acid or alkaline conditions or to contact with heavy metals and especially their soluble salts. The metabolism liquid at harvesting is at least 95 per cent water; the 5 per cent solids present may contain as much as 0·25 per cent or as little as 0·01 per cent of penicillin itself, as can be calculated from the figures in the Table.

The process of penicillin manufacture up to the stage of harvesting—separation of the mould mycelium from the metabolite liquid—will depend upon which of the two main types of mould is to be used as the biosynthetic agent. Of the many strains of penicillium examined since 1941, extremely few have been found suitable for purposes of large-scale production;

TABLE

PRODUCTION OF 10^9 UNITS OF PENICILLIN

PERIOD	EXPERIMENTAL*	SURFACE CULTURE	
		EARLY	RECENT
MEDIUM	Synthetic (modified Czapek-Dox)	Semi-synthetic (with "corn steep liquor")	Improved semi-synthetic (with "corn steep liquor")
Units per millilitre of metabolism fluid	10	50	200
Units per milligram of solids in metabolism fluid	0·2	1	4
Units per milligram of finished product	50	200	1,000
Concentration of fluid to finished product	1 : 5,000	1· 4,000	1 : 5,000
Weight (kilograms) per 10^9 units of finished product	20	5	1
Loss in processing %	60	50	40
Volume of liquid per 10^9 units of finished product (gallons)	56,000	9,000	2,000

* The figures in this column are of necessity only rough estimates.

some, indeed, produce very small or undetectable amounts of penicillin. The producer strains fall into two main types: the one, which includes the original Fleming strain, growing and producing penicillin preferentially on the surface of suitable solid or liquid media and the other giving more abundant yields of the antibiotic when grown beneath the surface of a liquid medium. Recently a strain of *P. chrysogenum*, a different species from Fleming's original *P. notatum*, has been used in large-scale production. The first type was used in England and the United States of America up to 1944 and the second type has gradually replaced the first in American factories and is now used exclusively in most of them. In Great Britain it is now also ousting the surface-growing strains and will doubtless completely supersede them in Great Britain also. The newest large British penicillin factories are designed solely for the deep (tank) fermentation process.

The time lag shown in the British procedure is entirely a product of wartime exigency. All information about the merits and special difficulties of submerged culture was transmitted by American technicians to their British colleagues and it was abundantly clear that its use involved problems insoluble in Great Britain under the conditions prevailing during 1942–1944, however great the advantages of deep fermentation over the current processes.

Large-scale surface culture is in effect a multiplication of the number of units used on the laboratory scale. The capacity of the individual unit, from 1 to 2 litres, is only a few times greater than the laboratory Erlenmeyer (conical) flask of 250 to 1,000 millilitres. The multiplication of the number, as distinct from the size, of units brought in its trail tricky problems of organization, handling and partial mechanization, but problems that could be faced and were solved even under the worst war conditions in England.

On the other hand, large-scale deep fermentation in vessels of more than 2,000 gallons capacity—some of even over 10,000 gallons—involved entirely new technical problems of plant design and control. These problems were also solved, thanks to the energy and skill of American chemical engineers. In Great Britain energy and skill had to be expressed in the effective use of plant that was in part "ersatz" and largely improvised and of labour that was largely "directed" and almost entirely unskilled.

In tank fermentation the sterile medium—from 2,000 to 10,000 gallons of it or more—after inoculation must be kept agitated, in order to break up the mycelium into aggregates small enough to filter, and aerated with sterile air; submerged growing strains as well as surface growers are obligatory aerobes. Both of these operations themselves require special plant and skilled control and must be conducted under aseptic conditions. The losses involved through contamination of even one tank by a penicillinase-producing organism might be considerable. The combination of agitation, aeration and asepsis—the three A's of deep fermentation in penicillin production—called for new plant design and construction which American technologists supplied, beginning in 1943. Now we are able to compete and friendly rivalry between British and American penicillin production efficiency has become possible.

From what has been written above it will be clear that nothing more than the broadest outlines of deep fermentation can be given here on the basis of British experience, although some interesting data are to be found in American publications. As already mentioned, the later stages of penicillin production, after harvesting to packing, are largely independent of the earlier ones and may be identical for both methods of culture.

The stages from preparation of medium up to harvesting are described for the multiple small unit procedure except where otherwise stated. It is necessary, however, to emphasize that an attempt will not be made to allot the credit for the great improvements that have been made in penicillin production since it was first undertaken on a manufacturing scale. Especially under wartime conditions there was an extensive interchange of technical information and only those with a vested interest in priority claims can possibly be concerned with discovering the "true and onlie begetter" of any particular improvement.

Preparation of medium

In general, media have been based upon the well known Czapek-Dox solution, although there have been innumerable variations in

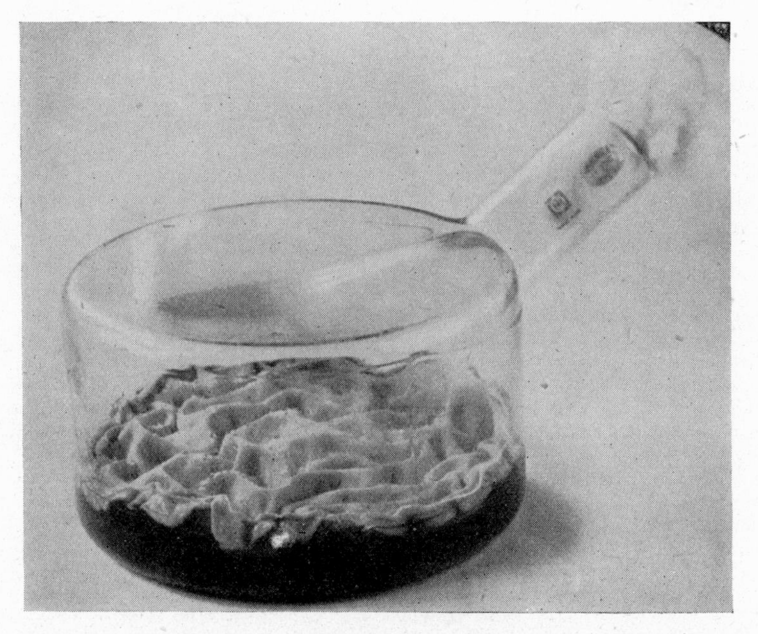

FIG. 13.—Penicillin flask—resistance glass vessel used in multiple small unit production by surface culture and in growing master-cultures for inoculation

(*Glaxo Laboratories, Ltd.*)

the nature and quantity of the ingredients used. The most important improvement took place when it was discovered that the concentrated liquors obtained from steeping maize, called "corn steep liquor" in the United States of America, contained a substance that markedly stimulated the production of penicillin. As far as is known all media used today for penicillin production contain "corn steep liquor". The precise nature of the stimulating substances present is not established. According to the nature of the fermentation process to be used the medium will be held either in tanks or in individual unit vessels. For multiple small unit production wide-necked Winchester bottles of 2 litres capacity, pint and quart milk bottles and a specially designed penicillin flask (see Fig. 13) have all been successfully used. The latter was made under wartime conditions on a very large scale indeed and over 300,000 have been produced by leading British manufacturers of resistance glassware. These flasks are easy to handle, fill, empty and clean. After the unit vessels have been thoroughly cleaned and rinsed, the requisite amount of medium is run in by means of semi-automatic apparatus that delivers a reasonably constant volume.

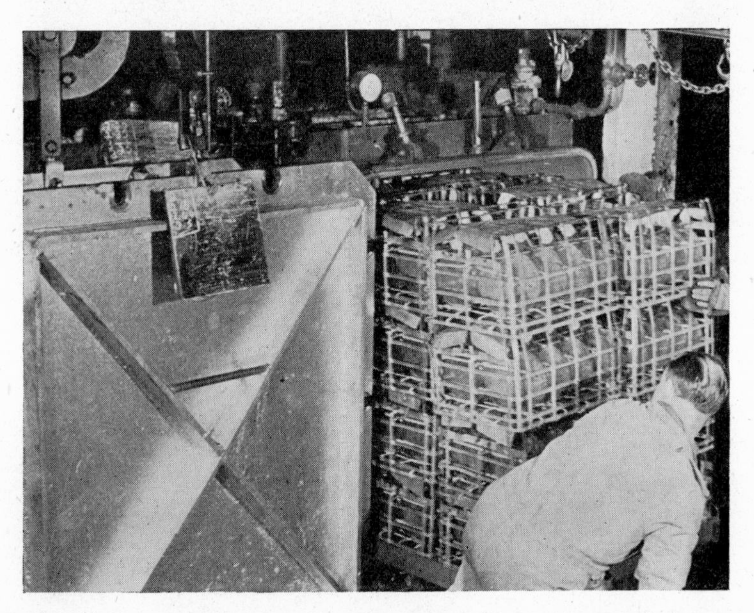

FIG. 14.—Sterilization—loading flasks filled with culture medium into steam autoclaves

(*Glaxo Laboratories, Ltd.*)

Sterilization and cooling of medium

Penicillin flasks are held in metal baskets or skips which are carried on trollies to steam sterilizers of the autoclave type. There they may be inserted on the trollies or after off-loading, according to the design of the sterilizer. A typical plant used for this purpose is shown in Fig. 14. After sterilization the flasks and contents have to be cooled in air or by carrying them in the metal skips through water with the temperature so adjusted that the flask contents reach the incubating stage at the desired incubator temperature. A set-up for the mass cooling of penicillin flasks is shown in Fig. 15.

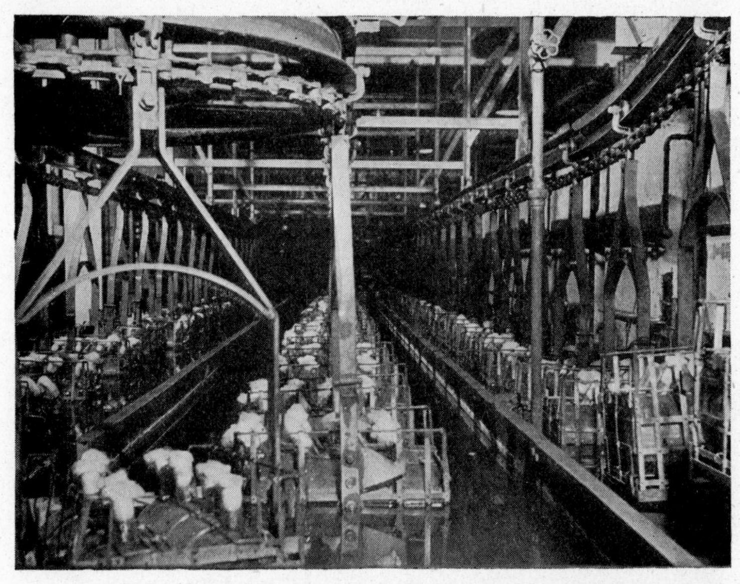

FIG. 15.—Cooling sterilized penicillin flasks—the flasks in metal skips are carried on an "endless chain"

(*Glaxo Laboratories, Ltd.*)

Preparation of spore suspensions and inoculation

Safeguarding of the parent penicillium culture is one of the most serious responsibilities in penicillin production. Various devices have been used both for the storing of spores and for the preparation of massive cultures. The system may be envisaged as a radial one. In a central laboratory a trained mycologist will carefully tend his basic strain, making sure that it remains uncontaminated and an active penicillin producer and also, as far as possible, of genetic uniformity. From this strain he will produce a number of subcultures and these will be distributed to the manufacturing units. These in turn will produce further subcultures in sufficient quantity to permit inoculation on the necessary scale. For this purpose suspensions of spores are made with a suitable wetting agent in order to secure uniform distribution and a simple semi-automatic pipette, delivering an approximately constant volume of suspension, can be used for inoculating the cooled vessels under aseptic conditions (see Fig. 16). Another system, in which milk bottles are inoculated on large movable racks, is shown in Fig. 17. In tank culture a single adequate inoculation of each vat is effected.

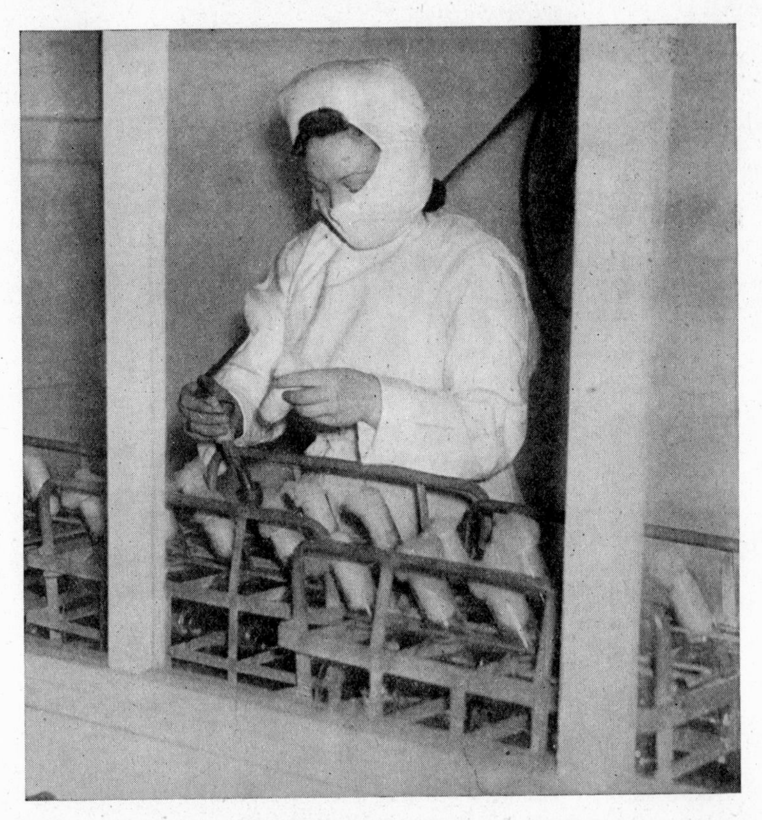

FIG. 16.—Inoculation—individual flasks "sown" with spore-suspension, prior to transfer on roller conveyor to incubators

(*Glaxo Laboratories, Ltd.*)

Incubation

The exact time and temperature of incubation are not independent variables; indeed they depend upon each other as well as on the particular strain of penicillium in use and the composition of the medium. Time and temperature must be predetermined by experiment and careful control. Fig. 18 shows the inside of a large-scale incubator in which the operation is carried out in penicillin flasks. It will be noticed that batches from different days are incubated simultaneously; this has a dual object. First it secures a continuous flow to the preceding and the subsequent operations; secondly it enables the heat given out by rapidly metabolizing mould to be largely used in supplying heat to other batches at an earlier stage of incubation. In some factories inoculation is carried out in the incubator itself, a spray-gun or other suitable appliance being used.

Deep fermentation

In this process, sterilization, cooling, inoculation and incubation are all carried out in the same vessel, of which batteries may be assembled in one factory. (See Figs. 19, 20.)

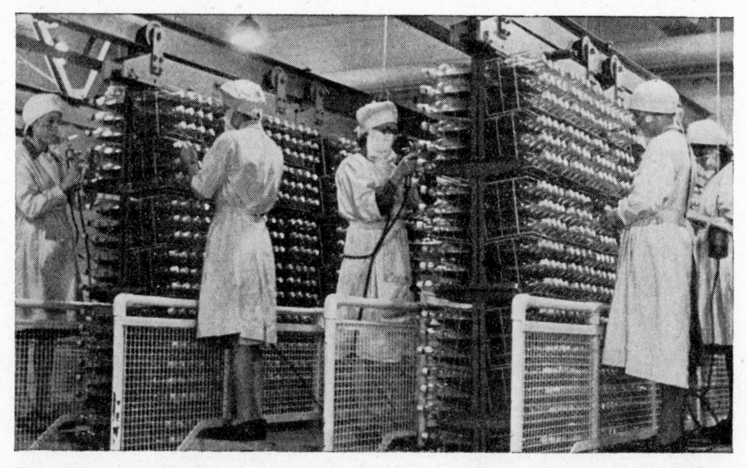

FIG. 17.—Inoculation room—milk-bottles in tiers are "sown" with spore-suspension and then carried to incubators

(*Wellcome Foundation, Ltd.*)

Harvesting

After incubation the liquid beneath the mould mycelia is simply poured away from the mould into tanks from which it is pumped to overhead containers with the minimum delay in order to avoid the risk of bacterial contamination. In tank culture filtration from the broken-up mycelia is necessary.

Concentration

Concentration is for the most part based upon the facts discovered by Raistrick and his colleagues and confirmed by all subsequent workers. It depends primarily on partition between water and a suitable organic solvent. Under slightly acid conditions the penicillin passes into the latter; at neutrality or with slight excess of alkali it remains in or passes into the aqueous phase.

By suitable adjustments of pH and choice of solvents, and sometimes in combination with a charcoal adsorption stage (Fig. 21), a concentration is reached many times that of the original metabolite solution at harvesting (Fig. 22). The aim is to produce a concentrated solution containing about 10 per cent of solids

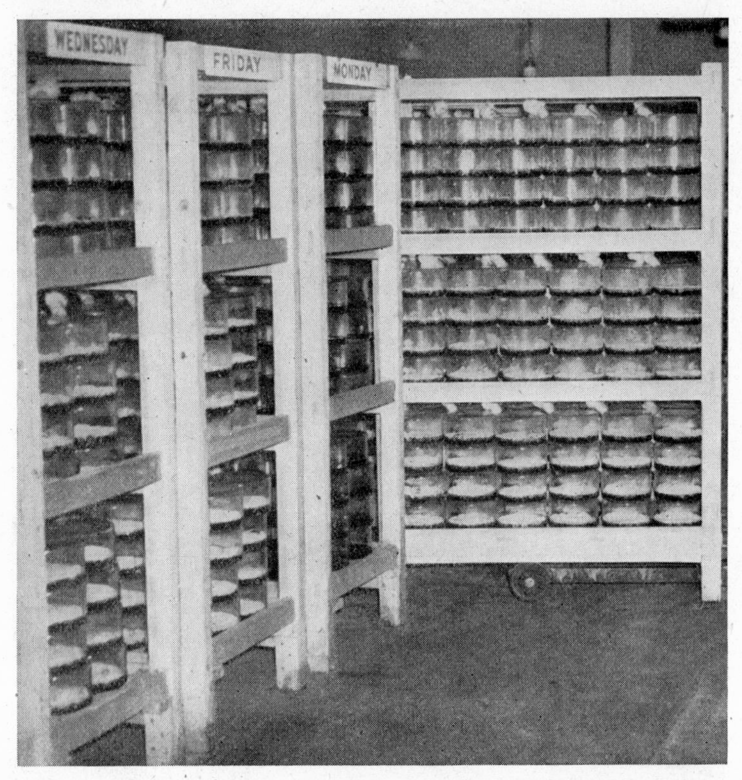

FIG. 18.—Incubation—view of large incubator for penicillin production in multiple small units

(*Glaxo Laboratories, Ltd.*)

suitable for drying. The activity of these solids will vary partly with the titre of the metabolite solution, as is indicated in the Table. The yellow colour of penicillin is due mainly to the pigment chrysogenin—isolated and analysed by Raistrick—and persists even in relatively concentrated penicillin preparations. These and other contaminants can best be removed by chromatographic methods.

Drying

Of the various methods available for drying liquids containing 10 per cent of solids, some are ruled out because of the chemical nature of penicillin and the necessity for maintaining aseptic conditions throughout manufacture. Only two methods have been

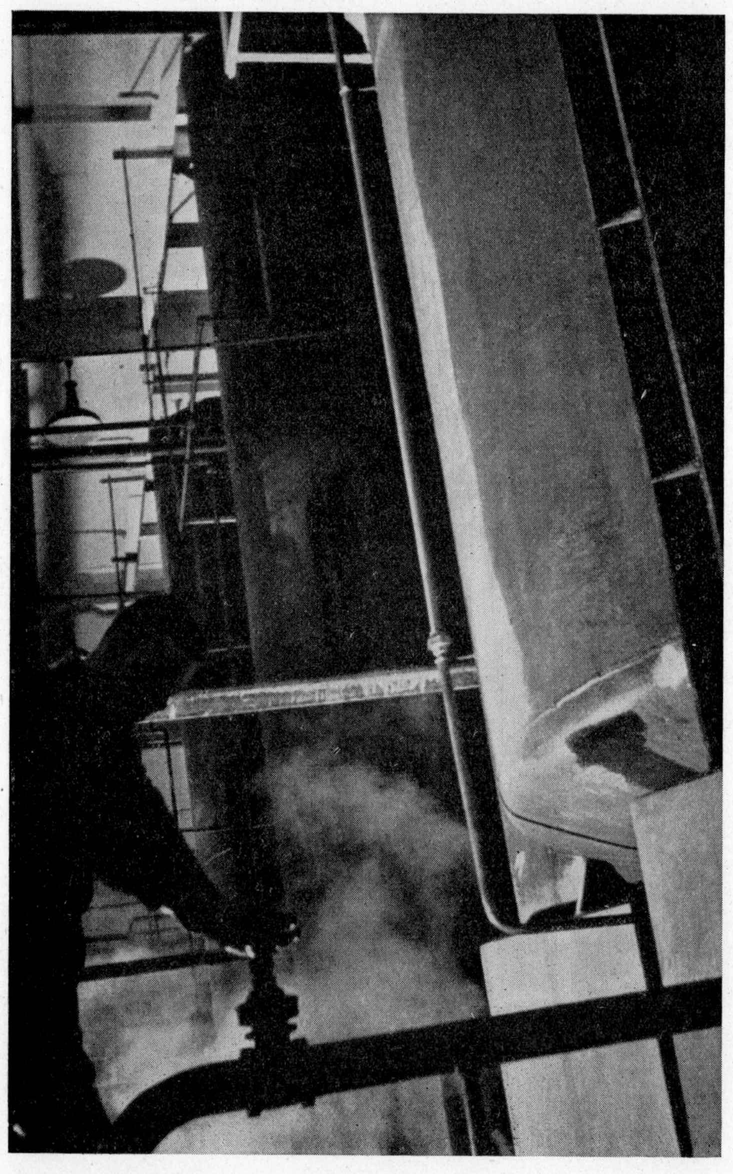

FIG. 19.—Deep fermentation—lower section of large vertical fermentation vats for deep culture

(*Glaxo Laboratories, Ltd.*)

found practicable, spray drying and freeze drying. The former has certain disadvantages but small quantities of penicillin have

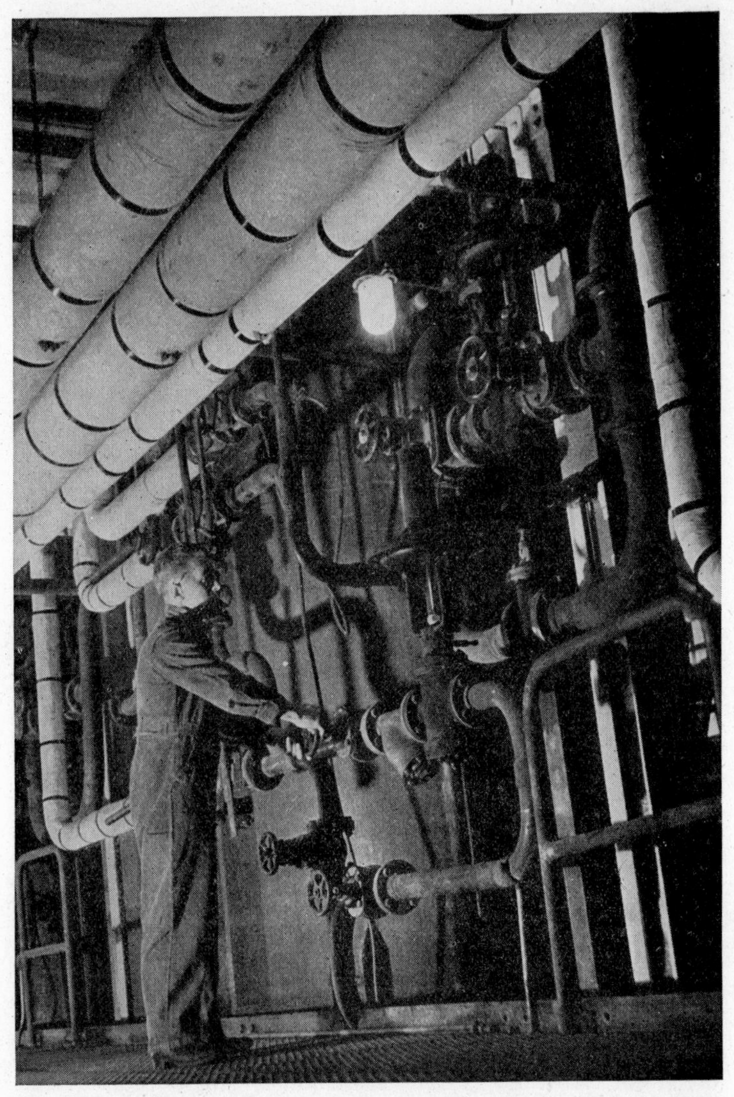

FIG. 20.—Deep fermentation—middle section of large vertical fermentation vats for deep culture

(*Glaxo Laboratories, Ltd.*)

been prepared experimentally by this means. Freeze drying, although presenting some serious technical difficulties and considerable expense in the erection of suitable plant, has the outstanding advantages that (1) the temperature is never raised above atmospheric, (2) that aseptic conditions can with care be strictly maintained through the whole process and (3) that the final product has a "flash" solubility to give a completely bright

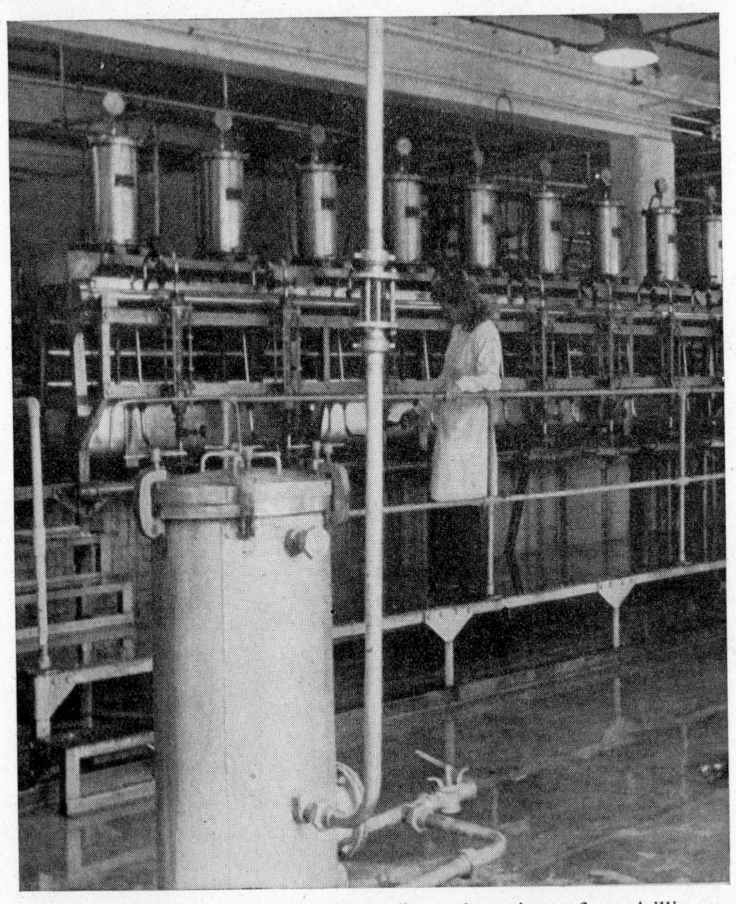

FIG. 21.—Concentration—meta-filters for adsorption of penicillin on charcoal and elution with aqueous acetone
(*Wellcome Foundation, Ltd.*)

solution not showing any deposit on standing, provided it remains uncontaminated. Freeze drying, similar in principle to the procedure used during the war for human plasma, has been carried out in bulk. The resultant powder is stored in intermediate bulk containers and then weighed under aseptic conditions into the final vial. Bacterial contamination at this stage is avoided by the usual precautions, but it is not always easy, particularly with the less highly purified products, to prevent access of moisture with consequent more or less rapid hydrolysis and inactivation of the

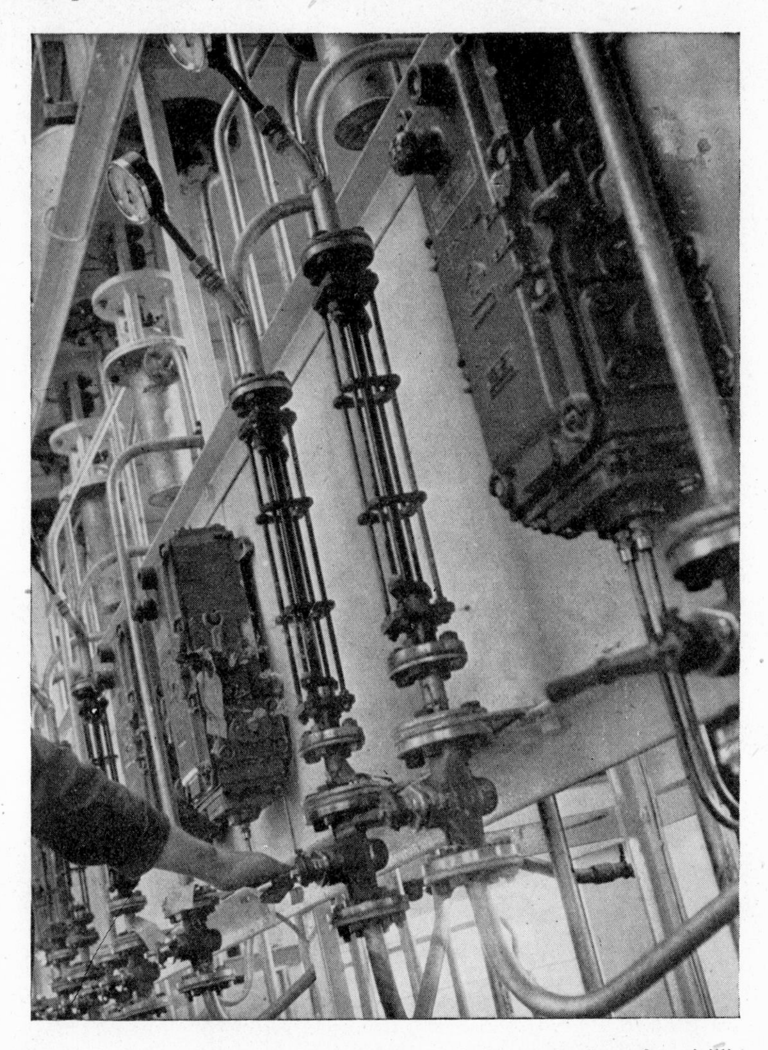

FIG. 22.—Extraction—control panel for regulating extraction of penicillin with suitable solvent

(*Glaxo Laboratories, Ltd.*)

penicillin. There is little doubt that the best method of freeze drying is that which involves filling the intended final vial with the 10 per cent solution and drying it there. The vials are held in trays, each containing 50 or 60, and are supplied with the requisite amount of solution, based on accurate assay, by means of a fine adjustable micro-burette and then dried in apparatus in which the water is volatilized direct from ice by reducing the pressure to a fraction of a millimetre of mercury. Fig. 23 shows

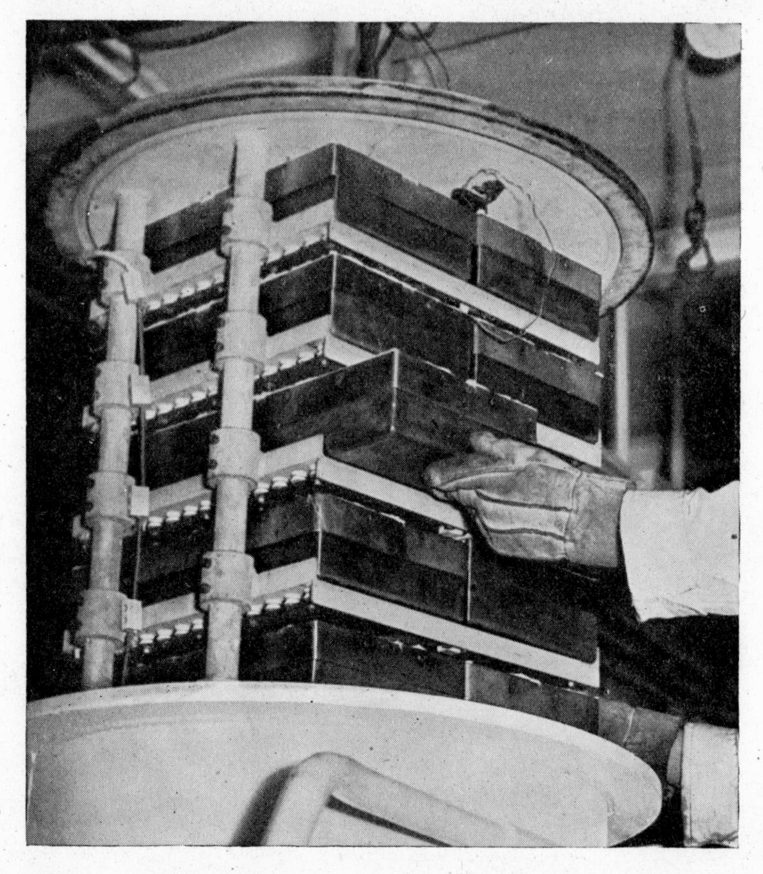

FIG. 23.—Freeze-drying—part of plant for drying penicillin concentrate in vials containing standardized quantities for direct use

(*Glaxo Laboratories, Ltd.*)

part of the type of equipment used. After drying, the vial is capped with rubber and tinfoil—the latter to prevent access of moisture which is possible through even the highest quality rubber caps.

SUMMARY

The above brief account of penicillin manufacture by the two current methods has perforce avoided mention of the great number of highly technical problems that had to be and were solved more or less *ambulando*. At all stages in the process of manufacture, whether the labour employed is skilled, semi-skilled or unskilled, strict supervision by a qualified scientific staff of chemists, microbiologists and engineers is the essence of the contract. As in other industries there is an increasing use of automatic control instruments for such purposes as the regulation of *p*H, the recording of refrigeration temperatures and the counting and labelling of each unit pack. With the resulting increased mechanization, although the number of hands involved becomes less, there has to be an increase both in the skill of the operatives and in the technical knowledge of the staff in control of production.

REFERENCES

[1] Clutterbuck, P. W., Lovell, R., and Raistrick, H. (1932) *Biochem. J.*, **26**, 1907.
[2] Coghill, R. D. (1944) *Chem. Eng. News*, **22**, 588.

PHARMACY OF PENICILLIN

By H. Berry, B.Sc., Ph.C., Dip. Bact. (Lond.), F.R.I.C.
Professor of Pharmaceutics, University of London

GENERAL CONSIDERATIONS

Penicillin is now included in the British Pharmacopoeia which defines it as the anti-infective acid produced when *Penicillium notatum* or related organisms are grown under appropriate conditions on or in a suitable culture medium, converted into the sodium or calcium salt.

Penicillin is also controlled by the Therapeutic Substances Act and regulations made under this Act govern the conditions of manufacture, its assay, standards of purity, packing, labelling and the sale of all preparations of it intended for parenteral injection. The Pharmacopoeia has adopted the standards included in the Act and has also included specifications for injections, creams, ointments and a lozenge.

Penicillin (B.P.) is issued as the sodium or calcium salt and must pass (a) tests for freedom from abnormal toxicity, (b) tests for freedom from pyrogens, (c) tests for sterility. It is packed in sealed containers which must state on the label (1) penicillin (sodium salt) or penicillin (calcium salt), (2) the total number of units in the container, (3) the minimum number of units per milligramme of the penicillin. Both penicillin salts are issued by manufacturers in rubber-capped vials each containing 100,000, 200,000, 500,000 or 1,000,000 units of dry salt (1,000,000 units equals one mega unit).

The Pharmacopoeia requires penicillin salts with a potency of not less than 300 units per milligramme and the Act forbids penicillin of lower potency than this to be issued or used for making preparations. As issued by manufacturers, samples of both salts vary in potency from 300 to about 1,400 units per milligramme, when they are light brown or pale yellow powders or scales. Pure sodium penicillin is now available as a white powder with a potency of 1,666 units. The calcium salt has not yet been obtained in such pure form.

Penicillin of low potency is unsuitable for parenteral injections as the impurities present are liable to cause reactions on injection, such as pyrexia or urticaria, and also cause trouble in the preparation of oily injections. For parenteral injections, the British Pharmacopoeia requires penicillin containing not less than 900 units per milligramme. The lower unitage material between 300 to 1,000 units per milligramme is quite suitable for preparing creams, ointments, lozenges and other preparations for topical use.

It should be noted that penicillin is prescribed by units, and although two vials may each contain 100,000 units, the actual weight of salt in each may vary because the salts vary in potency and purity, i.e., the number of units per milligramme. The declaration of potency on the label is an expression of the degree of purity of the material.

REGULATIONS GOVERNING THE DISPENSING OF PENICILLIN

Any pharmacist who wishes to prepare parenteral injections of penicillin must first obtain a licence from the licensing authority of the Ministry of Health[1], unless he is engaged under a hospital authority and a sale is not involved.

The regulation does not apply to the dispensing of parenteral injections on a prescription under the National Health Insurance Act but the terms of service of this Act require the dispenser to hold such a licence. The Ministry of Supply has made an Order[2] which directs that a pharmacist can only supply any preparation of penicillin (for parenteral or topical use) on the prescription of a registered medical or dental practitioner, signed by that practitioner with his usual signature, specifying the name of the patient for whose treatment it is given and stating the amount of the substance. The prescription can only be dispensed once unless repetition is stated on it. The prescription must be retained by the pharmacist who must mark the prescription each time it is dispensed with his name and address and date of dispensing.

PROPERTIES OF PENICILLIN

(1) It is highly bactericidal to certain organisms in their growing phase. The organisms swell and lyse. It is specific in its action, being ineffective against certain organisms, mainly Gram negative ones.

(2) Its activity is maintained in the presence of blood, serum, pus and large numbers of bacteria; it does not injure leucocytes and is non-toxic either locally or systemically.

(3) It is rapidly excreted into the urine and it is necessary, therefore, by various devices, to maintain its concentration during treatment.

(4) It is thermolabile; its thermostability being maximal when the substance is dry and minimal when water or moisture is present. The sodium salt is very hygroscopic and more liable to decompose during storage than the calcium salt. The calcium

salt is more suitable in the manufacture of dry preparations of penicillin such as tablets and lamellae and for insufflation powders.

(5) Whereas aqueous solutions of penicillin are unstable, oily suspensions of the dry substance should be relatively stable.

(6) Acids or alkalis decompose it. The optimum *p*H for stability in aqueous solution is 6 to 6·5, whilst a practical range is about *p*H 5·5 to *p*H 7·5.

(7) Certain heavy metallic ions such as copper, lead, mercury and silver tend to decompose penicillin and contamination from these metals must be avoided in the preparation of aqueous solutions. Their effect may be negligible in oily or fatty media. Oxidizing agents cause decomposition.

(8) Penicillin is quickly inactivated by the enzyme penicillinase which is excreted by certain bacteria when growing in aqueous solutions of penicillin. Penicillinase has the stability and reactions of enzymes and is destroyed in aqueous solution by boiling for 10 minutes. It is unlikely to be produced by bacteria in oily media. Non-sterile samples of distilled water may contain penicillinase and if such water is used for the preparation of penicillin solution it must be previously boiled and cooled to destroy any enzyme present.

(9) Certain pathogenic bacteria may develop resistance to penicillin. This can occur during clinical treatment with the drug. Underdosage may be a contributory factor and it is therefore important that penicillin preparations of doubtful potency should not be used.

Stability and storage

The most important factor influencing the stability of penicillin is water or moisture, the presence of which increases the effects of heat and *p*H. Moreover, decomposition by penicillinase can occur only in the presence of water. Therefore great care should be taken that moisture is not admitted when resealing a container of penicillin after removing some of its contents. This is particularly important with the sodium salt. In the dry condition, penicillin should be stored in well sealed containers at as low a temperature as possible, not above 15° C. Tablets of penicillin are probably more stable than the powder but they should be stored in a cool place at as low a temperature as possible—not exceeding 15° C. Reports on the stability of penicillin give varying results which are probably derived from data based upon the use of samples of varying degrees of purity. There are indications that the stability increases with the degree of purity. It is stated[3] that pure sodium penicillin in the dry condition is stable under conditions of heating to 100° C. for 2 hours, whilst samples of ordinary commercial sodium penicillin lose considerable potency at 56° C.

The stability of penicillin in various solutions

The stability of penicillin in aqueous solution is conditioned by temperature and *p*H. At *p*H 6·5 or when buffered at that *p*H, solutions are at their maximal stability. Such solutions will deteriorate and stock solutions should be stored in a refrigerator at about 4° C., when they may be reasonably expected to remain stable for one week without requiring restandardizing. There will, however, be considerable potency left after these periods which may be extended as the purity of penicillin is increased.

Suspensions of dry calcium penicillin in oil or in any fatty medium, provided water is not present, should be as stable as penicillin in powder. Such suspensions should retain full potency at room temperature over a period of 6 months. The sodium salt, because of its hygroscopicity, is not suitable for this purpose and would be much less stable. There are indications that rancidity in a vegetable oil inactivates penicillin although exact experimental results are lacking.

Phosphate buffers are effective in preserving aqueous solutions of penicillin although the degree of protection appears to vary with the sample of penicillin and the concentration of the buffer. Thus it was shown[4] that one sample lost only 5 per cent of its activity in phosphate buffer when heated to 100° C. for 15 minutes, whilst 50 per cent was lost in aqueous solution under the same conditions. A warning is given against the use of boric acid buffers for penicillin because of the toxicity when applied to wounds[5].

Phosphate buffered solutions of penicillin should not be injected nor should they be used for spray solutions. They may be used in penicillin creams.

Care must be taken when penicillin is prescribed in isotonic dextrose solution for if the latter is sterilized by autoclaving, its *p*H may drop to about 4·0 and such a solution may cause a rapid inactivation of the penicillin. Unless such a solution is used immediately after preparation, it would be advisable to sterilize the dextrose solution by filtration.

The compatibility of penicillin

(1) It is compatible with the sulphonamides when mixed as dry powders, but it is inactivated rapidly in aqueous solutions of the sodium compounds of the sulphonamides because of their alkalinity.

(2) It is not inactivated by certain antiseptics which are useful adjuncts in aqueous preparations of penicillin, to inhibit the

development of micro-organisms insensitive to penicillin, including those which produce penicillinase. Recommended for this purpose are chlorocresol (*p*-chloro-*m*-cresol) 0·1 per cent, phenoxetol[6,7] (ethylene glycolmonophenyl ether) 1–2 per cent, the alkyl esters of *p*-hydroxybenzoic acid and *p*-chlorophenol[8], and chlorbutol.

(3) It is claimed to be compatible with iodized oil[9], thymol, eucalyptol, menthol, oil of wintergreen, neoarsphenamine[10], heparin[11], salts of atropine, cocaine and physostigmine, procaine hydrochloride and amethocaine hydrochloride. The *p*H of any of these solutions must be taken into account and should they be compounded in acid or alkaline media then inactivation may occur. Thus penicillin is compatible with adrenaline and ephedrine, but acid solutions of adrenaline (epinephrine U.S.P.) such as the solution of adrenaline hydrochloride or solutions of adrenaline tartrate will inactivate it.

(4) It is not inactivated by aqueous solutions of sodium alkyl sulphate such as occur in many emulsifying waxes (Lanette Wax SX) used for preparing aqueous creams[6].

(5) It is incompatible with heavy metal ions such as lead, mercury, copper and silver. When the metals do not ionize as simple ions, as in phenyl mercuric nitrate or acetate, inactivation does not occur.

(6) It is incompatible with strong ethyl or methyl alcohols, including industrial methylated spirit. Weak alcoholic solutions such as 25 per cent ethyl alcohol do not inactivate it.

(7) It is inactivated to a greater or less extent by compounds containing R–S–H groups such as cysteine or thioglycollates. Cysteine has been recommended for inactivating penicillin prior to testing for the sterility of its solutions.

(8) Penicillin is stated to be not as stable in glycerin as in water, although further experimental evidence would seem desirable. It may have been due to the sample of penicillin used.

THE DISPENSING OF PENICILLIN

Penicillin may be administered parenterally by intravenous, intramuscular or intrathecal injection and, at the moment, is preferred to oral administration because of the loss of potency by the latter route. It is also applied topically to wounds, burns and skin infections as creams or ointments.

Parenteral injections

The problem in parenteral injections is how to maintain a sufficiently high bacteriostatic systemic level as penicillin is so rapidly excreted by the kidneys. Many different devices have been employed to produce this level without using excessively large and frequent doses. Thus benzoic acid[12] or *p*-amino-hippuric acid have been incorporated in the solution, with a certain amount of success, in order to slow down the rate of excretion.

Attempts have been made to design a preparation from which the penicillin would be slowly released on injection. The most promising of these appears to be a suspension of calcium penicillin in oil, containing bees wax, given as an intramuscular injection. Two preparations have been tried, one containing arachis oil[13] and the other ethyl oleate. The latter has the advantage of providing a less viscous preparation and easier to fill into the syringe, but arachis oil would appear, on balance, to give better the desired reservoir action. Comparative tests with both preparations show that the ethyl oleate suspension gave a blood concentration of penicillin as high as that of a similar strength aqueous solution but the concentration fell rapidly. The arachis oil suspension gave a lower concentration but maintained that concentration for a longer period and it did produce reservoir conditions so that one injection only might suffice. The British Pharmacopoeia has now made this preparation official.

Aqueous solutions of penicillin for intravenous, intramuscular and intrathecal injection are usually prepared in physiological solution of sodium chloride and occasionally in sterile isotonic dextrose solution. In the latter case, care must be taken that the dextrose solution has not become unduly acid as a result of autoclaving. The British Pharmacopoeia includes two parenteral injections, one a solution in physiological saline and another as a suspension in oil.

Injectio Penicillini (*B.P.*) (Injection of Penicillin, B.P.).—Injection of penicillin for intravenous, intramuscular or intrathecal injection is prepared by dissolving the contents of a sealed container in non-pyrogenic physiological solution of sodium chloride. When no strength is specified by the prescriber then an injection containing 20,000 units per millilitre shall be dispensed. The sodium or calcium salt may be used as they are therapeutically interchangeable, but the potency should not be less than 900 units per milligramme. When several doses of the injection are required in the same container then the solution must contain 0·1 per cent of chlorocresol as a bacteriostatic to prevent the growth of any penicillin-resistant organisms. Solutions for intrathecal injection must not contain chlorocresol and must be dispensed in single dose containers.

Solutions for intravenous injection (particularly intravenous drip solutions) must not contain chlorocresol if the volume dose exceeds 15 millilitres.

Any of these aqueous solutions of penicillin should not be stored longer than 7 days and should be kept at a temperature not exceeding 4° C.

As the preparation of these solutions involves the aseptic transference of the penicillin to the saline, strict aseptic technique must be used, including all the precautions of air conditioning of the laboratory or cabinet. Particular emphasis on aseptic precautions must apply to the preparations of intrathecal injections where contamination with such a penicillin-resistant organism as *Ps. aeruginosa* (*B. pyocyancus*) may be very dangerous. It should be remembered that infection with this type of organism may also lead to a rapid inactivation of the penicillin.

A warning is given[14] concerning the possibility of inactivation of penicillin by some samples of rubber tubing used in the drip apparatus. If this is suspected the rubber tubing should be processed by boiling in very diluted sodium hydroxide followed by boiling in diluted hydrochloric acid and then well washing with boiled distilled water until it has a neutral reaction.

Injectio Penicillini Oleosa (*B.P.*) (Oily Injection of Penicillin).—Oily injection of penicillin is intended for intramuscular injection only. The strength is 125,000 units per millilitre. It is prepared as follows.

Calcium penicillin		12,500,000 units
White beeswax		4·5 grammes
Arachis oil	to	100 millilitres.

Melt the wax in the arachis oil and sterilize by heating at 150° for one hour and at the same time allow the solution to filter through filter paper. Cool. Using aseptic technique incorporate the penicillin in the sterile base by trituration in a sterilized mortar; distribute into sterilized containers and seal.

Whilst oily injection of penicillin should be stored in a cool place it should retain its potency for at least six months at room temperature.

The preparation should be warmed to blood heat for several minutes and shaken before drawing it into a warmed syringe.

It should be labelled with (a) the name of the injection, (b) the number of units per millilitre, (c) "For intramuscular use only".

Sodium penicillin, because of its hygroscopicity, is not as suitable as the calcium salt for this preparation. The calcium salt used should have a potency of not less than 900 units per millilitre.

PREPARATIONS FOR TOPICAL USE

These comprise creams and ointments; tablets, lozenges and pastilles; eye drops, eye ointments and lamellae; spray solutions for wounds, nose and throat; powder for the insufflation of wounds; snuffs; inhalations; solutions.

Creams and ointments

Creams in the form of oil-in-water emulsions are in general use for the treatment of superficial wounds, burns and various skin infections. Ointments with a greasy base or compounded as water-in-oil emulsions are also used for skin infections.

These forms of application have a wide clinical use because they afford a means of slowly releasing penicillin at the site of infection. A wide range of potency is employed varying from 200 to 1,000 units per gramme.

There is a wide choice of base, which is determined first by the therapeutic use of the preparation, and secondly by the pharmacological necessity of producing a stable preparation. Aqueous creams of the oil-in-water type are very convenient for wounds and burns because they are miscible with water and wound exudates; they do not dry on the wounds or the dressing. Such aqueous preparations are, however, unstable and at room temperature their maximal life does not exceed 7 days. Moreover, such preparations, unless kept sterile or protected with some bacteriostatic, may become infected with organisms producing penicillinase. This can develop because of the water present and may cause rapid inactivation. Non-aqueous oily bases containing dry calcium penicillin and not containing water will remain stable at room temperature for 6 months. While not so suitable for application to wounds, they are suitable for most skin infections, unless the fatty base is contra-indicated, as in the case of lesions of the acne type when an aqueous cream should be used.

The usual type of aqueous cream is one prepared as an oil-in-water emulsion incorporating paraffins and using Lanette wax SX as the emulgent. The paraffins prevent the cream drying hard on the wound and dressings. The use of Lanette wax SX has been criticized[15] as some samples when autoclaved develop acidity which tends to inactivate the penicillin. Care must be taken not to exceed the time and temperature stated.

The British Pharmacopoeia now includes two aqueous creams of the oil-in-water type; one a sterilized cream not containing added bacteriostatic and intended for the treatment of superficial wounds and burns and the other contains 0·1 per cent of chlorocresol and is intended for skin infections, minor wounds and burns. Both creams contain 500 units per gramme.

Cremor Penicillini Sterilisatus (*B.P.*) (Sterilized Penicillin

Cream).—This cream is prepared according to the following formula.

Sodium or calcium penicillin	50,000 units
Lanette wax SX	7·0 grammes
Hard paraffin	5·0 grammes
Liquid paraffin	41·0 grammes
Sterilized water	47 millilitres.

This produces a thick cream. The Pharmacopoeia permits the quantities of hard and liquid paraffin to be varied or omitted, or soft paraffin to be added, in order to produce creams of different consistence. A pourable cream may be made by using Lanette wax SX 3·5 grammes, liquid paraffin 15 grammes and sterilized water 81·5 millilitres. In preparing the cream the Lanette wax SX and the paraffins are melted together with gentle heat and transferred to a wide-mouthed screw-topped bottle and cooled to about 60° C. Forty millilitres of the sterilized water warmed to about 60° C. are added, the bottle closed and shaken to emulsify. The bottle is placed in an autoclave and heated to 115° C. for 30 minutes, then removed and cooled to about 60° C. Then a solution of 50,000 units of sodium or calcium penicillin in the remainder of the sterilized water is added, the bottle closed, shaken vigorously and rapidly cooled.

Sterilized Penicillin Cream is intended for the treatment of surface wounds and extensive burns. Because it does not contain a bacteriostatic other than penicillin, it is liable to become infected with penicillin-resistant organisms, and, consequently it is preferable to dispense it in bottles containing sufficient cream for one application only. It should be handled and applied aseptically by trained persons and should not be applied by the patient.

Because it contains water it will lose potency on storage and should, therefore, be freshly prepared. It may be kept in a refrigerator at about 4° C. for 7 days without serious loss of potency.

Cremor Penicillini (*B.P.*) (Penicillin Cream).—The basis for this cream is similar to that for the sterilized cream except that it contains 0·1 per cent of chlorocresol as a bacteriostatic. Permission is given for variation in the paraffin content in order to produce a variation in consistence.

The Lanette wax SX and the paraffins are melted together with gentle heat, transferred to a wide-mouthed-screw-topped bottle or pot and cooled to about 60° C. The distilled water is heated to about boiling point for 5 minutes (to destroy any penicillinase), the chlorocresol is dissolved in the hot water, and the solution cooled to about 60° C. Fifty thousand units of sodium or calcium penicillin are dissolved in this solution which is then added to the warm base in the container. The latter is closed, shaken vigorously to emulsify and rapidly cooled. This cream is suitable for the treatment of skin infections where an aqueous preparation is indicated. Because it contains chlorocresol, no penicillinase-producing organism will develop in it and it is a preparation which can be applied by the patient himself as no aseptic precautions are necessary in handling it. Because it contains water it will lose potency on storage. It should be issued freshly prepared in a quantity for not more than 7 days' treatment. The patient should be instructed to keep it in a cool place.

Unguentum Penicillini (*B.P.*) (Ointment of Penicillin).—This is prepared as follows. It contains 500 units per gramme.

Calcium penicillin	50,000 units
Ointment of Wool Alcohols	100 grammes.

The base is first heated to about 110° C. for one hour to drive off any water and then cooled. The penicillin is triturated with a little of the base and then the remainder is incorporated. The Pharmacopoeia directs that the ointment should be stored in a well closed container protected from moisture. It is best dispensed in a collapsible tube. Sodium penicillin is not as suitable as the calcium salt for this preparation because of its hygroscopicity. This ointment is suitable for the treatment of skin infections in which the use of an oily base is not contra-indicated.

Because it does not contain water, the ointment is much more stable during storage than the cream. It should retain its potency for about 6 months at room temperature and, from the point of view of economy, should be preferred to the cream.

An ointment with a base of Eucerin LM[16] (which is similar to hydrous ointment B.P.) has been recommended. This will give a water-in-oil emulsion but such an ointment will not have the same stability during storage as the official ointment.

If it is desired to have an anhydrous greasy base[6] which is water-miscible, then a base of the following composition is suitable: Ointment of Wool Alcohols 50 grammes, Lanette wax SX 20 grammes, liquid paraffin 30 grammes. Such an ointment could be removed by washing with warm water. Because it does not contain water it should be stable for about 6 months.

Penicillin and phenoxetol cream.—This cream has been used for the treatment of wounds having a general infection including *Ps. aeruginosa* which is insensitive to penicillin. It can be prepared by the method described for sterilized penicillin cream but including 2 per cent of phenoxetol. The cream has the same stability as the penicillin cream. It should be freshly prepared and may be kept at 4° C. for 7 days. It will have the advantage that the growth of infecting organisms will be inhibited by the phenoxetol and therefore there is no risk of inactivation by penicillinase.

Oculentum Penicillini (*B.P.*) (Penicillin Ointment for the Eye).—This is prepared with the basis directed for Oculenta B.P. Calcium penicillin should be used in preference to the sodium salt and water should not be incorporated. It contains 1,000 units per gramme.

Calcium penicillin	100,000 units
Yellow soft paraffin	90 grammes
Wool fats	10 grammes.

Melt the soft paraffin and wool fat together and sterilize the mixture by heating to 150° C. for one hour and at the same time filter through coarse filter paper. Cool. Triturate the penicillin with a little of the sterile base in a sterilized mortar using aseptic precautions. Incorporate the remainder of the basis and dispense in small sterile collapsible tubes.

Whilst this ointment should be stored in a cool place, it should retain its potency for at least six months at room temperature. Care should be taken to use only a good quality soft paraffin.

Other preparations

Trochiscus Penicillini (*B.P.*) (Lozenge of Penicillin).—Each lozenge contains 500 units of calcium penicillin and is prepared as a compressed tablet with the precaution that water does not come into contact with the penicillin during the process. Dry small hard granules of lactose or sucrose, or a mixture of these are first prepared with suitable binding agents; the calcium penicillin powder is mixed with these and the mixture compressed into tablets each weighing about 1 gramme. The lozenges are directed to be stored in airtight containers in a cool place. Their stability should be about 4 months. They are intended to be sucked and not masticated.

The following unofficial preparations are prescribed:

Tablets.—These are supplied as sterile tablets, usually containing 10,000 units per tablet. Tablets containing the sodium salt must be carefully protected from moisture during storage. These tablets are useful for preparing small quantities of solutions or other preparations.

Eye drops.—These should be freshly prepared from sodium or calcium penicillin in a 1·4 per cent solution of sodium chloride and containing 0·03 per cent of chlorocresol. The solution should contain 1,000 units per millilitre and should be dispensed in an eye-drop bottle. The solution should retain its activity for 7 days if stored in a cool place.

Lamellae.—Lamellae should be prepared as compressed tablets from calcium penicillin and a lactose base. The official glyco-gelatin base is unsuitable because of its water content. Each lamella should contain 500 units.

Spray solutions.—Spray solutions for the skin, nose and throat should be freshly prepared from the sodium or calcium salt in physiological saline and usually contain 1,000 units per millilitre.

Insufflation powder.—For wounds and burns insufflation powder should be prepared sterile. It is made by mixing sterile sulphathiazole and calcium penicillin aseptically and dispensing in narrow-mouthed screw-capped bottles. The sulphathiazole is sterilized by heating to 150° C. for one hour. The mixed powder should contain 5,000 units per gramme for wounds, and 500 units per gramme for burns. Sodium penicillin is unsuitable for this purpose because of its hygroscopicity. Sterile lactose as a diluent for calcium penicillin has given good results. With care the lactose can be sterilized by heating to 150° C. for one hour but it is advisable to first dry it at 100° C. This will prevent subsequent caking. Dried human serum has also been used as a diluent instead of sulphathiazole. It must be prepared from sterile liquid serum and cannot be sterilized in the dry condition.

Snuff.—This is prepared with a basis of dextrose, using calcium penicillin. The strength may be 100,000 units in 11 grammes of dextrose.

Inhalation.—The use of aqueous solutions of calcium penicillin, 80,000 units per millilitre, is recommended[17]. The solution is atomized as a mist in a Collinson inhaler actuated by oxygen pressure. Adrenaline (epinephrine) and penicillin inhalant is described and the following formula recommended: solution of adrenaline 0·1 per cent, 2 millilitres; physiological saline solution, 50 millilitres; sterilized water to 100 millilitres; calcium penicillin, 10,000 units per millilitre of the above solution.

This solution must be made freshly because of the acidity of the adrenaline solution, or alternatively two stock solutions may be prepared containing the adrenaline and penicillin respectively and mixed just prior to use.

The inhalation is atomized by oxygen pressure from an inhaler.

REFERENCES

1 Therapeutic Substances Amendment Regulations, 1946 (S.R. & O. No. 467); also see *Pharm. J.* (1946) **156**, 296.
2 Ministry of Supply. Control Order (S.R. & O. 1946 No. 731); also see *Pharm. J.* (1946) **156**, 328.
3 Randall, W. A., Welch, H., and Hunter, A. C. (1945) *J. Amer. pharm. Ass.*, **34**, 110.
4 Pulvertaft, R. J. V., and Yudkin, J. (1945) *Nature*, **156**, 82.
5 Pfeiffler, C., Hallman, L. F., and Gersh, I. (1945) *J. Amer. med. Ass.*, **128**, 266.
6 Berry, H. (1946) *Pharm. J.*, **156**, 161.
7 Berry, H. (1944) *Lancet*, **2**, 175.

[8] Meleney, F. L., Pulaski, E. J., and Colonna, F. (1946) *J. Amer. med. Ass.*, **130**, 121.
[9] Romansky, M. J., Dugan, D. J., and Rittman, G. E. (1945) *Science*, **102**, 255.
[10] Jones, T. R. L., and Maitland, F. G. (1945) *Brit. J. ven. Dis.*, **21**, 65.
[11] Martin, P. (1944) *Brit. med. J.*, **2**, 308.
[12] Bronfenbrenner, J., and Favour, C. B. (1945) *Science*, **101**, 673.
[13] Romansky, M. J., Murphy, R. J., and Rittman, G. E. (1945) *J. Amer. med. Ass.*, **128**, 404, and *Bull. U.S. Army med. Dept.*, **81**, 43.
[14] Cowan, S. T. (1945) *Lancet*, **1**, 178.
[15] Gough, J. B., Still, M., and Wozencroft, C. J. H. (1945) *Lancet*, **2**, 91.
[16] Murray, D. S. (1945) *Lancet*, **2**, 544.
[17] Mutch, N., and Rewell, R. E. (1945) *Lancet*, **1**, 650.

PHARMACOLOGY OF PENICILLIN

By L. P. Garrod, M.D., F.R.C.P.
Professor of Bacteriology, University of London

The behaviour of penicillin in the body differs from that of the sulphonamides in several ways; two are fundamental and account for the far greater difficulty of its administration. The first of these difficulties is its instability in acid solution, which results in the loss of the greater part of any dose administered by mouth. This obstacle can be overcome by some form of parenteral injection, which is readily accomplished, since penicillin is highly soluble, innocuous to any tissue even in concentrated solution, and quickly absorbed into the circulation. The second and more serious difficulty is that whereas the renal excretion of sulphonamides is relatively slow, that of penicillin is exceedingly rapid. An initial concentration in the blood, much greater than that necessary for therapeutic effect, falls steeply, sinking below the therapeutic level within about 3 hours of giving a conventional dose. In order to overcome most infections which are treated with penicillin it is necessary to maintain a therapeutic level in the blood—a concentration, that is, which will inhibit the growth of the responsible micro-organism—for at least several days, and often for a week or 10 days. Treatment in exceptional circumstances must be even more prolonged than this, but whatever the duration, its effect must be continuous and a therapeutic blood level must be maintained at night as well as during the day.

The history of penicillin therapeutics is one of efforts to secure this condition dependably and regularly, with the least possible discomfort to the patient, with economy in the use of penicillin, and without placing an undue burden on those responsible for its administration.

The original method used at Oxford[1] was that of continuous intravenous injection, which was abandoned owing to the frequency of thrombosis in the vein. This complication was due largely to impurities in the drug, and present-day penicillin of good quality can be given without this difficulty[2], the blood level being kept more constant by this method than is possible by any other. The procedure adopted by Florey and his colleagues[3] was that of intramuscular injection of single doses at intervals usually of 3 hours. This method has been more widely employed than any other system of administration and is still by far the commonest choice if only because of its simplicity. Another alternative is continuous intramuscular infusion. The behaviour of penicillin has to be considered therefore when given by single spaced injections and when infused continuously.

Intermittent injection

Three routes are possible for intermittent injection: (1) the intravenous route, which produces a maximum blood level immediately; (2) the intramuscular route, which produces a maximum

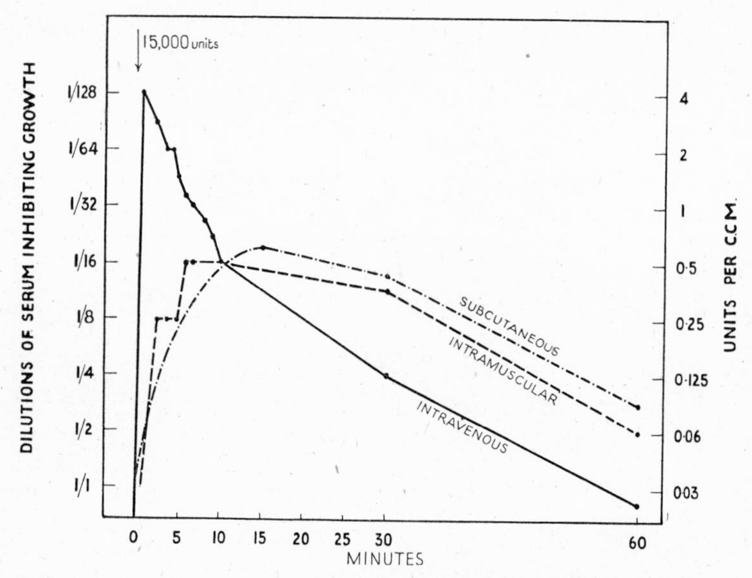

FIG. 24.—Bacteriostatic power of serum following injection of 15,000 units of penicillin intravenously, intramuscularly, and subcutaneously. (Fleming, Young, Suchet and Rowe) [4]

blood level within a few minutes; (3) the subcutaneous route, which is followed by rather slower absorption. In the studies of Fleming and his colleagues[4] (see Fig. 24), the effects of these three routes of injection are compared. It has sometimes been found, possibly when the subcutaneous injection was made into less vascular connective tissue, that the highest blood level attained by this route was reached more slowly and was lower than that following intramuscular injection, thus giving a more flat and extended curve. Penicillin is, therefore, rapidly absorbed into the circulation. If all of the drug remained there, the dose required to produce a therapeutic concentration in the blood adequate for many purposes—for example, 0·05 unit per millilitre—in an adult of average weight would be only 350 units. But renal excretion follows close on the heels of absorption, and to compensate for this rapid wastage it is necessary to give at least 50 times this amount. Penicillin therapy, as Florey has stated, is like trying to keep up the water level in a bath with the plug out. Assuming that the blood must be kept constantly bacteriostatic, it is important to know for how long this condition is secured after doses of different magnitude. The findings of two different groups of workers on this point are as illustrated (see Figs. 25 and 26). From these it is clear that dose and duration of effect are not directly proportional—doubling the dose does not by any means double the effect—indeed, the greater the magnitude of the dose, the less is the prolongation achieved by any given addition to it. According to McAdam and others[5], the lengths of time for which 3 different doses will maintain an

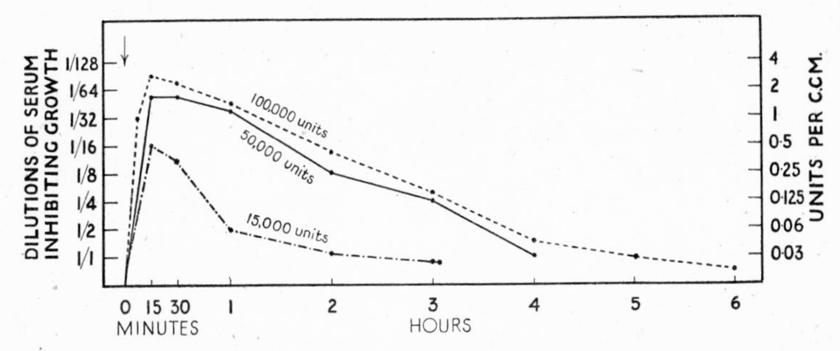

FIG. 25.—Bacteriostatic power of serum following intramuscular injection of 50,000 and 100,000 units of penicillin. Result with 15,000 units included for comparison. (Fleming, Young, Suchet and Rowe)[4]

adequate blood bacteriostasis to the standard H strain *Staph. aureus* are 10,000 units for 2 hours (120,000 units *per diem*), 25,000 units for 3 hours (200,000 units *per diem*) and 100,000 units for 4 hours (600,000 units *per diem*).

The figures in parenthesis give the total amount used daily when each of these doses and intervals is adopted; it is clear that small doses at short intervals are more economical, and the most economical system of all is continuous infusion. These authors were able to maintain the blood bacteriostatic by means of a continuous intramuscular infusion at the rate of 100,000 units in 100 millilitres of solution a day.

The immediate rise in blood level following a single intramuscular injection to 1 unit per millilitre or more, although it is transient, has been thought to have some value in promoting the diffusion of penicillin into the tissues. There is no proof that the wide fluctuations produced by intermittent infusion have this effect, and in spite of the large mass of clinical data now available, there appears to be no evidence that intermittent administration is superior to continuous infusion.

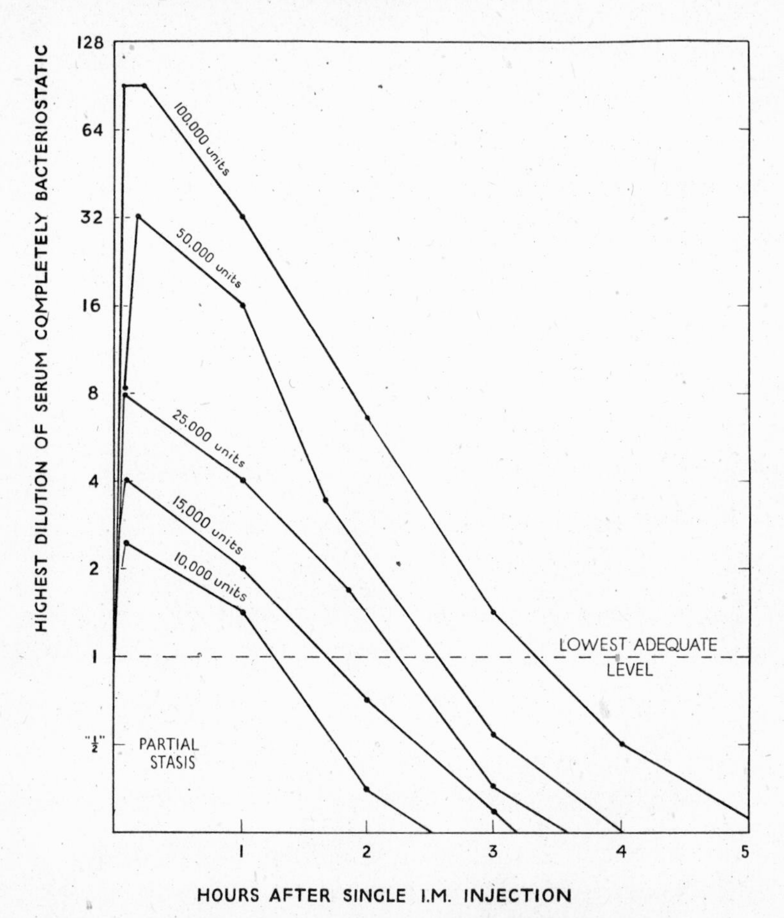

FIG. 26.—Average results of bacteriostatic estimations of serum after single intramuscular injection. (McAdam, Duguid and Challinor)[5]

The results of giving a series of doses at very short intervals have been studied by Fleming and his colleagues[4] and are as illustrated (see Figs. 27 and 28). Four intravenous injections of 15,000 units every 10 minutes forced the blood level up to over 30 units per millilitre, and this was followed by the passage of urine containing 400 units per millilitre. Intramuscular injections of the same dose every 15 minutes kept the blood level steady at about 2 units per millilitre. When administration was stopped the blood level fell just as it did after a single injection. It therefore appears that the capacity of the normal kidney to excrete penicillin is unlimited for practical purposes; hence a cumulative effect cannot be achieved. It has been claimed that 5 injections at hourly intervals during the evening enable patients to be left undisturbed at night[6], but the experimental findings quoted do not support this.

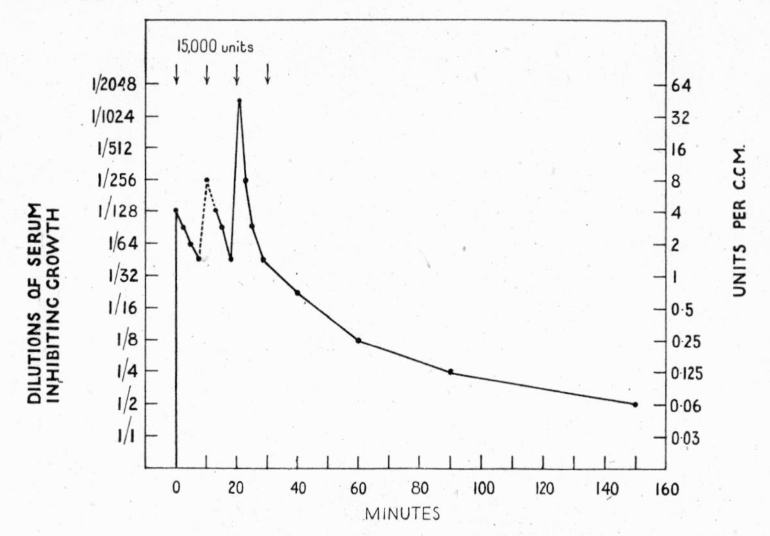

FIG. 27.—Result of rapidly repeated intravenous injections of penicillin. (Fleming, Young, Suchet and Rowe)[4]

Subcutaneous injection has been disregarded owing to the pain caused by it with earlier and grossly impure penicillin. This objection no longer has the same force, and the method is worthy of reconsideration, particularly since the slower absorption which follows should tend to prolong the maintenance of an effective blood level. Of 32 men given 15,000 units subcutaneously, 30 of them still had a measurable level in the blood after 2½ hours, whereas when the same dose was given intramuscularly it was found that the blood level was maintained in only 7 out of the 13 patients[7].

Continuous infusion

Continuous infusion of penicillin solution at a constant rate, whether intravenous or intramuscular, maintains a constant level in the blood. The relationship between the dose given and the level attained may be seen from the following table, which includes the findings of several authors.

Dose in units per hour	Result in units per millilitre of blood	Author
3,750	0·06	Fleming and others[4]
4,700	0·125	
7,000	0·25	
10,000	0·10–0·40	Goerner and others[2]
20,000	0·23–0·35	
25,000	0·50	
40,000	1·0	
100,000	2–3	Smith and Harford[8]

All these findings refer to intravenous injection with the exception of the last-named, which was obtained by continuous intramuscular drip. There is very little evidence relating to the blood levels produced by a given dose administered continuously by different routes. According to Bloomfield and others[9], 100,000 units daily maintains the blood level at 0·05 unit per millilitre if infused subcutaneously and at 0·1 unit per millilitre if infused intravenously. Hirsh and Dowling[10] assert that the intramuscular route maintains a higher level than the intravenous route. These statements, although not directly contradictory, are difficult to

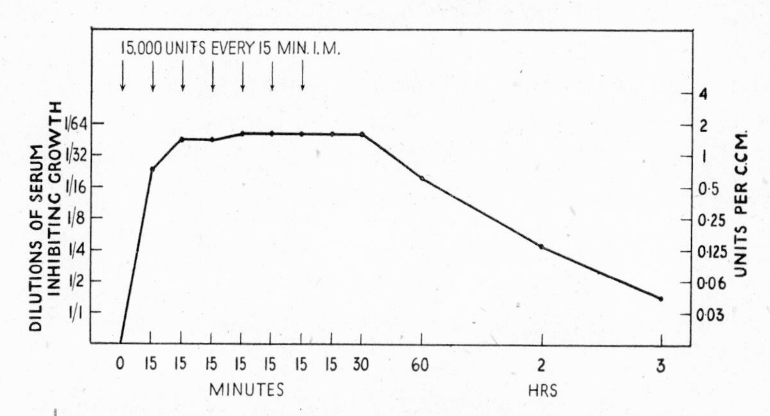

FIG. 28.—Result of rapidly repeated intramuscular injections of penicillin. (Fleming, Young, Suchet and Rowe)[4]

reconcile. There is no apparent reason why penicillin running directly into a vein should produce an effect differing from that of penicillin reaching the circulation in a few minutes *via* the tissues, and the probability is that the route makes little difference. Nor does it appear that the volume of fluid in which the daily dose is dissolved affects the result; this varies from a litre or more by the intravenous route to 100 millilitres or less intramuscularly.

Distribution in the body

The distribution of penicillin in the body after absorption was carefully studied by Florey and his colleagues[1] at an early stage in their work. A large proportion of the quantity administered appeared in the urine, and penicillin was also readily detected in the bile for several hours ; a small amount was found in the saliva, but none in the cerebrospinal fluid, lacrimal secretion, or pancreatic juice. Excretion in the bile, observed by these workers in the cat and in the rabbit, has been confirmed in man by Rammelkamp and Helm[11], who found the concentration in the bile to be higher than that in the blood. These general findings were confirmed by Rammelkamp and Keefer[12], who also studied the partition of penicillin in the blood between cells and plasma ; they found that less than 10 per cent was contained in the erythrocytes. A more detailed study of the distribution of penicillin in different tissues and organs, including the eye, has since been made by Struble and Bellows[13]. Penicillin traverses the placenta ; it has been demonstrated in the foetal circulation when a large dose has been given shortly before birth to the mother[14].

Diffusion takes place from the blood into serous sacs. The conditions governing this transfer are not clear—whether an equilibrium is reached and maintained between the content of the blood and that of a serous effusion, or whether the content of an effusion is only that of the fluid transuding or exuding from the circulation to form it ; probably the former explanation is correct. The point is practically immaterial, since infected effusions are best treated by injecting penicillin directly into them, by which means a far higher concentration is achieved than can possibly be attained by the systemic route. Absorption into the circulation follows, its rate apparently depending on the volume of the effusion and the state of the lining membrane. It is rapid from a normal serous cavity[15], but slow from such a collection as an empyema, in which an effective concentration may persist for several days. Absorption from a serous cavity is retarded if penicillin is being administered systemically at the same time[16].

Penicillin in the cerebrospinal fluid

The inability of penicillin to pass into the cerebrospinal fluid is by far the most important gap in its distribution in the body. This has been the subject of repeated observations culminating in the extensive study made by McDermott and Nelson[17], who examined the cerebrospinal fluid of 70 patients under treatment, and found a trace of penicillin only in fluids obtained after intramuscular injection in a single dose of 300,000 units or more, producing a blood level of 10 units or more per millilitre. There are several observations suggesting that some diffusion takes place through the meninges when they are acutely inflamed, but this should not be relied upon for the treatment of meningitis. The intrathecal injection of penicillin solution, first practised by Fleming[18], and subsequently studied by Cairns and his colleagues[19, 20], is safe and highly effective. A single dose of 4,000 units will maintain an adequate level in the cerebrospinal fluid for 24 hours. It appears to diffuse with remarkable facility; not only does it appear in the lumbar fluid after injection into the lateral ventricle, but injection by the lumbar route ensures a substantial concentration in the fluid bathing the brain and even, as a rule, in the ventricular fluid. It should be noted that although intrathecal injection is imperative for the treatment of meningitis, infective processes in the substance of the brain and cord can be attacked through the circulation. The successful treatment of neurosyphilis by intramuscular injection is evidence of this.

Not all of the penicillin administered by any route can be accounted for. Rather more than half is excreted in the urine, and some must be lost in the bile, but a certain proportion, probably about 30 per cent, disappears. There is no evidence that any tissue, even the liver, has any specific action in breaking down penicillin. On the other hand, it is common knowledge that penicillin contained in blood, if kept, loses its activity. Bigger[21] has studied this and demonstrated a marked loss of activity when penicillin is added to serum or blood and kept at 37° C. Whatever process accounts for this, it is presumably the same as that which occasions loss in the body.

Renal excretion

About 60 per cent of parenterally injected penicillin is excreted in the urine. The greater part of an intravenous or intramuscular dose escapes in the first hour, and diminishing quantities thereafter, a small amount still being found several hours after it has ceased to be detectable in the blood. The concentration attained in the urine is high. If the very moderate daily dose of 100,000 units is being given, the concentration in an output of 1,500 millilitres will be about 40 units per millilitre. For any urinary infection not due to a highly penicillin-resistant organism, penicillin should, therefore, be an excellent urinary antiseptic. Helmholtz and Sung[22] find that the average concentrations required to inhibit the growth of strains of *Str. faecalis* and *Proteus vulgaris* obtained from infected urines are 3 and 8 units per millilitre respectively. Even these organisms, which are usually classed as penicillin-resistant, are therefore susceptible in this special situation.

Excretion is tubular, and can be retarded by the simultaneous administration of certain other substances which are excreted by the tubules, such as *p*-aminohippuric acid. It is also retarded by nephritis and other lesions impairing renal function. This form of delayed excretion has been repeatedly demonstrated[4, 12], and a blood level as high as 10 units per millilitre has been observed in patients with grossly damaged kidneys after some days of treatment with ordinary doses. In the presence of almost complete suppression of urine, a single injection of 45,000 units has been known to maintain the blood bacteriostatic to *Staph. aureus* for 4 days[23]. It is important in nephritic patients under penicillin treatment to assay the blood concentration from time to time, since it is likely to be found that small doses at longer intervals than usual will suffice. It is also possible, though not known, that very high concentrations maintained for a long period may be harmful.

In the earliest days of penicillin treatment Florey and his associates extracted penicillin from patients' urine and re-administered it. Penicillin so obtained is purified by traversing the body, and thus of better quality than the cruder manufactured products. This procedure has since been neglected, but there is much to be said in its favour as long as any scarcity persists.

Prolongation of therapeutic effect

In the interests of both economy and the patient's comfort there would be much advantage in any procedure which secured a more prolonged effect from each dose of penicillin. Several methods of achieving this have been proposed, all of which act in one of two ways: they either obstruct renal excretion or bring about slower absorption from the site of injection.

Delayed excretion.—It has already been mentioned that nephritis causes delayed excretion, and that in the presence of any impairment of renal function, blood level assays should be done in order that the system of dosage may be regulated accordingly. It may be found that a single moderate dose maintains in a nephritic patient a therapeutic blood level for 6 or 8 hours instead of perhaps less than 3 hours.

Excretion by the healthy kidney can be delayed by administering certain other substances which are excreted *via* the tubules. The first of these to be suggested was Diodrast (diodone)[24]; the most thoroughly investigated has been *p*-aminohippuric acid. Studies of the action of this substance[25, 26, 27, 28], first in dogs and lastly in patients, have shown that when considerable quantities are given continuously—so that its concentration in the blood is kept at 10 milligrams per 100 millilitres or more—the renal excretion of penicillin is retarded. A single dose remains in the blood longer, and continuous injection maintains a considerably higher blood level. *p*-Aminohippuric acid has no toxic effects. It has to be administered parenterally, and the additional trouble of injecting two substances instead of one probably accounts for its not being generally used. The diminishing importance of the economy motive in America, where the output of penicillin has increased enormously, is another explanation of this. Benzoic acid has also been used in this way[29]; it is converted in the liver to hippuric acid, which has the same effect.

Delayed absorption.—When a solution of penicillin is injected intramuscularly, the greater part of it is absorbed within a few minutes. If this process could be retarded, a continuous and prolonged moderate blood level should result, instead of a sharp rise to a high level followed by a rapid fall. Undoubtedly the most effective means of retarding the process is to suspend finely pulverized solid penicillin in oil, as first suggested by Romansky and Rittman[30, 31], who devised it for the treatment of gonorrhoea by a single injection. The improved preparation now in use contains 300,000 units of highly purified calcium penicillin (potency about 1,000 units per milligram) in 1 millilitre of peanut oil containing 4·8 per cent of beeswax[32]. The subcutaneous injection of 1 millilitre of this compound maintains an assayable blood level for 20 hours in the majority of patients[33]. Absorption following intramuscular injection is more irregular and often more rapid. This preparation is exceedingly stable, and histological studies show that the oil is disposed of by phagocytosis and causes no undesirable tissue reaction.

Various other procedures have been suggested for delaying absorption when ordinary solutions of penicillin are injected. As would be expected, subcutaneous injection is followed by rather slower absorption than intramuscular injection. The pain which injection caused when the crude penicillin of earlier days was used is no longer a serious objection. The substitution of 5 per cent glucose for saline as the vehicle[34], and the addition of adrenaline (epinephrine U.S.P.)[35], are both said to delay absorption somewhat. Another vasoconstrictor, Neo-synephrine hydrochloride, has been recommended[36], with or without the addition of 20 per cent of gelatin. The application of an ice bag to the site of injection has also been advocated[37].

Oral administration

The instability of penicillin in acid media, and consequent loss in the stomach of the greater part of a dose given by the mouth, naturally caused this route of administration to be disregarded during the early period of scarcity. It now seems that oral administration of about 5 times the intramuscular dose will usually produce the same effect. The conditions governing absorption, and the efficacy of various methods designed to protect the penicillin against gastric acid, are not yet altogether clear. From the earliest stages of this study[38], the results have been much more erratic than those of parenteral injection, particularly when penicillin is given after a meal; absorption is more regular from the fasting stomach[39]. It is greater, as would be expected, in patients with achlorhydria[39]. Absorption is comparatively slow, continuing well into the second hour after administration; a rather more prolonged effect may therefore be obtained from each dose.

A great variety of vehicles has been suggested with a view to countering the destructive effect of gastric acid. Neutralizing substances added to an ordinary watery solution of penicillin include calcium carbonate[40], aluminium hydroxide[41], magnesium hydroxide[42], trisodium citrate[43], disodium hydrogen phosphate[44] and basic aluminium aminoacetate[45]. The penicillin has been enclosed in capsules[46, 47], and suspended in various oils[48, 49, 50], or mixed with raw egg[51, 52]. It is impossible to pronounce judgment on the relative efficacy of these different proceedings. According to Finland and others[39], who have studied this subject more extensively than most of the authors quoted above, 61 patients with gonorrhoea and 7 with pneumonia were treated by the oral route, and various proprietary capsules were tried containing oil suspensions or buffer materials. A simple aqueous solution gave results as good as any of these; a suspension of aluminium hydroxide seemed to improve absorption slightly. Among the preparations used by Bunn and his colleagues[53] in the normally successful treatment of 45 cases of pneumonia was a simple solution in iced water; it is of course possible that the hypochlorhydria often associated with severe acute infections may aid absorption in such patients.

Oral administration is therefore perfectly feasible if expenditure at the rate of, for example, 600,000 units a day, is justified. Finland takes the view that it should be used only in infections due to highly sensitive organisms. He would not include even staphylococcal infections in this category, and adds that very severe infections of any kind call for treatment by the more dependable parenteral route.

Other routes of administration

It is not within the purpose of this chapter to discuss various methods of applying penicillin locally, but it should be mentioned that any such method results in some degree of absorption; since the amounts used are usually small, this is of little consequence. It has been shown that if a highly concentrated penicillin solution is nebulized and inhaled, absorption takes place in the lungs, thus producing both a systemic and a local effect[54], Small doses administered by this route, usually by intubation or intratracheal injection, have been found useful for the purely local treatment of bronchiectasis, and larger doses have been inhaled to combine a systemic with a local effect.

Absorption from infected cavities.—A much more useful procedure is to combine local and systemic treatment by injecting a large dose of penicillin into an infected cavity. Florey and Heatley[15] have shown that if 120,000 units of penicillin are injected into an empyema cavity after aspiration, a therapeutic level of penicillin is maintained in the blood for 24 hours. A similar although less prolonged effect followed injection into an abscess, an infected joint, and into the theca. It is necessary that the cavity should be infected—that is, absorption is rapid from the normal pleura—and presumably the duration of effect depends also in part on the volume of the effusion. This is a very convenient method of treating patients who have large collections of pus. These authors also point out that a large intrathecal evening dose of penicillin given to patients with meningitis will maintain a systemic as well as a local effect during the night, and thus enable them to be undisturbed by intramuscular injections. Highly purified penicillin is necessary if a large dose is to be given by this route.

Absorption from the intestine.—Duodenal intubation, although it evades the gastric acid barrier and thus permits absorption, is not a feasible procedure in practice. Rectal administration is inefficient because penicillinase is produced by some of the bacteria in the lower bowel, and much of the penicillin is destroyed by it. Some absorption follows the administration of very large doses by rectal suppository[55], but the results are altogether too variable for any reliance to be placed on this method.

Toxic effects

The most miraculous property of penicillin is its harmlessness to the mammalian body, contrasted as it is with an unexampled lethal effect on certain bacteria. Fleming has shown that by a rapid succession of intravenous injections the concentration in the blood can be forced up to a level 1,000 times greater than that necessary for therapeutic effect[4]. Lourie and his colleagues[56], by giving enormous doses for the ambulatory treatment of syphilis, have obtained even higher levels, but in no case has any harm resulted. This is in striking contrast to the behaviour of all other chemotherapeutic agents, most of which have to be given in doses approaching the toxic level, and sometimes surpassing it, in order to achieve their full effect.

Appreciation of the full extent of this contrast has only become possible as penicillin of greater purity has become available. That crude culture filtrates were non-toxic to animals was shown by Fleming in his original work[57]. The early products of extraction obtained by Florey and his associates were tested on various living cells *in vitro* as well as in the whole animal and finally in man, every test showing that in concentrations necessary for therapeutic action penicillin had no demonstrable serious toxicity[1]. As purification proceeded further, the lethal dose for mice increased, showing that even such toxicity as had been demonstrable by giving large doses was due mainly to impurities[58]. For all practical purposes, penicillin of good quality has no toxicity at all. Dosage is limited not by the fear of ill effects, but only by the need for economy.

Acute toxicity in animals.—In Great Britain and the United States of America penicillin is subjected to an official test of toxicity in mice before being marketed. Unsatisfactory results are due to the presence of impurities; for instance, 90,000 units per kilogram body weight of a sample containing only 90 units per milligram were lethal when injected intravenously in mice, whereas 250,000 units per kilogram of a sample containing 500 units per milligram were not[59]. Although the products of different manufacturers almost invariably pass the prescribed test, their lethal dose varies widely. The toxicity of penicillin salts of a high degree of purity is due almost entirely to the cation, that is, pure sodium penicillin is scarcely more toxic than sodium acetate containing the same weight of sodium[60]. The order of toxicity of different salts of penicillin, dependent entirely on the cation, is sodium (least toxic), lithium, ammonium, strontium, calcium, magnesium and potassium (most toxic)[61]. All have the same therapeutic activity. Although the calcium salt is 6 times more toxic than the sodium, this need occasion no alarm, since the lethal dose for a 60-kilogram man would be over 10,000,000 units.

The actual cause of death in animals given an overdose of penicillin has not been determined. Guineapigs are more susceptible than mice.

Toxic manifestations in man.—These are all of a minor nature. There is no recorded instance of any damaging effect on the bone marrow, liver, kidney or other organs which may be affected by chemotherapeutic agents of other kinds.

One of the first toxic manifestations to be observed was thrombophlebitis resulting from continuous intravenous infusion, necessitating frequent change of vein. This appears to have been due mainly to impurities. Present-day penicillin has been given by this route with much less trouble[2]. Most commonly complained of has been the pain caused by injections; the admixture of 1 per cent procaine hydrochloride (Novocain) has been advocated to prevent this. It is common knowledge that painful injections are caused by cruder products, and elaborate tests with the different types of penicillin varying in potency from 175 to 1,127 units per milligram have shown that the amount of pain caused varies inversely with the degree of purity[62]. Good penicillin can be injected subcutaneously—a more painful route than the intramuscular—without complaint from the patient[7]. Various other subjective sensations which have been described are inconstant and of little consequence.

There is no doubt that treatment with certain batches of penicillin for several days can cause fever. This can be highly misleading, because the temperature chart may appear to indicate an increase in dose, whereas in fact the proper course may be simply to stop treatment. There is no need to do this if the continuation of treatment is considered necessary. Fever of this kind occurs commonly during administration by continuous intramuscular infusion, and is associated with inflammatory changes at the site of injection, particularly when this site is not changed every 2 days, as it should be. A purulent or semi-purulent effusion may form, and although the pus sometimes contains a penicillin-resistant organism such as *Ps. aeruginosa*—in which case the explanation is obvious—more often than not it is sterile. In such cases the continued infusion at one site of a concentrated solution of perhaps not highly purified penicillin presumably causes chemical damage to the tissues.

The most sensitive tissues to inferior penicillin are those of the central nervous system, and meningeal irritation, evidenced by a cerebrospinal fluid pleocytosis, has been frequently described following intrathecal injection. Such an effect should not deter further treatment if it is vital to continue it. The purer penicillin of the present day is relatively free from this disadvantage, and larger doses are being given with impunity. Excessive doses may damage the brain or cord; convulsions have followed injection into the lateral ventricle, and lesions of the cauda equina have resulted from lumbar injection[20].

There is abundant evidence that Herxheimer reactions may be produced in the treatment of syphilis. It is advisable to give a reduced dose during the first day or two of treatment in order to minimize them.

Sensitization phenomena.—Urticaria has been observed fairly often, and may occur at any stage of treatment. Various other skin conditions have been described, and a dermatitis may also follow local application. When such manifestations occur at a late stage in treatment, or particularly during a second course, it is natural to suspect that the patient has become sensitized. That sensitization can occur seems certain, but the mechanism is often obscure, and the erratic and infrequent incidence of the condition is unexplained. Sensitivity as demonstrated by skin tests has been observed in previously treated patients. Examples of this have occurred in a medical officer who dispensed penicillin[63], and in a man who had been "intimately exposed to moulds of various kinds for fifteen years"[64]. The chance inhalation of *Penicillium* spores is suggested as an explanation for the fact that 5 per cent of 144 normal subjects were found sensitive to the intradermal injection of pure penicillin[65]. Previous infection by fungi of other genera has been suggested as an explanation of abnormal reactions to penicillin. Some patients give such a history and react also to trichophytin (no control figures given)[66]. Sensitivity can be induced artificially by multiple intradermal injections[65]; an anaphylactic type of response has also been elicited, although very inconstantly, in guineapigs[67]. These findings are somewhat perplexing, but fortunately of no grave moment. It is rarely necessary to interrupt treatment by reason of such reactions.

REFERENCES

1 Abraham, E. P., Chain, E., Fletcher, C. M., Florey, H. W., Gardner, A. D., Heatley, N. G., and Jennings, M. A. (1941) *Lancet*, **2**, 177.
2 Goerner, Jessamine R., Geiger, A. J., and Blake, F. G. (1945) *Ann. intern. Med.*, **23**, 491.
3 Florey, M. E., and Florey, H. W. (1943) *Lancet*, **1**, 387.
4 Fleming, A., Young, M. Y., Suchet, J., and Rowe, A. J. E. (1944) *Lancet*, **2**, 621.
5 McAdam, I. W. J., Duguid, J. P., and Challinor, S. W. (1944) *Lancet*, **2**, 336.
6 Officer, R., Loewenthal, J., and Perry, J. W. (1944) *Med. J. Aust.*, **2**, 473.
7 Schneider-Green, J. E., and Houston, J. M. (1945) *J. R. Army Med. Cps*, **85**, 234
8 Smith, R. O., and Harford, C. G. (1945) *J. Lab. clin. Med.*, **30**, 502.
9 Bloomfield, A. L., Rantz, L. A., and Kirby, W. M. M. (1944) *J. Amer. med. Ass.*, **124**, 627.
10 Hirsh, H. L., and Dowling, H. F. (1945) *Amer. J. med. Sci.*, **210**, 435.
11 Rammelkamp, C. H., and Helm, J. D., Jun. (1943) *Proc. Soc. exp. Biol., N.Y.*, **54**, 31.
12 Rammelkamp, C. H., and Keefer, C. S. (1943) *J. clin. Invest.*, **22**, 425.
13 Struble, G. C., and Bellows, J. G. (1944) *J. Amer. med. Ass.*, **125**, 685.
14 Herrell, W. E., Nichols, D. R., and Heilman, Dorothy H. (1944) *J. Amer. med. Ass.*, **125**, 1003.
15 Florey, M. E., and Heatley, N. G. (1945) *Lancet*, **1**, 748.
16 Cooke, Jean V., and Goldring, D. (1945) *J. Amer. med. Ass.*, **127**, 80.
17 McDermott, W., and Nelson, R. A. (1945) *Amer. J. Syph.*, **29**, 403.
18 Fleming, A. (1943) *Lancet*, **2**, 434.

[19] Cairns, H., Duthie, E. S., Lewin, W. S., and Smith, Honor V. (1944) *Lancet*, **1**, 655.
[20] Smith, Honor V., Duthie, E. S., and Cairns, H. (1946) *Lancet*, **1**, 185.
[21] Bigger, J. W. (1944) *Lancet*, **2**, 400.
[22] Helmholz, H. F., and Sung, C. (1944) *Amer. J. Dis. Child.*, **68**, 236.
[23] Humphrey, J. H. (1944) *Nature*, **154**, 765.
[24] Rammelkamp, C. H., and Bradley, S. E. (1943) *Proc. Soc. exp. Biol., N.Y.*, **53**, 30.
[25] Beyer, K. H., Woodward, R., Peters, L., Verwey, W. F., and Mattis, P. A. (1944) *Science*, **100**, 107.
[26] Beyer, K. H., Flippin, H., Verwey, W. F., and Woodward, R. (1944) *J. Amer. med. Ass.*, **126**, 1007.
[27] Loewe, L., Rosenblatt, P., Alture-Werber, Erna, and Kozak, Mary (1945) *Proc. Soc. exp. Biol., N.Y.*, **58**, 298.
[28] Beyer, K. H., Verwey, W. F., Woodward, R., Peters, L., and Mattis, P. A. (1945) *Amer. J. med. Sci.*, **209**, 608.
[29] Bronfenbrenner, J., and Favour, C. B. (1945) *Science*, **101**, 673.
[30] Romansky, M. J., and Rittman, G. E. (1944) *Science*, **100**, 196.
[31] Romansky, M. J., and Rittman, G. E. (1944) *Bull. U.S. Army Med. Dept.*, **81**, 43.
[32] Romansky, M. J., and Rittman, G. E. (1945) *New Engl. J. Med.*, **233**, 577.
[33] Kirby, W. M. M., Leifer, W., Martin, S. P., Rammelkamp, C. H., and Kinsman, J. M. (1945) *J. Amer. med. Ass.*, **129**, 940.
[34] Armstrong, C. D., Halpern, R. M., and Cutting, W. C. (1945) *Proc. Soc. exp. Biol., N.Y.*, **58**, 74.
[35] Fisk, R. T., Foord, A. G., and Alles, G. (1945) *Science*, **101**, 124.
[36] Parkins, W. M., Wiley, Marjorie, Chandy, J., and Zintel, H. A. (1945) *Science*, **101**, 203.
[37] Trumper, M., and Hutter, A. M. (1944) *Science*, **100**, 432.
[38] Free, A. H., Leonards, J. R., McCullagh, D. R., and Biro, Barbara E. (1944) *Science*, **100**, 431.
[39] Finland, M., Meads, M., Ory, E. M., and Wilcox, Clare (1945) *J. Amer. med. Ass.*, **129**, 315.
[40] Seeberg, V. P., and Collen, M. F. (1945) *Science*, **102**, 225.
[41] Barach, A. L., Garthwaite, Bettina, Oppenheimer, Enid T., Forman, Joyce, and Osburg, Helen (1945) *Science*, **102**, 247.
[42] Welch, H., Price, C. W., and Chandler, Velma L. (1945) *J. Amer. med. Ass.*, **128**, 845.
[43] György, P., Vandegrift, H. N., Elias, W., Colio, L. G., Barry, F. M., and Pilcher, J. D. (1945) *J. Amer. med. Ass.*, **127**, 639.
[44] Charney, J., Alburn, H. E., and Bernhart, F. W. (1945) *Science*, **101**, 251.
[45] Krantz, J. C., Jun., Evans, W. E., Jun., and McAlpine, J. G. (1945) *Science*, **101**, 618.
[46] Burke, F. G., Ross, S., and Strauss, C. (1945) *J. Amer. med. Ass.*, **128**, 83.
[47] Ross, S., Burke, F. G., McLendon, P. A., and Porter, Bettie V. (1945) *J. Amer. med. Ass.*, **129**, 327.
[48] McDermott, W., Bunn, P. A., Benoit, Maria, DuBois, Rebeckah, and Haynes, Willetta (1945) *Science*, **101**, 228.
[49] Libby, R. L. (1945) *Science*, **101**, 178.
[50] Perlstein, D., Kluener, R. G., Liebmann, A. J., and Dorrell, I. (1945) *Science*, **102**, 66.
[51] Little, C. J. H., and Lumb, G. (1945) *Lancet*, **1**, 203.
[52] Heatley, N. G. (1945) *Lancet*, **1**, 590.
[53] Bunn, P. A., McDermott, W., Hadley, Susan J., and Carter, Anne C. (1945) *J. Amer. med. Ass.*, **129**, 320.
[54] Mutch, N., and Rewell, R. E. (1945) *Lancet*, **1**, 650.
[55] Loewe, L., Alture-Werber, Erna, and Rosenblatt, P. (1945) *J. Amer. med. Ass.*, **128**, 18.
[56] Lourie, E. M., Ross, A. O. F., Nelson, Rachel B., Collier, H. O. J., and Robinson, D. T. (1945) *Lancet*, **2**, 696.
[57] Fleming, A. (1929) *Brit. J. exp. Path.*, **10**, 226.
[58] Florey, H. W., and Jennings, M. A. (1942) *Brit. J. exp. Path.*, **23**, 120.

[59] Hamre, Dorothy M., Rake, G., McKee, Clara M., and MacPhillamy, H. B. (1943) *Amer. J. med. Sci.*, **206**, 642.
[60] Welch, H., Price, C. W., Nielson, Jean K., and Hunter, A. C. (1944) *J. Lab. clin. Med.*, **29**, 809.
[61] Welch, H., Chandler, Velma L., Davis, Ruth P., and Price, C. W. (1945) *J. infect. Dis.*, **76**, 52.
[62] Herwick, R. P., Welch, H., Putnam, L. E., and Gamboa, A. M. (1945) *J. Amer. med. Ass.*, **127**, 74.
[63] Barker, A. N. (1945) *Lancet*, **1**, 177.
[64] Welch, H., and Rostenberg, A., Jun. (1944) *J. Amer. med. Ass.*, **126**, 10.
[65] Rostenberg, A., Jun., and Welch, H. (1945) *Amer. J. med. Sci.*, **210**, 158.
[66] Cormia, F. E., Jacobsen, L. Y., and Smith, E. L. (1945) *Bull. U.S. Army Med. Dept.*, **4**, 694.
[67] McClosky, W. T., and Smith, M. I. (1944) *Proc. Soc. exp. Biol., N.Y.*, **57**, 270.

BACTERIOLOGICAL CONTROL OF PENICILLIN THERAPY

By Sir Alexander Fleming, M.B., B.S., F.R.C.P., F.R.C.S., F.R.S.
Professor of Bacteriology, St. Mary's Hospital, London

INTRODUCTION

Penicillin was born in a bacteriological laboratory and has grown up in close association with the laboratory. Bacteriological laboratory tests are of great value in controlling penicillin therapy. It has already been shown that while penicillin is very active against certain bacteria it is quite inactive against many others, and it would be mere waste of time and material to use it in infections by these insensitive organisms. During the administration, also, it is often helpful to estimate the penicillin in the blood to check the intake of the drug, and in the urine to check the excretion. These and other matters have to be dealt with in the laboratory. A large number of workers have devised methods for carrying out these investigations and it is impossible to detail all of them.

The methods described are those which have been found convenient and useful in practice, but often there are alternative methods which can give equally good results.

MEASUREMENT OF THE POTENCY OF PENICILLIN

It is not usual for hospital laboratories to make extremely accurate assays of penicillin. Under the Therapeutic Substances Act the manufacturers have to state the potency in units of penicillin in the container, and this is done in the most accurate manner possible for obvious economic reasons. We can, therefore, accept this standardization and, if it is at any time desirable to see that the penicillin is up to strength, it can be diluted until it should be 2 units per millilitre and then this weak solution can be titrated by one of the methods to be described.

There is as yet no satisfactory method of assay—it is always done by a measure of the bacteriostatic power of a penicillin solution on a sensitive organism. Many test organisms have been used; I originally used staphylococcus, Clutterbuck, Lovell and Raistrick used pneumococcus, the Oxford workers in 1940 used staphylococcus; since then streptococcus, *B. subtilis* and other organisms have been employed. The International Conference on the Standardisation of Penicillin, which met in London in 1944, recommended that staphylococcus should be the test organism—not any staphylococcus, but one of two strains which had been extensively used in the United Kingdom and United States for the purpose, and which had been shown to give consistent results with all known types of penicillin. These staphylococci can be obtained from the National Collection of Type Cultures under numbers N.C.T.C. 6571A and N.C.T.C. 6718.

The test is not an absolute one, for in this, as in all biological reactions, the absolute result may vary with the conditions of the test—it is a comparison of the result obtained with the unknown solution and obtained when a standard solution of penicillin of known strength is used under the same conditions. An International Standard is maintained at the National Institute of Medical Research in London and it is with this, or with another substandard corresponding with this, that all penicillin manufactured is compared.

Methods of assay

Assay is made by one of two main methods: (1) by measuring the distance through which the test organism is inhibited in an

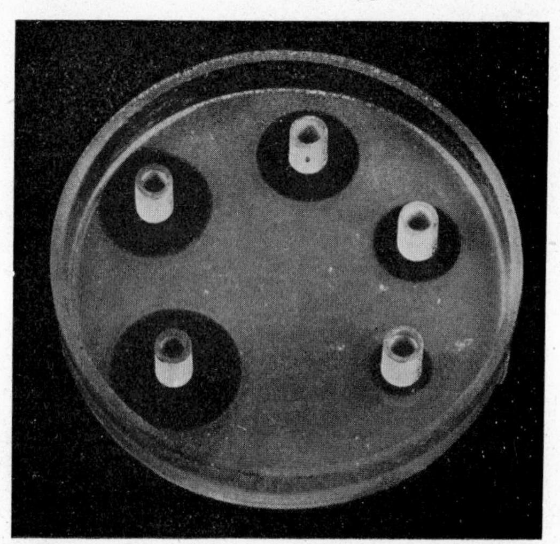

FIG. 29.—Assay plate. Test organism—staphylococcus. The cylinders contained 4, 2, 1, 0·5, and 0·25 units of penicillin per millilitre

(*Brit. J. Surg.*)

agar plate by penicillin solution; (2) by noticing the dilution of the penicillin solution which completely inhibits growth of the test organism in fluid culture.

(1) *Agar diffusion method.*—The first observations on penicillin showed that it was freely diffusible in agar and Fleming in 1929

used this as a means of measuring the sensitivity of different organisms to crude penicillin. When penicillin had been concentrated at Oxford, Heatley adapted this to a method of assay and by a control of all the factors the method gives a high degree of accuracy and is the one most commonly used by the manufacturers to-day.

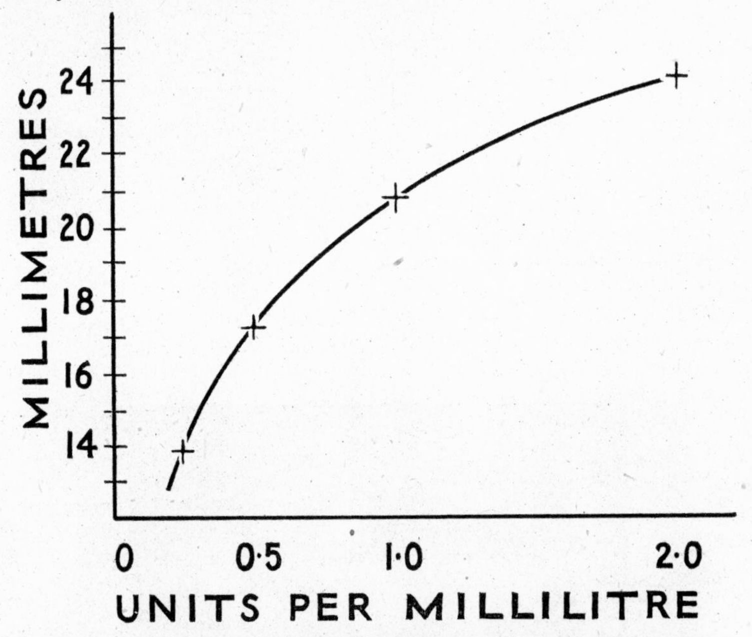

FIG. 30.—Typical curve relating diameter of zone of inhibition with concentration of penicillin solution causing it

Heatley's method[1, 2] consists in placing on an agar plate, which has been regularly seeded with staphylococcus, a number (4–8) of porcelain or glass cylinders (7 millimetres external diameter by 8–10 millimetres tall) in a ring towards the periphery of the plate. These must be made with their ends perfectly level and smooth so that they fit perfectly on the agar, making a seal which prevents the escape of fluid placed in the cylinders. Some of the cylinders are filled with dilutions of the penicillin to be tested and some are filled with known dilutions of standard penicillin. The plate is then incubated at 37° C. overnight and the diameters of the zones of inhibition of growth are measured (see Fig. 29). To obtain accurate results attention has to be paid to many details. The more important of these are given below.

(*a*) Inoculating the medium with the test organism. Melted agar is inoculated with a small amount of staphylococcus broth and is poured into the culture plate. As an additional refinement the plates may be poured in two stages: first a layer of sterile agar and then, when this solidifies, it is covered with another thin layer of the staphylococcus-infected agar.

(*b*) Pouring the plates. The culture medium should be of uniform depth. Frequently Petri dishes are irregular and these should not be used. Large flat dishes of plate glass, carefully levelled before the agar is poured, have been used.

(*c*) Filling the cylinders. These are filled almost level with the top. Small variations in the amount of fluid makes no appreciable difference to the result.

(*d*) Reading the results. The plate may be placed on a millimetre scale and the diameter of the zone of inhibition measured; or, greater accuracy can be obtained by a variety of mechanical devices, one of which is to project on a screen the enlarged image of the plate and the measuring scale.

(*e*) The establishment of a standard curve. Solutions of 2, 1, 0·5, and 0·25 units per millilitre are filled into cylinders on a staphylococcus-infected plate. For greater accuracy this is often done in triplicate or quadruplicate. After incubation the inhibition zones are measured and the curve is constructed. (See Fig. 30.) From such a curve the potency of any unknown penicillin solution can be calculated provided it produces a zone of inhibition within the limits of the curve.

(*f*) Potency of the unknown solution. From the shape of the curve it is clear that results will be most accurate when the distance of inhibition falls within the limits 0·25–2 units per millilitre. Dilutions of the unknown solution, therefore, should be made so that one or more of them fall within this limit.

The accuracy of the method has been given by Heatley and others as about ±15–20 per cent. By means of multiple estimations greater accuracy can be obtained.

Alternatives to cylinders.—The agar cup illustrated in Fig. 9 is in principle the same as the cylinder but in practice it is not so convenient when a larger number of estimations have to be done. In a laboratory, however, where cylinders are not available, the agar cup method may be used with equal success.

Discs of filter paper impregnated with measured volumes of solutions of penicillin have been used successfully (see Fig. 34).

(2) *Serial dilution method.*—The Oxford unit was originally described as that amount of penicillin which, when dissolved in 50 millilitres of meat extract broth, just inhibits completely the growth of the test strain of staphylococci. To titrate an unknown penicillin solution, dilutions of this and a penicillin solution of known strength are made in broth and each of these dilutions is inoculated with the test staphylococci. After incubation overnight the dilution which completely inhibits growth of the staphylococcus is noted in each case and by a simple calculation the strength of the unknown solution is arrived at.

Rapid methods of assay

In the manufacture of penicillin it is necessary to be able to obtain a rapid assay to enable the culture to be "harvested" at the proper moment. This has been done in a variety of ways, some of which are indicated.

(1) Turbidemetric methods[3]. By means of a photo-electric apparatus a curve of turbidity is obtained for broth inoculated with staphylococcus and containing known amounts of penicillin. The turbidity of the growth with an unknown penicillin in the same conditions can be estimated and the potency can be read off by the curve.

(2) Titrations have also been done using haemolytic streptococcus with blood as the indicator[4,5]. Results can be read in 3 or 4 hours if the proper conditions are observed.

Prévot[6] has used *Cl. perfringens* (*B. welchii*) as the test organism and diazine green (Janus green) as the indicator. If conditions are adjusted satisfactorily the results can be read in 2 hours.

Assay of penicillin creams and ointments

For clinical purposes a rough estimate is usually sufficient. A loopful of the cream or ointment is placed on a culture plate infected with staphylococcus. If after incubation there is a considerable zone of inhibition, it is clear that the cream is potent. If practicable, a control should be made with a freshly prepared product.

A measured volume of the cream can be well shaken in a suitable volume of water and, if time is allowed, the penicillin dissolves out into the water and can be titrated in the usual manner.

Assay of powders, snuffs and lozenges

A measured weight of substance is shaken up in a given volume of water and after sufficient time has elapsed for the penicillin to dissolve, the fluid is titrated in the usual way. (In the case of lozenges a lozenge should be crushed with pestle and mortar before the water is added.)

ESTIMATION OF PENICILLIN

Estimation of penicillin in blood serum

In 1943, I[7] described micromethods of assaying penicillin in blood serum. Micromethods are desirable as it is not always convenient to draw off repeatedly large quantities of blood from the patient.

Slide cell method.—Serial dilutions of the serum are made in 10 per cent normal human serum. This diluent is better than normal saline as it furnishes sufficient pabulum for the test organisms to grow no matter how high is the dilution of the patient's serum. These dilutions are conveniently made in 50 cubic millimetre quantities on a paraffined slide. To each of the dilutions 5 cubic millimetres (a small loopful) of a suitable dilution of a 24-hour broth culture of the standard test-staphylococcus is added. The infected serum dilutions are run into slide cells which are sealed with equal parts of hard paraffin and soft paraffin. The dilution of the staphylococcal culture should be such that

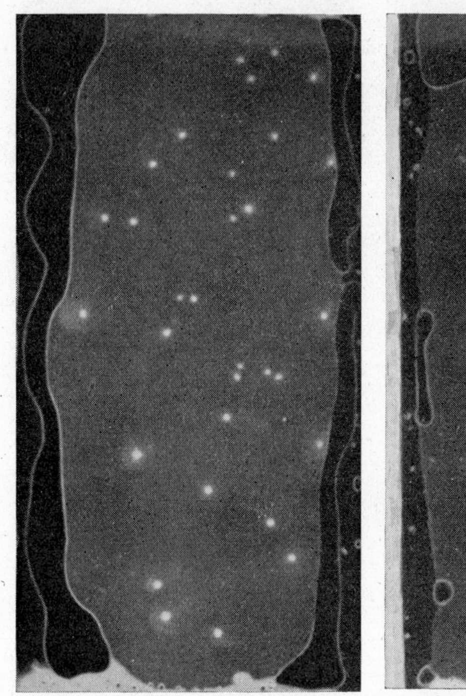

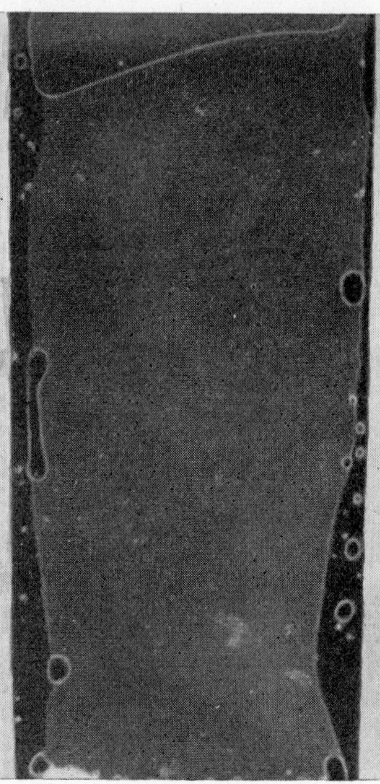

FIG. 31a FIG. 31b

Estimation of penicillin in serum by the slide cell method. (a) Staphylococci growing in patient's serum—before treatment. (b) No growth when sufficient penicillin in serum

there is a maximum of 50 colonies in each cell; it will vary with the profusion of the culture but with our stock medium a dilution of 1 in 40,000 has sufficed. (This is easily made by mixing 5 cubic millimetres of the culture with 1 millilitre of broth and then diluting 5 cubic millimetres of this in a second millilitre of broth.)

After incubation the staphylococci grow out into visible colonies in those serum dilutions which contain insufficient penicillin to inhibit growth. (See Fig. 31a.)

Heatley and Garrod[2] have used modifications of the slide cell method by making the dilutions in smaller quantities (about 10 cubic millimetres) on a slide. These are covered with small sterile coverslips, sealed with wax and incubated.

As sometimes there is some difficulty in seeing whether growth has occurred in the cells, I[8] suggested that a haemolytic streptococcus should be used with human blood as an indicator.*

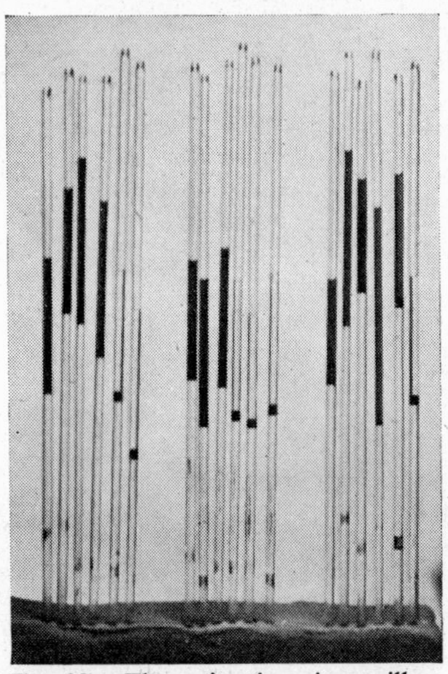

FIG. 32.—Three titrations in capillary tubes using streptococcus as the test organism and human blood as the indicator. The capillaries after incubation have been set upright in plasticine on a slide and the undissolved corpuscles have settled at the bottom. In each set the concentrations of serum from right to left are 1 in 2, 4, 8, 16 and 32, and the left-hand tube is a control

(*Lancet*)

If the streptococcus is not inhibited by penicillin in the patient's serum, it grows and haemolyses the blood, providing a good end point.

* In clinical work such as this, the nature of the test organism is not of as great importance as it is in the primary assay of penicillin in the factory. Staphylococcus was chosen as the test organism in the primary assay as it gave approximately the same result with the different types of penicillin. For clinical work the ideal method would be to test the potency of the blood serum on the actual organism which was infecting the patient, but this introduces difficulties which greatly outweigh the advantages. When a test organism other than staphylococcus is used, it can always be checked by using as a control a titration of a solution of the same batch of penicillin which was administered to the patient.

The dilutions of the test serum are made in 25 cubic millimetre volumes; each of these is mixed with 25 cubic millimetres of defibrinated human blood which has been infected with one loopful (about 5 cubic millimetres) per millilitre of a 24-hour broth culture of the test streptococcus. These mixtures are run into slide cells which are sealed and incubated. In order to avoid any killing of the streptococci by the blood itself, leucocytic action should be abolished. This can be done by (*a*) removing the leucocytes, (*b*) heating to 50° C. for 30 minutes, (*c*) using blood more than 2 days old, and (*d*) adding liquoid to a concentration of 1 in 2,000.

Capillary tube method[8]*: using staphylococcus as the test organism.*—Dilutions of serum are made as above, and infected with staphylococcus in the same way. The dilutions are then touched with the end of a sterile capillary tube held at a suitable angle. The fluid runs into the capillary and can readily be manipulated into the middle of the tube while the ends are sealed in a flame. The capillaries are then stuck horizontally in Plasticene on a microscope slide and are incubated in this position. The staphylococci develop into colonies along the side of the tube.

Capillary tube method: using haemolytic streptococcus as the test organism.—Dilutions of serum are made as before, but saline does as well as diluted serum for the purpose, since the blood which is added subsequently provides a good culture medium for the streptococcus. The dilutions are infected with $\frac{1}{5}$ of their volume of 50 per cent human blood which has been infected with one loopful per millilitre of a 24-hour broth culture of a suitable haemolytic streptococcus. This gives a blood content of about 10 per cent to the mixtures. The serum-blood-streptococcus mixtures are then placed in capillary tubes and incubated horizontally as above. Before reading they are allowed to stand vertically for about an hour when the undissolved corpuscles (if any) settle to the bottom. (See Fig. 32.)

This method gives a very good end point and it has an advantage over the staphylococcal method in that there is a much wider margin in regard to the amount of the inoculum.

In all these methods it is wise to put up a control series with serum to which has been added a known amount of penicillin (say 0·5 unit per millilitre).

The capillary tube method is preferred by some on purely technical grounds, as it avoids the preparation of slide cells and because the results are never spoiled by imperfect sealing. If reasonable care is exercised good results can be obtained by any of these methods.

Rammelkamp's method[9].—Veal broth 0·2 millilitre is placed in all but the first of a series of small test tubes. The same volume of fluid to be tested is added to the first two tubes. From the second tube 0·2 millilitre is carried to the next tube, and so on until a series of dilutions is made. To each tube is now added 0·5 millilitre of a 1 per cent suspension of erythrocytes in veal broth which has been infected with haemolytic streptococci (between 1,000 and 10,000 per millilitre). After incubation for 18 hours the tubes are examined for haemolysis, and a loopful of each of the cultures near the end point is streaked on a blood agar plate to check the sterility.

Heilman and Herrell[10] have compared the results obtained by them with Rammelkamp's and with my slide cell method. They found the latter to be more reliable in determining the actual concentration of penicillin in serum, and they were able to detect smaller amounts by the slide cell method.

Agar diffusion method.—When there is sufficient penicillin in the serum it can be assayed in exactly the same way as a penicillin solution by the use of an agar cup, or cylinder, on a culture plate planted with the standard test staphylococcus. This, however, is not sufficiently delicate to detect the small amounts of penicillin which can be assayed by the other methods described.

Estimation of penicillin in the cerebrospinal fluid

If the concentration is sufficient it may be done by the agar diffusion method as in the assay of penicillin solution or it can be done exactly as the titration of blood serum.

As there is usually a sufficient amount of cerebrospinal fluid, the penicillin content can be estimated by a simple serial dilution method in broth using staphylococcus as the test organism, as in the same method of assay of penicillin solution.

Estimation of penicillin in urine

With urine there is no need for micromethods as there is always an ample supply of test fluid. When a patient is receiving 100,000–120,000 units in 24 hours, the urine generally can be diluted to between 1,000 and 2,000 times before it loses its bacteriostatic power. In patients receiving 1,000,000 units a day the urine lost its bacteriostatic power only when diluted 15,000 times.

If the urine is sterile the assay can be done by the agar diffusion or serial dilution methods, in exactly the same manner as has been described for penicillin solutions.

If, as frequently happens, the urine is contaminated with non-sporing bacilli, a small sample may be heated to 60° C. for half an hour to destroy these, and then the titration may be carried out; or it may be filtered before titration.

Estimation of penicillin in pus

Usually only a relatively crude estimation is required, and this can readily be done by placing the pus in an agar cup or cylinder on a plate planted with the test staphylococcus, and comparing the area of inhibition with that around a similar cup or cylinder filled with a known strength of penicillin.

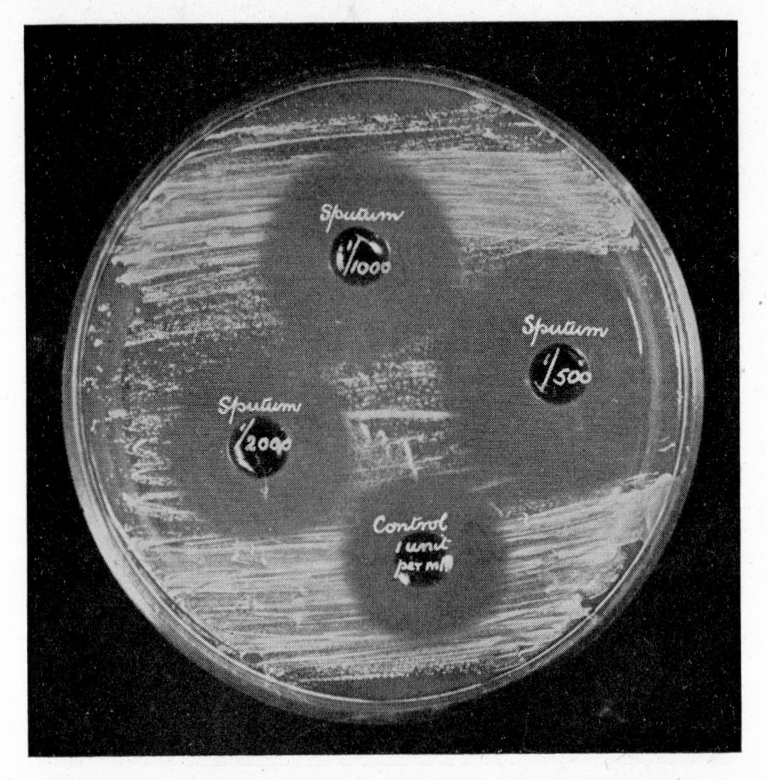

FIG. 33.—Assay of penicillin in sputum 12 hours after inhalation

Alternatively, the pus can be centrifuged, and the supernatant fluid can be tested in exactly the same way as blood serum (described above). If no satisfactory pus fluid can be obtained, a measured volume of saline can be added to the pus, well mixed, and allowed to stand for a short time to extract the penicillin. The mixture is then centrifuged and the supernatant tested.

Estimation of penicillin in sputum

In systemic treatment this estimation will have more academic than clinical importance, but after inhalation treatment penicillin may persist in the sputum for many hours and the concentration may be 1,000 units per millilitre or more. This means that it is far beyond the optimal concentration for placing in cylinders or agar cups in the agar diffusion method of assay. Dilutions in saline must be made, therefore, to bring the concentration down to that suitable for the test. The actual dilutions will vary with the circumstances and the expected result. Cylinders or agar cups on

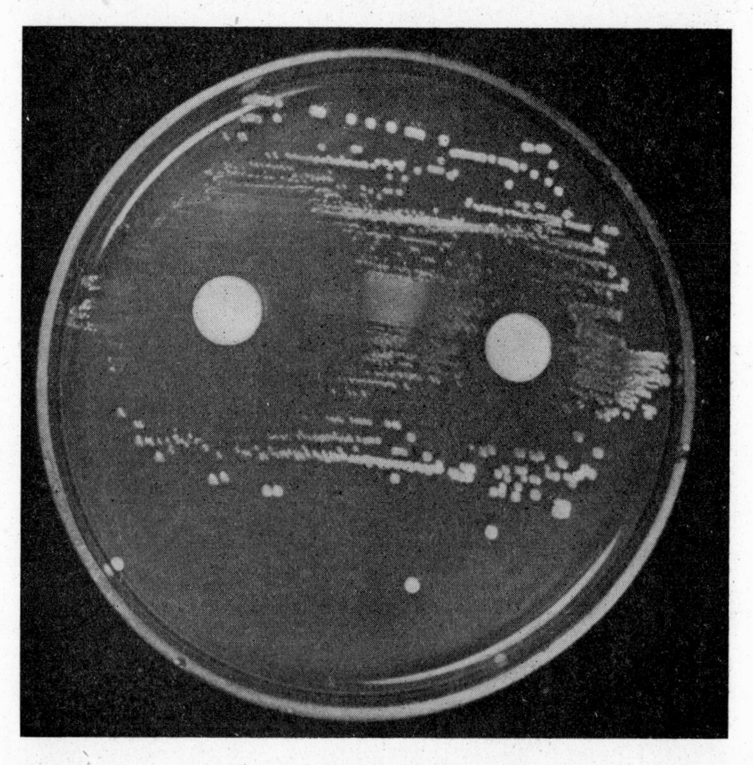

FIG. 34.—Test of sensitivity to penicillin in the primary culture. Penicillin solution 5 and 1 unit per millilitre placed on filter paper discs after the pus was planted on an agar plate

a staphylococcus-infected plate are filled with these dilutions, and as a control one cylinder or cup is filled with a 1 unit per millilitre solution of penicillin. In this way a fair estimate of the amount of penicillin in the sputum can be obtained. Fig. 33 shows the result obtained with sputum collected 12 hours after the inhalation of 90,000 units. In this case a dilution of 1 in 2,000 gave a rather wider ring than did the 1 unit per millilitre control. The sputum, therefore, contained over 2,000 units per millilitre.

Estimation of the penicillin-sensitivity of the infecting microbe

There are many methods of testing the sensitivity of a microbe which at once suggest themselves to a bacteriologist, and the actual method used will depend on the circumstances. As with the test of the potency of penicillin, they fall into two classes: a serial dilution method, or a measure of the distance to which a culture is inhibited on an agar plate. In both cases, if exact measurements are required, a control should be made with a standard culture of staphylococcus under exactly the same conditions.

Serial dilution method.—Dilutions of a standard penicillin solution are infected with the test microbe and after incubation the dilution which just inhibits growth completely is noted.

Agar diffusion method.—Here the technique varies with the circumstances.

(1) If a number of different microbes have to be tested the gutter plate method illustrated in Fig. 8 is the easiest. Penicillin in a strength of 5 units per millilitre should be mixed with an equal volume of agar and poured into the gutter. One of the microbes streaked across should be the standard staphylococcus with which all the others should be compared.

(2) If it is wished to test the sensitivity of a primary culture—as is often desirable in clinical work—2 cylinders are placed on the more thickly planted portion of the culture and these are filled with penicillin in a strength of, respectively, 5 and 1 unit per millilitre. (See Fig. 34). After incubation the size of the zones of inhibition are measured. For ordinary clinical purposes no standard is absolutely necessary but it is quite easy for any bacteriologist to streak the standard staphylococcus across the plate up to the cylinder and so obtain a control.

The cylinders may be replaced by agar cups or by blotting-paper discs. The cups are filled with penicillin (5 and 1 unit per millilitre), or the discs are soaked in the same solutions. Each worker may choose his method and once familiar with it he can obtain accurate results.

(3) Another method which was used by me in the early days of penicillin was to inoculate a culture plate in the ordinary way with the material and then carefully spread over one half of the plate 4 or 5 drops of about 5 unit per millilitre penicillin. This method is rather crude, but it is easy and it gives in most cases sufficient information for clinical purposes. It has the advantage that it permits the easy isolation of penicillin-insensitive microbes in the culture.

Morley[11] described a very convenient method. He prepared discs of filter paper each containing 1 unit of penicillin. These were freeze-dried and were kept in a screw-capped bottle with a drying agent. For use, one of them was placed on the primary culture plate and the area of inhibition was noted. The writer found that these discs retained their potency for 6 months at room temperature.

PENICILLINASE

Abraham and Chain[12] found that certain penicillin-insensitive organisms contained a substance—having the properties of an enzyme—which destroyed penicillin. This substance they called penicillinase. They found also that at least one penicillin-sensitive microbe, *M. lysodeikticus*, contained penicillinase, so its part in determining the resistance of the organism to penicillin is not entirely clear. Penicillinase can be extracted from the bodies of the organisms in a number of ways but it can be more easily prepared by simple filtration of a week-old broth culture of a suitable microbe—generally a coliform bacillus or *B. subtilis*.

Penicillinase is useful in that it can be used to neutralize the

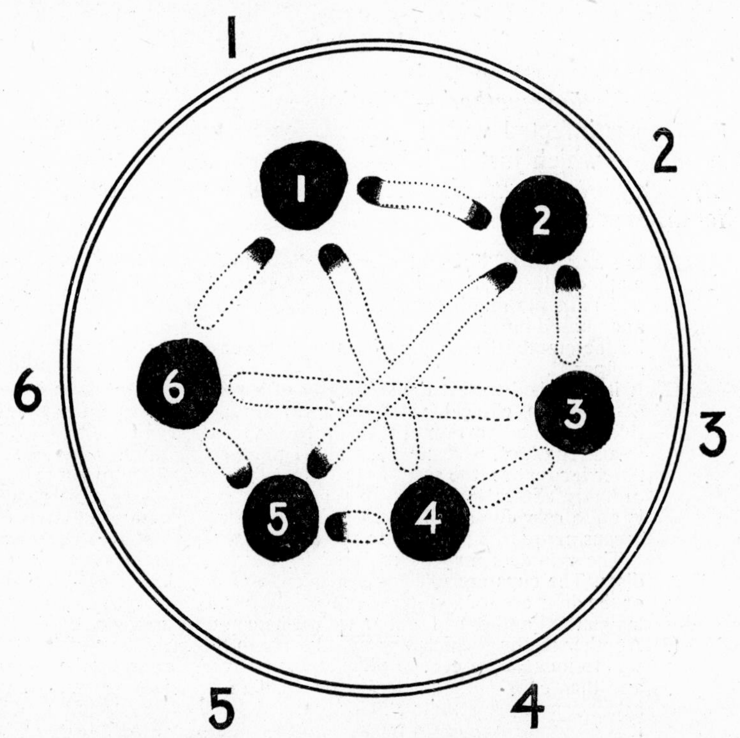

FIG. 35.—Simple method of discovering penicillinase producing bacteria. Bacteria (1 to 6) planted in spots on agar plate containing penicillin (2 units per millilitre). Staphylococcus then planted in streaks indicated by dotted lines. Penicillinase produced by 1, 2 and 5 allows staphylococci to grow around the colony

bacteriostatic power of penicillin in blood, pus, or other fluid, and so allow the development of bacteria in cultures which otherwise would be inhibited by the penicillin contained in the material.

It causes trouble in penicillin therapy in two ways, as follows.

(1) If penicillinase-producing bacteria are present in sufficient numbers in a lesion associated with penicillin-sensitive organisms, the latter may be protected by the penicillinase.

(2) If a penicillinase producer contaminates a penicillin pre-

paration (solution or cream) it can rapidly destroy its activity.

Method of ascertaining whether or not an organism is a good penicillinase producer

Possibly the simplest method is to plant the microbes to be tested in spots on a culture plate of agar containing 2 units

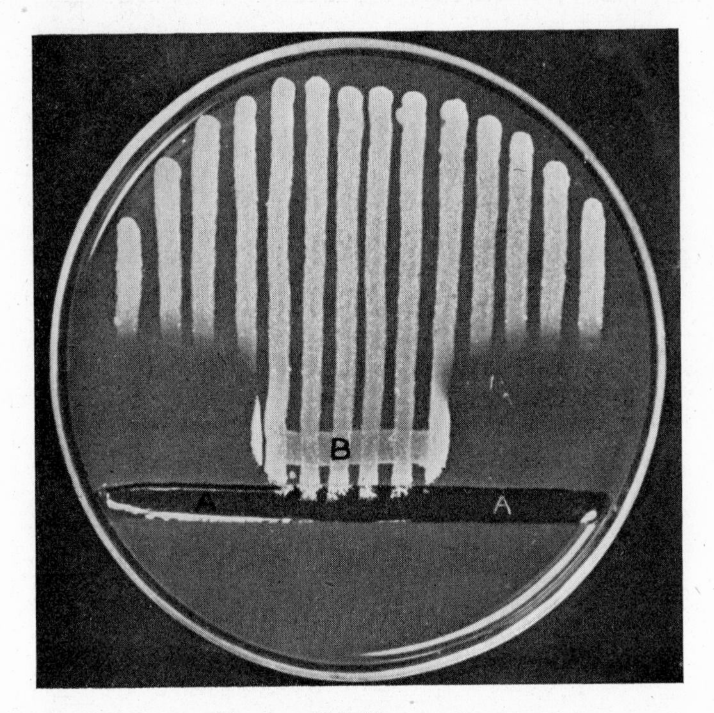

FIG. 36

Demonstration of the action of penicillinase on agar plate. Gutter A filled with agar containing penicillin 50 units per millilitre. Gutter B filled with agar containing penicillinase. Staphylococci then planted in streaks across the plate from Gutter A to periphery. The penicillinase diffuses out and allows the staphylococci to grow even on the agar in the penicillin gutter

per millilitre of penicillin. Five or 6 microbes can be tested on a plate. After 2 or more days' growth, staphylococcus is spread in streaks between the areas of growth. The penicillin in the culture medium prevents the growth of the staphylococcus except in the region where penicillinase, produced by the test bacteria, has destroyed the penicillin. Fig. 35 illustrates the result which is obtained.

Methods of demonstrating that penicillinase neutralizes penicillin

Titration.—Various dilutions of penicillinase are made and then an equal volume of penicillin is added and the tubes are infected with staphylococcus. The tubes containing the stronger concentrations of penicillinase will grow staphylococcus, but as soon as the penicillinase becomes so weak that it will no longer

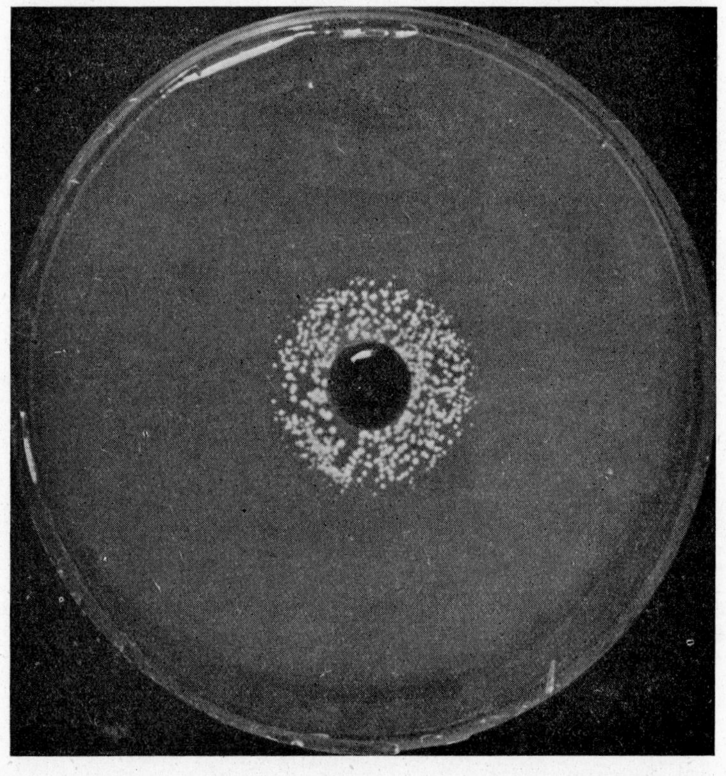

FIG. 37
Demonstration of the action of penicillinase on agar plate containing penicillin (2 units per millilitre). Whole surface inoculated with staphylococci and central cup filled with penicillinase. Growth only round cup where penicillinase diffused out and destroyed penicillin

neutralize the penicillin, growth is inhibited. There is a very sharp end point.

This method also determines the potency of penicillinase when known concentrations of penicillin are used.

Agar diffusion methods:—A great variety of experiments can be designed to demonstrate the antagonism of penicillin and penicillinase. Fig. 36 illustrates one of them.

Penicillin, 50 units per millilitre, is embedded in agar in gutter A across a plate. Penicillinase is embedded in a shorter gutter in front of this. Staphylococci are then streaked across the plate at right angles to the gutters. Fig. 38 shows the result after 24 hours' incubation. It is quite clear that the penicillinase has diffused out and neutralized the penicillin for a considerable distance.

Fig. 37 illustrates an even more dramatic exhibition of penicillinase. The medium is agar containing 2 units per millilitre

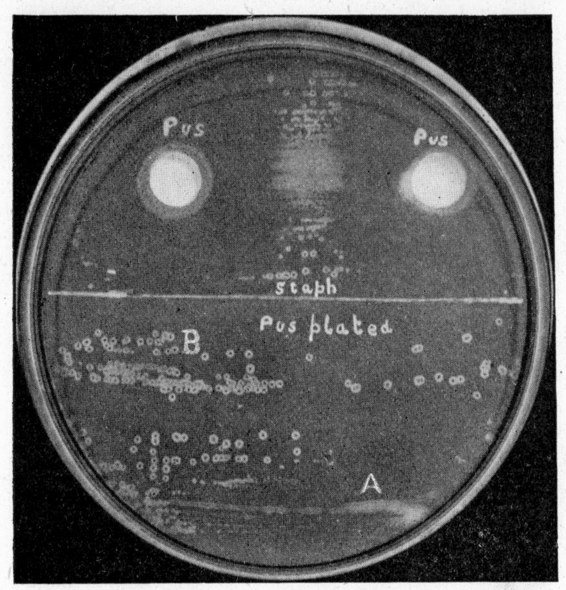

FIG. 38.—The upper half shows the bacteriostatic effect of penicillin contained in pus collected 24 hours after injection of penicillin into an axillary abscess. Test organism—staphylococcus. The lower half shows the same pus planted in the usual way commencing in region A and finishing in region B. In spite of the penicillin in the pus there is a considerable growth of staphylococcus in region B where the pus was most sparsely planted. (*Proc. R. Soc. Med.*)

of penicillin. The whole surface is inoculated with staphylococci, after which an agar cup is cut from the centre of the plate and is filled with penicillinase. There is growth of the staphylococci only round the cup where the penicillinase has diffused out and destroyed the penicillin.

Precautions to be taken in the culture of material from patients under penicillin treatment

The specimen may contain sufficient penicillin completely or partially to inhibit the growth of sensitive bacteria. This penicillin can be completely destroyed by penicillinase. If information concerning the nature of the treatment is available, a rough estimate of the possible amount of penicillin present may be made and an appropriate amount of penicillinase can be added. The fluid to be tested can be mixed with penicillinase before planting out or it may be spread on a culture plate and then sufficient penicillinase—more than enough to neutralize the penicillin in the specimen—can be spread over half of the plate.

Even when considerable amounts of penicillin are present in pus, cultures of sensitive organisms can be obtained if the specimen is inoculated sparsely on the culture plate (see Fig. 38).

REFERENCES

[1] Heatley, N. G. (1944) *Bio-chem. J.*, **38**, 61.
[2] Garrod, L. P., and Heatley, N. G. (1944) *Brit. J. Surg.*, **32**, 117.
[3] Foster, J. W. (1942) *J. biol. Chem.*, **114**, 285.
[4] Wilson, Ursula (1943) *Nature, Lond.*, **152**, 475.
[5] Rake, G., and Jones, Helen (1943) *Proc. Soc. exp. Biol., N.Y.*, **54**, 189.
[6] Prévot, A. R., and Ferly, A. (1946) *Bull. Acad. Méd. Paris*, **130**, 123.
[7] Fleming, A. (1943) *Lancet*, **2**, 434.
[8] Fleming, A. (1944) *ibid.*, **2**, 620.
[9] Rammelkamp, C. H. (1942) *Proc. Soc. exp. Biol., N.Y.*, **51**, 95.
[10] Heilman, Dorothy H., and Herrell, W. E. (1945) *Amer. J. clin. Path.*, **15**, 1.
[11] Morley, D. C. (1945) *J. Path. Bact.*, **57**, 379.
[12] Abraham, E. P., and Chain, E. (1940) *Nature, Lond.*, **146**, 837.

METHODS OF ADMINISTRATION

By W. Howard Hughes, M.D., B.S.

Assistant, Inoculation Department and Allergic Diseases Clinic, St. Mary's Hospital; Tutor in Bacteriology, St. Mary's Hospital, London

INTRODUCTION

Any description of the administration of penicillin is bound to be ephemeral since the methods now in use, devised during a war and with the need for strict economy constantly in mind, are rapidly being changed for other methods less complicated and tedious. The ideal preparation, from the point of view of both the patient and the doctor, would be one which would maintain a constant high blood level when administered by mouth, or failing that, when given once or twice in 24 hours. The ideal preparations at present available will not allow any such easy methods to be followed economically but developments are foreshadowed by the introduction of the oil and wax suspensions which may well render elaborate procedures unnecessary.

The methods and apparatus to be described have shown good results in the hands of a number of doctors and the equipment is readily obtainable.

SYSTEMIC ADMINISTRATION

Here the object is to introduce the penicillin so that it reaches the infecting organism through the blood stream and maintains an adequate concentration in the blood and the infected area continuously. This may be achieved in the following ways: (1) by injections given intravenously, intramuscularly or subcutaneously—each of these routes can be used for either intermittent injections or for continuous drip transfusions; (2) by inhalation; (3) orally.

CONTINUOUS ADMINISTRATION

The Table on page 64 shows that the most economical method of giving penicillin is by a drip transfusion, for which the intravenous route appears at first sight to be the most suitable as an immediate high blood level is achieved. There is the concomitant disadvantage that the veins are liable to thrombose, especially if the solution is made up in glucose or glucose-saline.

The intramuscular route is only slightly slower in giving high blood levels. It is not stopped by venous thrombosis but, alternatively, special precautions must be taken to keep the needle in the muscle and the volume must be kept small to prevent stasis from the accumulation of fluid.

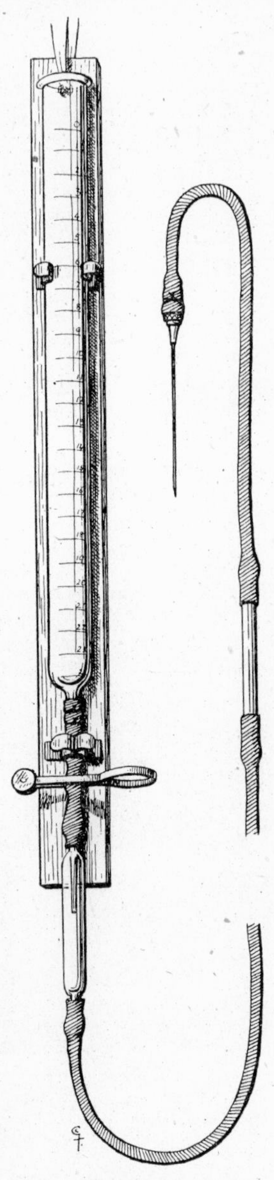

FIG. 39
Eudrip No. 1. A modification of the standard transfusion apparatus for continuous intravenous or intramuscular administration

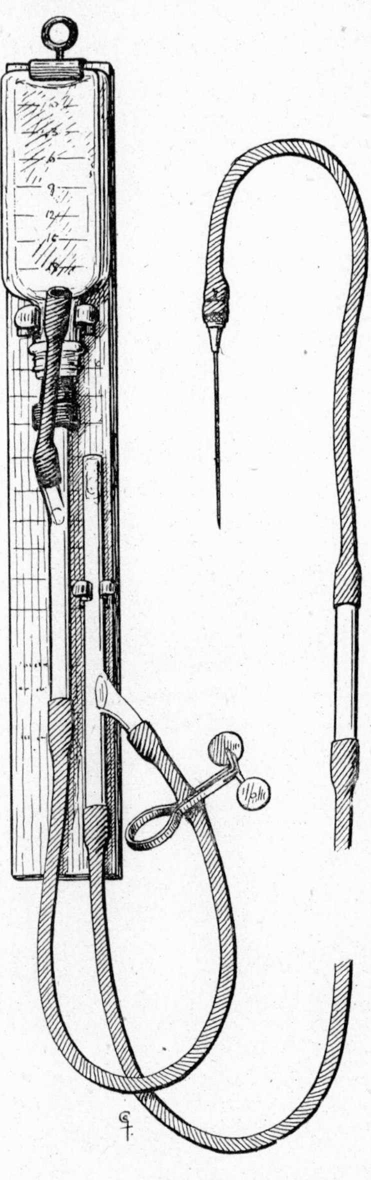

FIG. 40
Eudrip No. 3. A continuous drip apparatus giving simpler control than earlier models

The subcutaneous route was at first unpopular since the crude preparations caused pain and it was not easy to prevent accumulation of fluid in the tissues with consequent discomfort to the patient and irregular absorption. These disadvantages have been overcome by the use of local anaesthesia, purer preparations and the development of a method of administration—the clock drip—which uses really small volumes of fluid.

One type of apparatus now in use has been evolved from the standard transfusion apparatus which was used during World War II for giving either blood or plasma. This apparatus is known to most doctors. The standard apparatus can be used in its unmodified form but it will be found that it is difficult to prevent the flow from running so fast that the amount to be spread over 24 hours is used up before the time, and the advantages in economy that should be obtained from a drip transfusion are lost. Control is made simpler if a scale, indicating the correct amount that should have run after varying intervals, is attached to the side of the bottle; this may be made by drawing on the glass with a grease pencil or by sticking a strip of paper or adhesive plaster down the side.

The first modification of this apparatus, for the special purpose of giving penicillin, is shown in Fig. 39. A reservoir is provided which is narrower than the standard milk bottle and which is graduated; with this aid it is easier to control the flow to obtain a slow rate and it requires less attention for a shorter time. This apparatus, Eudrip No. 1, has been further modified to give the type of equipment illustrated in Fig. 40, which illustrates Eudrip No. 3. Eudrip No. 2 is similar. Whereas in the earlier model the reservoir was open at the top for filling and while in use was closed with a cottonwool plug, the others have an inverted bottle holding only 100 millilitres. To control this smaller volume there is a side tube added which contains a capillary tube through which the slow trickle of air allows the displacement of the fluid in the reservoir. Raising or lowering a second side tube will retard or accelerate the rate of the drip; it is also possible to refill the reservoir through this side tube without having to disconnect any part of the apparatus. In this model the scale is on the board which holds the reservoir.

The needles in use with this apparatus are either of the ordinary intravenous type—12 standard wire gauge is wide enough for solutions of low viscosity—or there is a special needle which is perforated at intervals and which may be used. The disadvantage of this latter type of needle is that it is not strong and may break at the holes; it has the theoretical advantage that it is less likely to be obstructed. A useful modification to any of these needles which are to be used for intramuscular drips is for them to be bent about half an inch from the mount through an angle of 30°. This enables the needle to be strapped to the skin with the point in the muscles and prevents the pull which may be uncomfortable to the patient, and also the tendency for the needle to be levered out of the muscle into the subcutaneous tissues by the pressure of the dressings.

An entirely different type of apparatus, the clock drip, designed by Last, is shown in Fig. 41. It consists of an electric clock which rotates a cage attached to a screw; this screw rests on the piston of a record syringe containing a strong solution of penicillin. The thread of the screw is such that 24 turns allow it to move $1\frac{1}{2}$ inches. The solution is made up in as much fluid as will fill $1\frac{1}{2}$ inches of the barrel of the syringe. The very small amounts of fluid are conveyed to the needle in the patient through Southey's tubes;

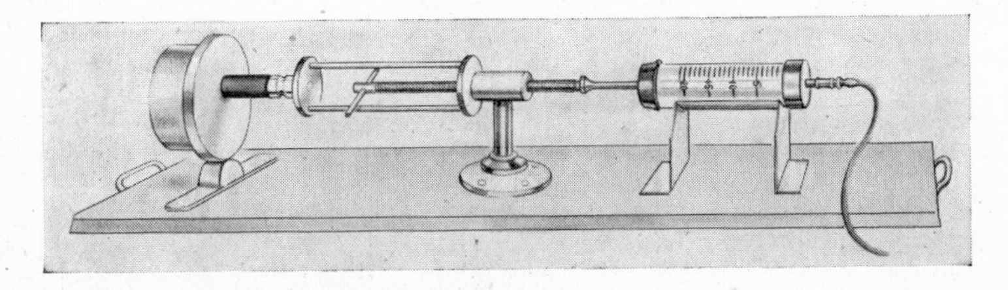

FIG. 41
The clock drip for continuous administration of small volumes of penicillin

there is a trap for bubbles next to the nipple of the syringe and an inspection chamber near the needle.

With the small amount of fluid in use it is unimportant whether the drip is being given subcutaneously or intramuscularly as fluid will not tend to accumulate and the absorption is regular.

With all methods of drip transfusion the chief difficulty arises from the blocking of the needle. This is frequently the result of a temporary interference with the flow in the tubing from pressure from either the patient's limb, the bedclothes, a cradle or while the patient is being moved to the operating theatre or the X-ray department. The pause in the flow permits the tissue fluids to seep into the needle and clot. With ordinary care it should be unnecessary to replace needles more often than once in 24 hours; under exceptional conditions the same needle can be kept in one site for as long as 3 days but there is no disadvantage in changing the site of the injection more frequently.

The second most frequent source of difficulty is the development of air locks in the tube. As with any transfusion it is most important to see that the final length of tubing from the needle to the drip chamber is full. This is made easier with the standard type of apparatus if the needle is attached to a short length of tubing, 1 or 2 inches, which can be disconnected from the rest of the apparatus to allow fluid to be sucked with a syringe, or allowed to flow by gravity into the lower portion of the tubing without any danger of displacing the needle. This small attachment may allow a temporary block in the needle to be cleared and intravenous or intramuscular transfusion re-established.

THE SITE OF INJECTIONS

When an intramuscular drip is to be given it will be found that the outer aspect of the thigh gives the patient the greatest freedom of movement and allows the apparatus to be inspected easily. It is important to protect the tubing from the weight of the bedclothes, for which purpose a cradle is used which can, with advantage, contain some form of heating in the winter. The tubing is usually led in from the bottom of the cradle in order to lessen the danger of its being trapped by the patient's arms, books, bed-tables or trays.

With the intravenous drip transfusion method it is usual to choose the leg veins as the site of injection. The usual antecubital veins are technically satisfactory but, since the drip is expected to continue for some days, restriction of the patient's movements is considerable and there is excellent justification for cutting-down on to the veins near the ankle and tying a cannula into them.

When the needle has to be changed because of blockage or other causes it is wise to change the site of the injection. The opposite thigh or a different position on the same side is suitable for the intramuscular drip while, for the intravenous, the opposite ankle is probably the best site.

For intermittent injections the technique is the same in giving penicillin as in giving any other drug. The amount to be injected is dissolved in sterile water or physiological saline and taken up in a sterile syringe. It will be found convenient if the concentration is such that the dose chosen is contained in 1·5 millilitres of the solution, and then if this amount is taken up in a 2 millilitre syringe it will be possible to add 0·5 millilitre of ½ per cent procaine hydrochloride or any other suitable local anaesthetic, when no appreciable pain will be experienced.

This precaution is worth while as some patients feel for some time the sting of the cruder preparations.

The site should be changed with each injection, otherwise it becomes sore and unnecessary pain is caused. The buttocks and thighs will usually provide sufficient sites but the upper arm and the chest can be used if the course is protracted. When the buttock is used the usual precautions against hitting the sciatic nerve should be taken as the concentrated drug in its present state is not without irritant effects. If the injection is made above and behind the line joining the ischial tuberosity and the great trochanter no danger need be feared.

INTERMITTENT INJECTIONS

Continuous administration has the disadvantage that not every patient likes to be attached permanently to the apparatus and the patient who is not too ill will often prefer to have 8 injections a day. With intermittent injections likewise there is not any complicated apparatus to prepare, sterilize or control and, while in the large and fully equipped hospitals there is not any difficulty in finding someone with the necessary skill to undertake this work, expert supervision is required and so the method is unsuitable for use in the small cottage hospital or in the patient's home.

It will be seen from the Table (see page 64), that the 3-hourly intermittent dose will give almost as economical results as the drip and it is not noticeably less effective; it has the disadvantage that the 3-hourly scheme of dosage itself is inconvenient in the patient's home, or where trained staff are not available at night, and it interferes with rest. It was devised to give the greatest measure of efficiency combined with economy at a time when supplies were strictly limited, but it is now possible to modify the scheme of doses so that the interval could be increased in the patient's interest. The following Table shows the scale of doses that must be used to give comparable results with increasing time intervals.

TABLE

Time in hours	Preparation	
	Aqueous solution (units)	Oil and wax suspension (units)
3	15,000	
4	30,000	
6	100,000	50,000*
8	150,000	100,000
10	200,000	120,000
12	300,000	150,000
18	500,000	250,000
24		300,000

* With the smaller doses the levels fluctuate and doses should therefore be of 50,000 units and over.

It will be noticed that the use of the oil and wax suspensions of penicillin will prolong the time of effective bacteriostasis. It has not been possible to show in this Table that there is also a more constant level in the blood, and there is not the same rapid rise and fall seen in the graphs for aqueous solutions (see Pharmacology).

The oil and wax preparation may not yet be generally available but when it is a dose of 120,000 units given at 8-hourly intervals

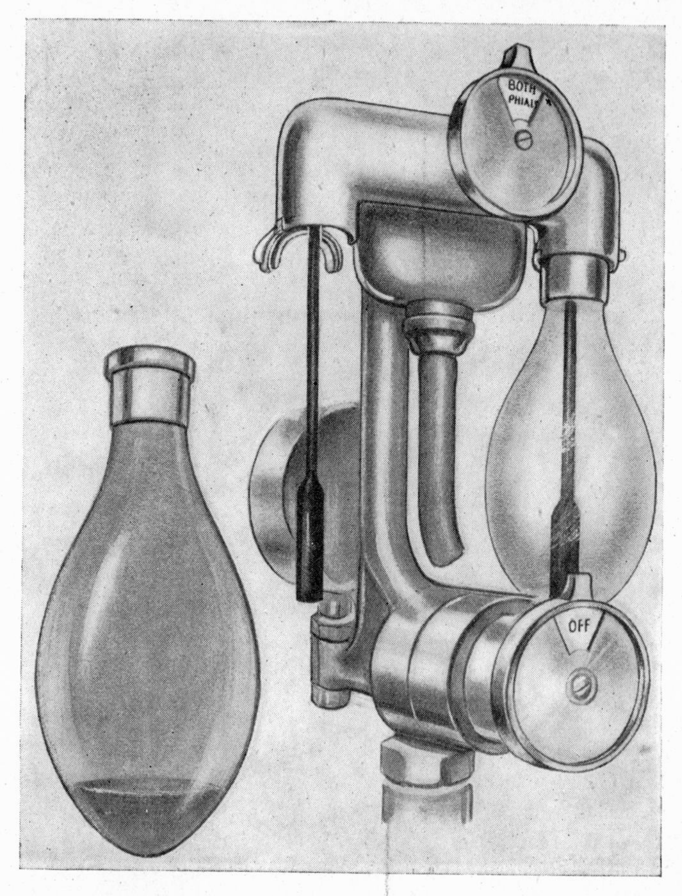

FIG. 42
The Collinson apparatus for administration of atomized penicillin

should solve some of the problems of the treatment of the ambulant patient or of the patient who cannot be transferred to hospital. While only aqueous preparations are in use a good night's rest should be encouraged by making the last dose 150,000 units. Such a dose given to the quiet patient will last from 10 or 11 p.m. until 6 or 7 a.m. the next day.

SYSTEMIC PENICILLIN BY INHALATION

During the investigation of the effects of penicillin by inhalation it was found that this route, while most suitable for certain respiratory diseases, was also efficient in giving a high blood level. This method could be used in general diseases. It has been restricted so far to respiratory conditions but there is no reason why its use should not be extended. The techniques suitable for the upper respiratory infections, dealt with later in this article and in the chapter on Otorhinolaryngology, are insufficient both for diseases of the lung alveoli and for systemic administration; for these purposes a special type of apparatus is desirable.

At first the drug was injected through the cricoid membrane or introduced through the anaesthetized larynx by a nasal catheter or a bronchoscope. While good results from these methods were reported, they were not very easily applied to large numbers of cases and frequent dosage was not possible. In general they are superseded by the use of vapours. Vapours have been produced in rooms by the use of apparatus of the aerosol type and patients have been allowed to inhale them. This method appears to be pleasant and effective but it is wasteful and is probably best reserved for respiratory diseases in infants; in older children or adults it is probable that the individual atomizer is better. The atomizer most commonly used is the Collinson, illustrated in Fig. 42. This, in its elements, consists of a jet of oxygen led through the penicillin solution to the patient who inhales it through a mask. The rate of flow is controlled by a tap and there is an alternative container which may have in it as a lubricant glycerin 0·5 millilitre and water 2·5 millilitres.

The vapour is filtered free of the larger particles and the remainder is led through a bag to the mask which is of the B.L.B. type. The patient inspires through the nose and expires through the mouth; if there is re-breathing into the bag through the nose there is a loss of efficiency. The dose of from 100,000 units to 500,000 units is dissolved in 3 millilitres of water and will be found to require up to half an hour to be absorbed. For respiratory conditions, in which the blood levels are of secondary importance, it will be found that inhibition of organisms can be maintained in the sputum with doses given twice daily. Should a high blood level be required it will be necessary to increase the frequency to every 4 or 6 hours depending on the size of dose.

It is not always necessary to use this type of inhaler as satisfactory blood levels and certainly good local results can be obtained with the ordinary hand atomizer used by asthmatics for adrenaline inhalations and for the proprietary antispasmodics. A typical example of these atomizers is illustrated. They are usually operated by hand and to be successful there must be a face mask (see Fig. 43). This is not usually designed for the nose alone, but it must, however, be used as though it were, so that the patient does

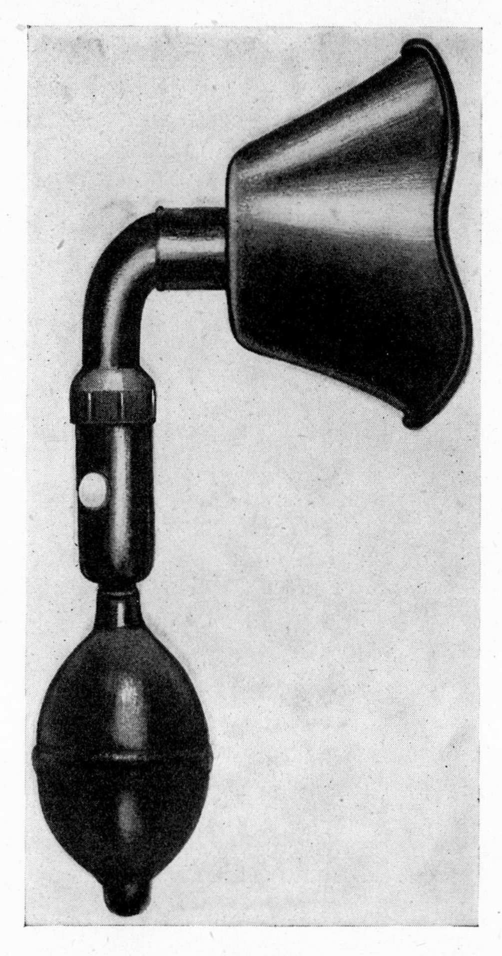

FIG. 43
Hand atomizer with mask suitable for either systemic administration or the treatment of lung conditions

not exhale the vapour any more than is necessary. The conscientious patient will manage to breathe in through the nose and out through the mouth but more mental concentration is necessary than with the Collinson mask. It is possible to substitute for the hand-operated bulb on some of these atomizers an electric pump which drives air through the solution. A foot pump from a car may be found to make the administration less tiring when an electric pump is not available.

ORAL PENICILLIN FOR SYSTEMIC CONDITIONS

The idea of giving penicillin by mouth is attractive, particularly when patients in general practice, or out-patients insufficiently ill to allow admission to hospital beds, are being dealt with. The reasons for distrust of this route are fully discussed in the chapter on Pharmacology (page 59). It will be appreciated that it is the least satisfactory route of administration and also the most costly, since the dose must be 5 times that which would give a more constant effect by injection. When it is decided to administer it by mouth there are several preparations available. It can be given with an enteric coating as a pill or capsule but there is, in our experience, a less degree of absorption with the coated than with the plain penicillin; with some coatings no absorption at all could be demonstrated. It can be given through a duodenal tube; and this is probably the most effective experimental method but it is less attractive to the patient than any injection. It may also be given simply as a draught with some alkaline suspension to neutralize the hydrochloric acid in the stomach. The various alkaline preparations are discussed in the chapter on Pharmacology (page 59). The mixture should not be given within 2 hours of a meal and it is better if meals are so spaced that the draught is taken 3 hours after one meal and one hour before the next.

THE RECTAL ROUTE

Various preparations in the form of suppositories and enemas have been suggested in the hope that there might be steady absorption of the penicillin from the lower bowel. It will be seen from the work on penicillinase that it is unlikely that there can be effective medication in any area where there are Gram negative organisms, and the rectal route can be regarded as quite useless.

LOCAL PENICILLIN

It will be readily appreciated, from a consideration of the facts given on the diffusion of penicillin into serous cavities, into the meninges and into abscesses, that it will require an enormous concentration and total dosage of penicillin in the blood stream to give adequate inhibitory levels in some localized foci. It appears that a dose of about 25 mega-units in the blood is required to give the same effect in the meninges as 500–1,000 units given directly into the theca. A high blood level may well have its place in a localized disease in preventing the formation of metastatic foci but the systemic route is not the most certain or most economical way of treating the localized condition. The treatment of many localized processes is dealt with fully in the appropriate clinical chapters, therefore it is necessary only to deal with the smaller septic conditions here.

LOCAL INFILTRATION AND INJECTION

Infiltration of the tissues around an abscess is intended to set up a barrier between the infected area and the normal tissues and, at the same time, to attack the organisms in the wall of the abscess. Should this be attempted it is particularly important to combine the drug with a local anaesthetic as the stretching of the inflamed tissues is painful; for the same reason the dose should be in a small bulk of fluid.

Injection into the abscess cavity is usually found to be as satisfactory as infiltration and it is easier and less painful. As much pus as possible should be drawn off before the penicillin is injected. If at first it is too viscid to pass through the needle, it will often be found that, after a day or two of treatment, it will be less viscid and can then be aspirated more easily. The strength of solution can be 1,000 units or more and this can be used to refill the cavity after the aspiration; the small axillary abscess will require from 0·25 to 2 millilitres and the treatment can be given daily.

LOCAL TREATMENT BY OINTMENTS AND CREAMS

The special techniques used by dermatologists are set out fully on page 317. The use of ointments and creams in prophylaxis and treatment of other conditions are described in the appropriate clinical chapters. Therefore it is necessary here to deal only with their use in minor conditions. If it is necessary to treat an open wound or a sinus which is draining it is difficult to maintain a concentration of the drug in solution in it and it will be found more satisfactory in practice to use a cream or ointment; this can be introduced through a wide needle into the sinus or spread on ribbon gauze and packed into it. Other suggestions for introducing these and similar preparations into the nasal sinuses are described on page 306.

LOCAL TREATMENT BY SPRAY

Earlier in the chapter the method of treating lung conditions was mentioned in connexion with the systemic administration of penicillin by inhalation. The Collinson inhaler and the other inhalation apparatus with masks are suitable for the treatment of local conditions of the bronchi or larynx. For conditions of the throat and nose it is possible to use any simple hand instrument.

LAMELLAE

The use of the special lamellae for ophthalmic conditions is dealt with on page 293.

LOZENGES

Lozenges are used extensively for mouth infections and act as far back as the tonsils. The technique of their use is important as success depends on it. The lozenge should be introduced into the buccal pouch and if possible forgotten. It will remain for 2 hours or more in the mouth during absorption. The tablet placed in the upper pouch at night will still be found after 7–8 hours' sleep. If results of any value are to be achieved it is imperative that the lozenge should be neither sucked nor bitten.

REFERENCE

Last, C. E. (1945) *Brit. med. J.*, **1**, 122.

PROPHYLACTIC USE OF PENICILLIN

By A. E. Porritt, C.B.E., M.Ch., F.R.C.S.

Surgeon, H.M. Household; Surgeon to Out-Patients and Assistant Director of the Surgical Unit, St. Mary's Hospital, London

and

G. A. G. Mitchell, O.B.E., M.B., Ch.M.

Late Adviser in Penicillin and Chemotherapy, 21 Army Group; Professor (Elect) of Anatomy, Manchester University

Except in the case of war wounds, large-scale prophylactic trial of penicillin has not yet been possible. MacGregor and Long[1] have suggested that the use of penicillin pastilles or lozenges might prove to be of value in preventing airborne infections and in limiting epidemics produced by penicillin-sensitive pathogens, for example, diphtheria. Knott and Blaikley[2] have shown that in a maternity hospital the persistence of staphylococcal and streptococcal carrier infections was reduced by about 50 per cent by the regular use of penicillin nose and throat sprays, and the benefit of any measure which reduces the incidence of micrococcal carrier infection does not require emphasis. The pastilles in common use each contain 500 Oxford units of penicillin; if they are placed in the buccogingival sulcus and are not sucked, they persist for 1½–2 hours, so that 8–10 pastilles, properly used, should last for a whole day. The solutions used by Knott and Blaikley contained 1,000 units of penicillin per millilitre and were applied by means of an all-glass atomizer. Both sides of the nose and throat were sprayed for about 1 minute every 3–4 hours.

The line between prophylaxis and therapy may be ill defined. This is exemplified in the case of acute ulcerative gingivitis. Thus Powell and Colquhoun[3], after the successful treatment of such cases with penicillin, recommended, in order to prevent recurrence, the subsequent use for a time of tooth powders or pastes containing penicillin.

It is obvious that there is scope for the prophylactic use of penicillin in venereal diseases, but so far records are not available of its employment for this purpose. Local and oral methods will ultimately be used in addition to, or in place of, the parenteral route. As with sulphonamides, the prophylactic use of penicillin in venereal diseases will carry the risk of breeding resistant strains, a matter of serious practical importance that cannot be dismissed lightly. There is one partially reassuring point in favour of penicillin: pathogens can develop a relatively great resistance to penicillin, but there is not any definite proof that an organism originally completely sensitive to penicillin has ever become completely penicillin-insensitive.

Once penicillin is freely available, its lack of toxicity and remarkable freedom from sensitivity effects[4] will favour its large-scale employment as an aerosol in operation theatres, hospital wards, labour rooms, cinemas, offices, factories and so forth. Streptococcal, staphylococcal, diphtheritic, pneumococcal, meningococcal and other infections might be lessened greatly by such measures. Its blandness will make it the favourite agent in the prophylaxis of neonatal eye infections.

Without doubt the advent of considerable supplies will also lead to the widespread use of penicillin as a prophylactic measure before, during and after operations and labour. Increasing supplies will hasten the day of the easier but relatively uneconomical methods of oral administration. Until then parenteral administration must be retained, using slow-release vehicles, intramuscular infusions, mechanically operated syringes, or other methods of giving intermittent injections.

All the above possibilities are either relatively or completely untried. We are on surer ground, however, when the prophylactic value of penicillin in preventing the occurrence of infection in war wounds[5] is considered, and there is no reasonable doubt that similar results will be obtained in civilian casualties.

PENICILLIN PROPHYLAXIS IN WAR WOUNDS

Owing to shortage of supplies in earlier campaigns, the precious drug had to be used mainly in therapy, and the first time penicillin was available in really adequate amounts for both prophylaxis and therapy was in the invasion of North-West Europe. Full advantage was taken of this favourable circumstance and from D-day onwards the basis of the penicillin policy in the 21st Army Group (the British and Canadian Armies invading Normandy) was prophylaxis. At least 100,000 men received penicillin treatment and the majority had the benefit both of prophylactic and of therapeutic administration.

All the dangerous pathogens commonly found in war wounds are penicillin-sensitive and if they are subjected to an adequate concentration of penicillin for a sufficient period of time the organisms should be inhibited or destroyed. It was therefore decided to exploit penicillin prophylactically at the earliest practicable stage and in the most effective manner possible. Plans were made to give casualties parenteral or local penicillin, or both, at the most forward surgical levels; once started, the penicillin was continued no matter how or where the patient went until such time as he had been evacuated from the battle theatre or until a surgeon had decided that the treatment could be terminated. Parenteral penicillin was not administered to the lightly wounded—it was reserved for the men with major wounds. The widespread use of parenteral penicillin at forward levels had not been attempted previously, and whereas in many wounds adequate prophylaxis may be provided by local applications, we are convinced that in the more severe and complicated wounds systemic administration in addition is essential for the securing of maximum protection.

The prophylactic dosages and methods of administration had to vary with circumstances; every official memorandum[6] emphasized that the lavish expenditure of any chemotherapeutic agent would not purchase an indulgence for therapeutic sins. After adequate primary surgery, penicillin powder (5,000 units of penicillin in 1 gramme of sulphonamide) was applied to the wound, and parenteral administration was initiated whenever it was considered to be necessary. Frequent injections could not be given in forward units working under great stress, as, for example, during a battle. To simplify matters, and to ensure that every patient requiring penicillin received it, large infrequent doses were allowed and recommended (90,000–100,000 units as soon as possible after the wound had been inflicted, followed by injections of 50,000 units at approximately 5-hour intervals on the line of evacuation). It was stressed that this was a relatively extravagant method justifiable only in difficult circumstances, and that in more favourable conditions, as would be the case in civil life, an adequate titre could be maintained by giving 15,000–20,000 units 3-hourly, or by the use of continuous injection methods (100,000–120,000 units *per diem*). Many "travelling" intramuscular infusions were employed on ambulances, planes and ships, but intermittent injection methods were used most often on the line of evacuation.

The recommendations were interpreted generously, a possibility which had been foreseen when the prophylactic policy was being framed, but the high rate of initial expenditure was justified by the handsome dividends which resulted. Reports from all sources commented on the marked absence of severe sepsis and the reduced incidence of all wound infections. This conviction was universal amongst those with much experience and although better methods, better conditions, better surgery, better communications and other factors played their part, few doubted that penicillin was the dominant factor in the control or the elimination of infection—formerly the greatest single problem in war surgery.

The clinical improvement was unquestioned and confirmation was provided by bacteriological investigations. In the Middle East Forces it was a rarity to get a report of "no growth" on the first wound swabs taken after admission of the patient to a hospital. Thus in a series of 100 consecutive cases investigated (1942) in No. 1 Orthopaedic Centre, Middle East Forces[7], a positive culture was obtained in every case and the following were the more important organisms isolated.

Streptococci	68 per cent (50 per cent haemolytic)
Staphylococci	58 per cent (46 per cent *Staph. aureus*)
Clostridia	28 per cent
Pyocyaneus	16 per cent
Proteus	14 per cent
Esch. coli	6 per cent

In all except 6 cases the infection was mixed, so that the above percentages merely give an indication of the incidence of various organisms in 100 consecutive cases. For purposes of comparison it is interesting to recall that in World War I haemolytic streptococci were the predominant pathogens and accounted for the majority of all severe wound infections[8].

In the British Liberation Army "no growth" cultures from wounds were common, whereas staphylococcal, and particularly streptococcal, infections were much less common. Thus 268 (48 per cent) out of 560 wound swabs taken from casualties, almost all of whom had received prophylactic penicillin, gave "no growth" on culture[9]. The more important organisms isolated from this series were as follows.

Staphylococci (coagulase +)	62	139 (25 per cent)
Staphylococci (coagulase −)	26	
Staphylococci (no details given)	51	
Str. haemolyticus	18	29 (5 per cent)
Non-haemolytic streptococcus	11	
Coliform bacilli	56	(10 per cent)
Clostridia	9	(2 per cent)

"No growth" reports were received in 268 (48 per cent) of all reports.

As in the Middle East Forces series mixed growths were the rule, and it should be stated that penicillinase was not employed in many of the cultures; a number of false negatives, therefore, probably were obtained. Nevertheless these laboratory findings confirmed the clinical impression that the great majority of the wounds were cleaner than were those commonly seen in former campaigns, and it is intriguing to consider the reasons why this was so.

Resuscitation, anaesthesia, primary surgery and postoperative care were more or less standardized long before the invasion of North-West Europe, and unorthodox procedures were not favoured in the British Liberation Army. The majority of the surgeons, anaesthetists and transfusion officers who landed in Normandy in June 1944, had not any previous experience of field surgery and therefore the balance was not tilted favourably by the weight of previous experience. Having been well grounded in a faith founded on the practical experiences of the Desert campaigns and having in their midst a small and select band of experienced veterans, their work was excellent, but was not any better than, for example, that achieved by their predecessors in the glorious 8th Army; their results, however, as judged by the condition of the wounds, were much better—despite the more dangerous nature of the terrain over which the battle was fought. Certainly both the climate and the diet were more favourable in France than they were in Libya, but neither had changed significantly between 1940 and 1944, yet the incidence and severity of wound infection had altered very appreciably. It is known too that woollen materials, when driven into wounds, are more dangerous than cotton materials, because they are more liable to harbour infection; to a certain extent this factor must have counterbalanced any advantage dependent on the more favourable climate.

Some commentators have assumed that variations in time-distance factors explained all the differences, having forgotten or having ignored the fact that men wounded in the same theatre of war in 1940 had shown no comparable absence of sepsis; and apart from this the assumption will not stand informed analysis. Two time-distance factors require consideration: (1) the interval between wounding and primary surgery; (2) the interval between primary and secondary surgery. These in turn are related to important subsidiary factors such as rest, frequency of dressings and so forth.

From the prophylactic viewpoint the first interval is the more important and it was not significantly different in the Middle East Forces, Central Mediterranean Force, or British Liberation Army theatres. On an average it was 12–14 hours.

The second interval was often prolonged in the Desert, especially in the earlier phases, and this probably explained the almost universal occurrence of moderate to severe wound sepsis. The long and exhausting journeys, the lack of rest, the frequency of pain, the difficulties of providing suitable invalid diet and sufficiency of fluids, and the irrepressible tendency to change dressings at each staging post all led to inevitable infection. At the time of Alamein, however, the front remained static for some time. Communications were good and lines of evacuation short, so that most casualties arrived in base hospitals within 2–4 days, after having received excellent forward treatment and the usual prophylactic course of sulphanilamide; as a rule, dressings had not been changed between the time of primary surgery and the arrival in hospital. It would, therefore, be most important for the purpose of comparison to know the condition of such wounds. They were all infected to a greater or lesser degree—yet these men were as well treated and had as easy and rapid a passage as had most of the wounded men in North-West Europe.

Air transport of casualties was used extensively in the 21st Army Group, chiefly in evacuating patients to the United Kingdom, but not in transporting patients from the battlefield to the forward surgical units a few miles behind. Thus air evacuation did not influence the more important time-distance factor from the prophylactic viewpoint—that between the reception of the wound and primary surgery. It might have influenced the interval between primary surgery and the secondary surgery performed in a base hospital, since from the time of Alamein onwards air evacuation was used increasingly between forward and base medical units. Analysis of figures from general hospitals in the 21st Army Group (October 1944–March 1945) showed that (1) 1,290 men had their wounds sutured within 1–7 days after they had been wounded and (2) that 863 men had their wounds sutured 8 days or more after they had been wounded. As it was the general rule to suture most wounds within 1–2 days after the men had been admitted to hospital, it is clear that about 40 per cent of the casualties did not reach a hospital where definitive surgery was possible until about a week or more after they had been wounded. From late 1942 onwards the average intervals in other theatres were not greater.

Little need be said about the missiles or the nature of the wounds. At one phase there were more mine injuries, at another more mortar wounds, at yet another a preponderance of shell or bullet wounds, but, taken all over, there were as many severe wounds in the North-West European theatre as anywhere else. The nature of missile or wound cannot be regarded, therefore, as a factor in the changing incidence of infection.

We have considered in turn the principal factors influencing the occurrence of infection in war wounds and have shown that they, alone or in combination, did not vary sufficiently between the beginning and the end of the war and between different theatres of operation to explain the marked diminution in the incidence of infection. About these facts there is no great divergence of opinion, but about another factor—chemotherapy—there is considerable difference of opinion. Most believe that penicillin is very valuable in both prophylaxis and therapy. Many hold that the sulphonamides, although less powerful, are also valuable, but whereas their therapeutic value is acknowledged universally, their prophylactic value is less certain. The evidence favours the view that they usually prevent spreading or generalized infections, but have no appreciable effect on the incidence or severity of local infections. This was well exemplified in the later Desert campaigns. By then the administration of prophylactic sulphanilamide was extremely efficient and although the spreading infections commonly seen in the presulphonamide phase were comparatively rare, the great majority of the wounds showed evidences of active local infection. In the 21st Army Group both penicillin and sulphonamides were freely available and there was a remarkable change for the better in the condition of the wounds. It was commented on by all with previous experience of war surgery, and it did not require faith for its appreciation. The one really new factor was the early and adequate exploitation of prophylactic penicillin and it must be accorded most credit for the dramatic improvement.

PENICILLIN VERSUS SULPHONAMIDES IN PROPHYLAXIS

An obvious question required an answer. Was any advantage gained by using sulphonamides in addition to the use of penicillin in prophylaxis? Once the latter was freely available it seemed to be unnecessary to give both if penicillin alone was equally effective, especially as the sulphonamides occasionally produced annoying or even dangerous complications. The majority of surgeons were satisfied from the appearance of the wounds that penicillin was a more efficient agent than any they had previously used, but officially more definite evidence was required before a general order was issued to replace prophylactic sulphonamide by penicillin.

A scheme was therefore instituted[10] whereby one out of each pair of Corps Casualty Clearing Stations ceased to use oral sulphonamide and employed penicillin only, whereas the other Casualty Clearing Station continued to use both. The routine prophylactic course of sulphonamide was 5 grammes daily for 5 days. In the 21st Army Group men with less serious wounds had local applications of penicillin powder, whilst all those with more severe wounds received parenteral penicillin in addition to the local application, as a prophylactic measure; the dosages and methods of administration have already been mentioned briefly. For the purposes of this investigation the small amounts of sulphonamide used as a diluent for the penicillin powder had to be ignored, but in the great majority these small amounts could not have produced any significant effect since 1–2 grammes of penicillin powder sufficed to insufflate all except very large wounds.

In parentheses we might state that at a later date penicillin diluted with dried plasma instead of sulphathiazole or sulphamezathine (sulphadimethylpyrimidine) was used in many cases; the results were not significantly different—confirmation that penicillin alone could produce as good clinical results as could penicillin plus sulphonamides.

The cards of all casualties were clearly marked "No S" if sulphonamides had not been given, and surgeons in the hospitals to which the patients were admitted were asked to compare the results in those who had received penicillin only and those who had been given both prophylactic penicillin and a sulphonamide. They placed the cases in 4 categories, depending upon the condition of the wounds when first examined in hospital: 0=without evidence of infection, +=slight infection, ++=moderate infection, +++=severe spreading infection.

In assessing results all relevant factors should be considered, such as severity of the wounds, degree of contamination, primary surgery, time intervals, and so forth, besides any chemotherapy employed. It was believed, however, that by getting a sufficient number of casualties with the same types of wound sustained in the same areas, these other factors would be minimized or equalized. This is a reasonable assumption, and as the numbers analysed exceeded 1,000 it is probable that they were representative and provided fair contrasts.

The Table gives the results compiled from the reports of 17 surgeons. The majority of the "penicillin only" group had received both parenteral and local penicillin. All the penicillin and sulphonamide group had had local penicillin powder plus the routine prophylactic course of an oral sulphonamide, and some had also received parenteral penicillin. The "sulphonamide only" patients had all been given an oral sulphonamide and most had had local applications in addition. The miscellaneous group

Agents	Total Cases	Degree of infection				Percentage 0 and +
		0	+	++	+++	
Penicillin only (parenteral and/or local)	497	298	165	28	6	93·1
Penicillin (parenteral and/or local) and oral sulphonamides	480	275	159	37	9	90·4
Sulphonamides only (oral and usually local)	157	74	41	25	17	73·2
Miscellaneous	43	19	16	7	1	81·4
Totals	1,177	666	381	97	33	88·9

had received only local applications, usually sulphathiazole with 1 per cent proflavine or Nuflav (a somewhat similar proprietary mixture).

The two last groups may be dismissed briefly. The number of severe infections was highest in the "sulphonamide only" group, but these were practically all in prisoners and it would be misleading to compare them directly with the others. The miscellaneous group consisted almost entirely of men with minor wounds.

Study of the main "penicillin only" and "penicillin and sulphonamide" groups shows that the former did not suffer from the absence of prophylactic sulphonamide, and the men escaped the unwelcome side-effects inevitably associated, in a proportion of cases, with sulphonamide administration.

As 0 and + infections are not readily differentiated clinically, they were both included when computing the percentages in the final column. For all practical purposes these may be regarded as clean wounds and in this series at least 9 out of every 10 wounds fall in this category. Only 15 out of 977 patients had infections classed as severe (1·5 per cent). This figure conveys an accurate picture of the results in casualties treated with penicillin.

The difference between the results in the two first groups is small, but it is significant that a higher proportion of the "penicillin only" group received parenteral penicillin. Thus in 126 "penicillin only" cases, 117 men had had both parenteral and local penicillin and 9 had local applications of penicillin alone, whereas in 152 "penicillin and sulphonamide" cases, 90 had received both parenteral and local penicillin and 62 had local penicillin alone. If these are a fair sample of the whole it suggests that the "penicillin only" group contained a larger proportion of men with severe wounds, as these were the ones more likely to receive parenteral penicillin. Thus the men with more tissue damage had less wound infection. This and similar observations in many other cases are the basis of our belief that parenteral in addition to local penicillin is essential in all the more severe wounds in order to ensure maximal protection and benefit.

APPLICATION TO CIVIL PRACTICE

The foregoing mass clinical experiment suggests that, when penicillin becomes freely available, it should be used as a prophylactic agent in all cases of potentially infected wounds.

In minor and more superficial wounds a local dusting with penicillin powder should suffice; it should be carried out as soon as the wound is first seen, and should be repeated, if necessary, at a subsequent dressing. For war wounds the penicillin powders employed contained 5,000 Oxford units per gramme, and sulphathiazole, sulphamezathine, or powdered plasma were commonly used as diluents. As the average wound in a civilian is treated more promptly and is less heavily contaminated than are war wounds, powders containing half the penicillin content mentioned above should provide adequate prophylactic cover. Powders with a strength of 500 units per gramme have given good results in practice, but it is probable that a higher unitage is desirable to ensure maximal safety.

The common practice of frequent change of dressings or inspection of dressings cannot be too strongly deprecated, and it is to be hoped that the free use of penicillin will do much to abolish this tendency.

In more severe wounds, and in particular in those with obvious contamination, both parenteral and local penicillin treatment should be used, but it must again be emphasized that penicillin does not replace surgery. Every case should receive the appropriate surgical treatment at the earliest opportunity and the use of antiseptics and antitoxins is supplementary to this procedure.

Owing to shortage of supplies oral administration is not yet a practicable proposition; for parenteral prophylaxis penicillin must therefore be given by the intermittent or the continuous injection method. The common methods and dosages at present in use are 3-hourly intramuscular injections of 15,000–20,000 Oxford units dissolved in 1–2 millilitres of sterile isotonic saline or distilled water, or 100,000–120,000 units dissolved in 100–500 millilitres of sterile isotonic saline and administered intramuscularly over a 24-hour period by means of one of the various types of apparatus for continuous administration (Eudrip III, modified saline-transfusion set and so forth). The penicillin may be given also by mechanically operated syringes, or may be incorporated in a slow-release vehicle, but these methods up to the present time have been mainly employed in therapy. Prophylactic administration should be started at the first available opportunity and should be continued until the satisfactory state of the patient's general and local condition shows that the danger of infection is past.

In frankly contaminated wounds, especially those liable to contain anaerobic organisms (for example, street accident cases), the initial prophylactic dose may be greatly increased—up to 100,000 units as a single injection, or 300,000 units by continuous infusion in the first 24 hours. The higher blood titre thereby obtained may produce an adequate penicillin level in tissues partially deprived of their blood supply. The fact must be emphasized again, however, that penicillin prophylaxis will not absolve the surgeon from the responsibility of employing every necessary surgical measure.

Whether or not sulphonamides should be used in conjunction with penicillin in routine wound prophylaxis must remain a matter of individual preference. Experience in a large number of cases in North-West Europe proved that penicillin alone gives adequate protection, and that the margin of safety is not appreciably increased by the coincident use of the potentially dangerous sulphonamides. It follows from this that sulphonamides can be justifiably withheld unless there arises a specific indication for their use.

Penicillin prophylaxis in other fields is still in its infancy, but there are excellent prospects that its use in one or other of the various ways mentioned at the beginning of this chapter will produce beneficial results in minimizing the possibility of infection or in preventing it altogether. And when pathogens do gain a foothold the early use of penicillin should do much to abort the infection or to limit its spread. It is to be hoped that the results of adequately controlled clinical experiments in this largely unexplored realm will soon be forthcoming.

REFERENCES

[1] MacGregor, A. B., and Long, D. A. (1944) *Brit. med. J.*, **2**, 686.
[2] Knott, F. A., and Blaikley, J. B. (1946) *Brit. med. J.*, **1**, 349.
[3] Powell, R. P., and Colquhoun, J. (1945) "Penicillin in the Treatment of Acute Ulcerative Gingivitis". *Penicillin Therapy and Control in* 21 *Army Group*, p. 267.
[4] Mitchell, G. A. G. (1945) "Reactions and Complications in Penicillin Therapy". *Penicillin Therapy and Control in* 21 *Army Group*, p. 249.
[5] Porritt, A. E., and Mitchell, G. A. G. (1945) "Factors Influencing the Occurrence of Infection in War Wounds", "Penicillin and Sulphonamides in Prophylaxis". *Penicillin Therapy and Control in* 21 *Army Group*, pp. 13, 21.
[6] 21 Army Group Memorandum on Surgery No. 5: Penicillin (May, 1944); No. 8 (Aug., 1944); Memorandum on Penicillin Therapy in 21 Army Group (Feb., 1945), etc.
[7] Mitchell, G. A. G. (1943) *Investigation of War Wounds. Penicillin. A Preliminary Report to the War Office and the Medical Research Council on Investigations Concerning the Use of Penicillin in War Wounds.* War Office A.M.D. 7/90D/43, p. 42. London.
[8] Fleming, A., and Porteous, A. B. (1919) *Lancet*, **2**, 49.
[9] Porritt, A. E., and Mitchell, G. A. G. (1945) "The Results of Wound Closure Using Penicillin and Contrast Agents". *Penicillin Therapy and Control in* 21 *Army Group*, p. 152.
[10] 21 Army Group, Memorandum on Surgery, No. 8 (Aug., 1944).

GENERALIZED INFECTIONS

By R. Vaughan Hudson, F.R.C.S.
Surgeon, Middlesex Hospital, London

GENERAL CONSIDERATIONS

Three years have elapsed since a grant of penicillin by the Medical Research Council made it possible to treat and follow up 400 cases of every type of penicillin-sensitive infection. The contrast of clinical experience in the unaided treatment of acute infection, first supplemented by the use of the sulphonamides after Domagk's discovery, and now with penicillin as a consequence of Fleming's discovery, has been a fascinating experience.

In the untreated, the progress of the disease depends upon the resistance of the host, for without aid he must rely on his own natural resources to localize infection and to neutralize the hostile organisms and their deleterious effect upon his tissues. More often than not, part of the battlefield in which this devastating combat is waged has to be sloughed out and discarded by the host. In this lonely and unassisted fight with disease the result can be measured in terms of tissue sacrifice, impairment of function, and the time-consuming loss of social and economic life.

The result of the battle is not always clear cut. Some patients, in spite of complications, recover completely; on the other hand, in a considerable number there develop later in life indefinite periods of ill health and changes in connective tissue which suggest that still somewhere in the body organisms of low grade are fabricating a toxin. Of more interest and difficulty in treatment is another group of patients who never fully recover the health experienced prior to their illness; they appear to exist in symbiosis with the causative organism and to have periodic and varying exacerbations of the original infection. At times pus is formed which is found to be sterile, but on other occasions it contains the original causative organism of the disease.

In employing the chemotherapeutic agents it has been noteworthy that the tendency to render the patient and the organism "symbiotic" has increased. It is as if, although the fire of the infection has been damped down, smouldering ashes still present can be fanned into flame in the immediate or the remote future. Observations strongly suggest that this chemotherapeutic effect is mainly dependent upon the size of the dose and the duration of treatment, and it has been possible to show that a recurrence is roughly proportional to the degree of underdosage and, in surgical cases, to the type of ancillary surgery employed.

In the choice, therefore, of a chemotherapeutic agent, the size of the dose and the duration of treatment is of the utmost importance. The determination of the clinician should be to cure the patient quickly and completely with the minimum of tissue sacrifice and so that there is little likelihood of further recurrence, since, in the "symbiotic", the natural resistance of the patient appears to be arrested and further treatment with specific chemotherapeutic agents to be less effective, for these exercise their function as an assistant to the natural resistance of the patient.

In instituting specific therapy, the time factor is not only of supreme importance as a prophylactic but also is a prophylactic in the prevention of complications in the early stages of acute infection. Owing to the triviality of the initial lesion the patient quite naturally relies on his own imperfect knowledge and does not seek medical aid unless infection is spreading or a complication has occurred. On the other hand, disastrous consequences have occurred owing to inapropriate interference, most particularly when injudicious trauma by a needle or the knife has been applied to a spreading infection; in surgical procedures the implantation of infection in clean wounds or the scattering of organisms from infected sites or lesions is not uncommon. There appears to be, therefore, a considerable opportunity for the education of the layman in simple correct first-aid measures for the home and the factory, and for surgeons to make more use of prophylactic chemotherapy when they are dealing with infected or potentially infected areas of the body.

When the effect of penicillin was first witnessed, the change in the patient was so remarkable that it was difficult to believe in it; so rapid were the initial changes that it was as if a motor car which was rushing downhill out of control, through the agency of some unseen power had suddenly been put into reverse and was climbing backwards to halt on the brow of the hill. The release of the unseen agent still enabled the experience to be repeated, for its effect had to be maintained for some considerable time while the car was slowly backed to permanent safety.

In 1943, a boy of 8 years of age was admitted in coma with head retraction and meningism; there was an effusion into the right knee joint and a swollen and inflamed lower right leg. The blood culture provided a heavy growth of *Staph. aureus*; although the X-ray picture was negative, a diagnosis was made of osteomyelitis of the shaft of the tibia, and penicillin treatment was begun. In 3 days the boy was sitting up to eat a reasonable meal and was attempting to do a little painting; 3 days later, through a $\frac{1}{4}$-inch incision, a large cold abscess was drained from the peri-osseous soft tissue; in a further 6 days the discharge had ceased, the small temporary drain was removed, and the incision was healing over. Surrendering to his pleading—for he was a cheerful, tough and very normal little boy—permission was given for him to sit up in a wheel chair, and in a month from the day of his admission he had to be restrained from racing the chair round the wards.

The institution of the correct chemotherapy can begin to reverse the process of infection and to inaugurate healing only from the state arrived at by the tissues ravaged by the infective agent. Assistance can start to operate, therefore, only at the particular stage of the disease. When chemotherapy is applied before the onset of complications there will not be any complications; when complications have already occurred further complications will not arise, but recovery must begin under a load of added difficulty.

It was quickly recognized that failure to obtain a satisfactory clinical result was the fault not of the drug but of the clinician, and the best methods of obtaining success appeared to be worthy of intensive study; there were deaths, there were failures and there were disappointments, but behind them, it was perceived, lay certain truths and principles of therapy. As time went on it was found that a guaranteed result could be achieved in a given time, provided that the organism was penicillin-sensitive, that the size of the dose, the interval between doses and the duration of treatment were correct, that the clinical management of the case was precise, and that the patient was not *in extremis* before treatment was begun.

The remarkable property of penicillin proved to be its specificity. This virtue was due to its bactericidal and bacteriostatic action and its power of perfusion into infected tissue; the fortress harbouring the organism was crumbled and was pervaded by the advancing tissue cells, and at each phase of progress both egrants and inhabitants were destroyed. In this combat the penicillin "mercenaries" proved to have little side-effects upon the engager.

Up to the present time, because of the idiosyncrasy of the patient or because of some injurious compound in the agent itself, penicillin therapy has not had to be prematurely stopped, although in 6 per cent of cases reactions identical with serum reactions of a major or minor quality have been experienced. These properties are entirely different from those of the sulphonamides, to the action of which many people are becoming increasingly sensitive, and in severe infections it is often a race between the final cure of the disease and the necessity for the cessation of treatment because of the toxic effects of the drug. Within reason, therefore, penicillin can be applied in large doses and for a long period of time.

In weighing the choice between one chemotherapeutic agent and another, the ease of administration of the sulphonamides has to be balanced against the more difficult administration of penicillin, the only objection to which, up to the present time, is the necessity for parenteral administration. Provided, however, that these minor difficulties of administration can be overcome, the results are better than are those obtained by use of the sulphonamides; they are more rapid and more certain, and are attended by less moral and physical illbeing, and organisms resistant to sulphonamide therapy respond if they come within the penicillin-sensitive group.

THE INFECTION

The cases received in our research clinic were of a complicated nature and therefore, in the great majority of infections, were not a true index of the results obtained by more simple methods. It was striking, however, that in a large percentage of cases the complications had arisen from a simple lesion—the infection of a clean operation wound or the result of trauma to, or surgical procedure in, an already infected site. It was occasionally found that an attempt had not been made to prove the type of organism which had caused the infection, or to make a clinical diagnosis of the cause of infection.

Diagnosis

A clinician is the first to admit that clinical diagnosis is of the greatest difficulty and that laboratory facilities are not always readily available, but precise and specific therapy can be instituted only when both the clinical diagnosis and the causative organism have been established. In all infections there is at some point a portal of entry; in many cases the portal is obvious—in fact so obvious that its presence may be brushed aside as unlikely—but in others it is concealed, and deliberate and repeated search has to be made before it is discovered. That clinician is fortunate who has available a reliable pathologist and facilities for X-ray diagnosis. In such a case the isolation of the organism and its sensitivity to the varieties of chemotherapeutic agents can be assessed in the laboratory, and in X-ray examination the common sites of undiscovered lesions and their metastases in generalized infections sooner or later can be detected, since they lie so often in the lung fields and in bone. The opportunity for repeated X-ray examinations during treatment also proves to be of the utmost value.

In the assessment of laboratory reports certain points have to be remembered. The presence of a collection of pus implies the existence of a cavity, and it is the effect of systemic penicillin upon the wall of the cavity that demonstrates its virtue, since it is in the wall of the cavity that the living and striving granulation is encompassing small abscess cavities and avascular infected tissue. Pus from the cavity which is reported to be sterile is not an indication that the wall of the cavity has been freed of the causative organism. The continuation of the cavity due to the presence of the sterile pus maintains the toxaemia of the patient and prevents the collapse of the cavital walls, and the evacuation of pus allays the toxaemia and permits the full cooperation of penicillin and surviving tissues to deal efficiently with the infected avascular tissue containing the causative organism. The continuation of therapy is the last factor in obtaining the result, but time must be allowed for the process to become complete.

The organism captured from the surface is not always the organism which has gained entry to the tissues of the host, and absolute reliance, therefore, cannot in all cases be placed on the laboratory report on the surface organism. In this respect it is well to remember that although penicillin-insensitive organisms may be the apparent predominant feature, these may be only contaminants and the causative organism may belong to the penicillin-sensitive group. If this penicillin-sensitive organism be destroyed, the secondary invaders, more often than not, die out. On the other hand, penicillin-insensitive organisms may be the cause of the infection and pyogenic penicillin-sensitive organisms may be acting as secondary invaders or contaminants. In this case the cure of the secondary organisms, although it improves the patient's condition, will not enable the lesion to heal because of the persistence of the insensitive group. Disappointments and difficulties have been particularly experienced in the presence of an underlying causative organic lesion; in imperfect resolution of the infection, therefore, the possibility of the presence of an underlying carcinoma, a tuberculous lesion, a leukaemia and, in surface lesions, a chronic skin disease, should be suspected. The presence of such lesions is not an indication for withholding penicillin therapy, but it constitutes a necessary factor in the assessment of prognosis and of future therapy directed to the persistent lesion; without such knowledge disappointment will occur if the persistence of the lesion continues, for it will invite reinvasion by further organisms at an early or a later date.

These facts are mentioned because the patient may well ask what the issue of therapy will be should he submit to it, and whether or not the disease for which he is being treated will recur again. So far, it has been the experience that the immunity of the patient to his hostile organism is not lowered, and although recurrences have taken place they are unusual unless a persisting constitutional or organic lesion encourages reinfection.

Aim of therapy

Before he decides to begin therapy the clinician will ask himself, How far has the infection proceeded and how is the patient responding to it? His therapy can be regarded as an assistant to a patient in whom the infection has already been localized and it can be used to relieve pain and to slough out more rapidly the dead tissue; the clinician has, as well, the opportunity of employing the drug by a "knock-out" method with the deliberate intention of localizing and sterilizing the lesion. If the latter effect is intended, then it must be borne in mind that a high degree of concentration of penicillin must be maintained for a long period of time in order that it may reach organisms enmeshed in stubborn infected avascular tissue, and that even the surgeon is unable to remove all dead tissue and all organisms, and that therefore treatment must be carried on until it is considered that the residual infected avascular tissue has been neutralized and rendered fit for absorption by the patient's tissues.

Institution of therapy

In clinical practice it may be extremely difficult to determine whether penicillin administration should be begun forthwith or whether precious time should be lost while laboratory proof of the cause of the infection is awaited. The line of conduct was taken that if the life of the patient was not unduly endangered by delay, it was much wiser to attempt, by every possible means, to obtain evidence of the causative organism before treatment was started. On the other hand, if the clinician from his experience considered that his clinical diagnosis were reasonably certain and that the life of the patient would be endangered by delay, penicillin therapy was begun; this, however, did not excuse the clinician from making every attempt to obtain the organism while treatment was in progress. If the organism were not present in the blood stream then, more often than not, an abscess was formed either at the portal of entry or at some other site, and the organism could be cultured from pus or from a piece of slough. Should therapy have to be instituted before the organism had been identified, the clinical behaviour of the patient was used as the yardstick of response. When the clinical response is satisfactory the clinician can feel confident that he is dealing with a penicillin-sensitive organism; when the dosage is correct and a satisfactory clinical response is not obtained, the clinical diagnosis is probably incorrect. An answer should be obtained to such anxious questioning within 3 days of the start of therapy; lack of response should make the clinician realize that therapy has belied the diagnosis and indicates that continuation of treatment is unlikely to improve the condition of the patient. Considerable information can be obtained by repeated clinical observation, and cases can be conducted to a certain safe conclusion by clinicians stationed remote from, or bereft of, the advantages of laboratory or X-ray diagnostic aid.

Two phases in therapy

In therapy there are two phases. The first is the initial control of the infection, the sterilization of the blood stream, the arrest of the spreading inflammation, and the localization of the infection to the portal of entry and the sites of metastases; this is the easier and the shorter of the two and is governed by the size of the dose and the time interval between doses. The second phase depends upon the duration of treatment; it is longer and more difficult, and requires patience and fine judgment, for it consists in the continued control and management of the residual focus or foci of chronic infection already induced and held in check by the penicillin.

This final management of organisms lying in infected avascular tissue is the whole difficulty in the final cure of the patient—which so often is impossible to obtain with the sulphonamides—for if inadequate treatment has been given, a revitalizing of the remaining efficient organisms will certainly occur and they will again reinvade the tissues of the host. Such a recurrence is a disaster to clinician and to patient for although a second course of treatment may be—and usually is—successful, the proceeding is time-consuming and distressing for patient and clinician alike. There is as yet no definite evidence that organisms can become penicillin-resistant, but experience in the past tends to show that this is a real possibility and is an added argument for adequate therapy.

The first phase.—The first phase of successful therapy and the most striking evidence of its success is the improvement in the clinical condition of the patient and the relief of pain. The fever may drop by crisis but more usually does so by a step-ladder type of lysis; in a few patients a degree of pyrexia persists and remains until the course of penicillin has been completed. More often than not, the pulse rate does not follow the temperature chart as it does in the spontaneous recovery of patients who are unassisted by chemotherapy. The wellbeing of the patient is the index of success, and if the pulse rate is higher than expectation it is probably an indication of the amount of tissue damage inflicted by the disease process prior to the beginning of specific therapy. It is an indication, therefore, of the wisdom of going slow in convalescence in order to give time for the repair and remodelling of damaged tissues.

In surface lesions the colour changes are striking. In the abrupt halt of the spreading tide of infection, there is a rapid fading of the acute scarlet vasomotor dilatation and consequently a rapid diminution of the erythema and redness of inflammation, which turns to a faded—but still oedematous—bluish type of lesion. Within a short time the residual focus is distinguishable and the amount of avascular infected dead tissue is apparent.

The second phase.—Decision now has to be made on the length of time during which therapy will have to be maintained, and on how much assistance should be afforded by surgery. From observations made on patients it would appear that, provided that treatment is adequate, a small amount of pus can be absorbed, the cavity collapses and the infected avascular tissue within its wall gradually fragments, liquefies and is dealt with by the host. As a result, in the course of time tissue damaged beyond repair is removed and tissues capable of repair bear no trace of the noxious assault, fibrosis is minimal and the area is supple and elastic. At other sites pus is formed in greater amounts, usually painlessly and insidiously, and the cold abscess tends to track along the natural lines of least resistance to some point on the surface. A close watch for pus formation is imperative because it may form extremely rapidly. The condition becomes one of particular urgency when the presence of pus threatens a closed tract or cavity such as the theca, the pleura and the meninges, or any site at which its rupture in a spontaneous attempt at escape might prove to be disastrous to the patient.

Tension pain or the presence of a low-grade and persistent toxaemia, or a stationary period in the clinical improvement in the patient, is strongly indicative of a persistent toxaemia due to concealed pus, and the condition should redouble the efforts of the clinician to discover the whereabouts of the pus. Provided, however, that pain is lessening, the general condition of the patient is improving, the whereabouts of the pus is known and it is ascertained that the pus is tracking to an accessible site, it is in general a wise plan to wait for the abscess to point so that its evacuation is possible without the traverse of intact tissue.

Adjuvant measures

On account of the importance of the collapse of the cavity it has been the experience that, when possible and as soon as is appropriate, it is wise to remove infected tissue or provide adequate drainage by means of a small incision so that the escape of sloughs and inspissated material too large to pass through the lumen of a needle, is permitted. The aspiration of pus and the reinstillation of penicillin will prove to be uniformly successful only when the effusion is thin and the cavity is maintained in a collapsed condition and is emptied reasonably quickly. The instillation of penicillin in a cavity in which drainage is adequate, is usually unnecessary, and is often unwise when systemic therapy is being maintained, since it is extremely difficult to prevent secondary penicillin-insensitive organisms from gaining an entry. In the cure, therefore, of the lesion which has spontaneously ruptured or has been deliberately opened by the surgeon, every effort must be made to permit adequate drainage and to discourage secondary infection by use of methods and application of dressings which do not neutralize the penicillin in the tissues at the mouth of the opening.

Convalescence

In convalescence it has been found to be satisfactory to permit movement provided that this is painless and graduated, for when the tissues are free of active infection movement is safe and function is more rapidly regained. On the other hand, friction and massage in the early stages of convalescence tend to further the recrudescence of the infection. Severe infections which have been successfully treated have still taken toll of the patient. As was the case before the day of chemotherapy, the wasting, the hepatic and renal damage, the myocardial and muscular weakness have still to be assisted by appropriate methods before recovery is final and complete.

Rat-bite fever

In 1943 Lourie and Collier[1] found that penicillin was curative in experimental mouse infections due to either *Spirillum minus* or *Streptobacillus moniliformis*; in 1944 this was confirmed by Heilman and Herell[2].

It is of value to recognize that there are certain clinical differences between rat-bite fever caused by *Sp. minus* and that caused by *Streptobacillus moniliformis*. Altemeier, Snyder and Howe[3] pointed out that in *Sp. minus* infections there is local swelling, pain and a purplish-red discoloration which develops into a chancre-like ulcer, with a regional lymphangitis and lymphadenitis, from one to three weeks after the bite. A large macular or papular rash usually presents itself. The blood cultures are negative. There is a polymorphonuclear leucocytosis and secondary anaemia. The Kahn reaction tends to become positive at the end of the fourth week but the Wasserman reaction is negative.

In rat-bite fever due to *Streptobacillus moniliformis* the wound heals readily and the patient presents a healed and usually painless scar, but 2 to 3 days after the bite constitutional changes are marked. There is severe arthritis with or without a myositis and painful nodules of some size may be found in the muscles. The blood culture is negative. The Wasserman and Kahn tests are also negative but a polymorphonuclear leucocytosis together with a secondary anaemia is present.

Of the two infections, that due to *Streptobacillus moniliformis* is the more common. It is important to remember that the infection may be conveyed not only by the bite of a rat but also by the bite of a cat; although the subject is usually an adult it is by no means uncommon for an infant to be the victim.

The *Sp. minus* responds to arsenotherapy but the *Streptobacillus moniliformis* is resistant. As a consequence of the experimental evidence penicillin was successfully employed in man by Kane[4] in Great Britain, by Robins[5] in the United States of America in 1944 and later further successful cases have been described by Altemeier, Snyder and Howe[3], Wheeler[6] and Weber and Favour[7]. Wheeler has shown that in man both these causative organisms are penicillin-sensitive.

Weil's disease.—In 1944 Alston and Broom[8] also demonstrated experimentally that *Leptospira icterohaemorrhagiae* was penicillin-sensitive and Lloyd Hart[9] described a case in which his patient appeared to benefit from penicillin; the organism disappeared from the urine. Cross[10] in 1945 described a case of Weil's disease in an airman of 35 years of age who was successfully treated with penicillin and an antiserum. His recovery appeared to be due to the administration of penicillin.

In treating infections caused by these organisms there appears to be a necessity for continuing treatment from 7 to 10 days and employing a dosage in accordance with that used in other penicillin-sensitive infections.

Summary of dosage

At this stage our experience in dosage can be summarized. It has to be borne in mind, however, that the interpretation of the clinical and pathological changes taking place in one patient are true only of the particular dose employed, and that comparative results of therapy are possible only when the same dosage is employed in a series of patients at the same stage of disease. The length of time taken to obtain negative cultures, the duration of stay in hospital and the eventual freedom from recurrence, on the average will not be the same with small doses as with large doses when a large series of comparable cases are analysed. It is with full recognition of these facts that a suggested basic table of dosage of proved success is given; in certain infections, longer experience may lead to modification of the size of the dose and of the time interval between doses.

Experience has shown that a certain number of cases could be treated with success with as low a dose as 5,000 units administered 3-hourly by intramuscular injection if treatment were continued over a long period of time. It was, however, only with doses of 20,000 units producing an average blood level of 0·09 unit per millilitre, that results became more uniform. In order to test the matter further, in a series of parallel cases of every type of infection the results were compared with those in which the dose had been raised to 60,000 units with an average of 0·23 unit per millilitre. With this increased dose the patient's stay in hospital was shortened because of a more rapid control of infection, an increased rate of healing and a greater preservation of tissue. The duration of treatment depended to a considerable extent upon the site of the infection; the average minimum duration of days of treatment at the 60,000 level was, broadly, as follows.

Uncomplicated gonorrhoea	1
Vincent's angina	2
Erysipelas, impetigo	3
Carbuncles, cellulitis and adenocellulitis	5
Breast abscesses	7
Otitis media and mastoiditis	8–10
Sinusitis, pulmonary lesions and meningitis	10–12
Complicated septicaemias	12–21
Endocarditis	21–28

The exceptions to the 60,000 dose are found, possibly, in cases of uncomplicated gonorrhoea; 30,000 units administered 2-hourly for 5 doses can be employed as suggested by Lloyd Jones[11]. In boils, carbuncles and purely cutaneous lesions a 3-hourly dose of 20,000 units appeared to give as good results as did one of 60,000 units. Certain types of infection are not included in this broad scheme of dosage: in actinomycosis, for example, 60,000 units given 3-hourly for 21 days provided the only apparent cure—and this in an early case of the cervical type—but similar doses and shortened duration of treatment, or this same dose, failed in the remaining 5 cases.

In diseases of the eye and of the skin prolongation of the 3-hourly dose of 20,000 units or the raising of it to 60,000 for as long as 21 days failed to cure 5 cases of subacute exacerbation of intra-ocular chronic infection, and 10 of 15 secondarily infected lesions of the skin.

In osteomyelitis a 3-hourly dose of 60,000 units was found to be superior to one of 20,000 units, but in spite of the favourable results it is not considered that, in the majority of cases seen late in the course of the disease, the duration of 10–12 days' treatment is long enough and will prove to have established a permanent cure.

An account of a few representative cases may be of assistance to the clinician. It should be remembered, however, that some of these cases were under treatment while we were searching for the correct size of the dose and the correct duration of treatment; the results of this search are the reason for, or the proof of, the suggested basic dosage; they illustrate also the limitations of the sulphonamides, and the manner in which organisms gain entry, invade and affect the patient, as well as the way in which metastases occur and can be managed and controlled.

TYPES OF CASE

Boils and carbuncles

Of 35 cases in which the patients were ill enough to require admittance to hospital, in 18 the lesion had been localized; in 13 the infection was rapidly spreading, contiguous structures were imperilled and the threat of metastases was ever present. In these 31 cases the assistance afforded by penicillin controlled the infection and enabled the sloughs to separate and be discharged spontaneously, or permitted these to be lifted out by dressing forceps; surgical interference was thus rendered unnecessary. By the third day of treatment pain had been completely relieved, and by the seventh day—on the average—the sloughs had separated. In 4 further cases the inflammation was spreading and metastasis had already developed; 2 patients who were moribund on admission died, and 2 severely ill patients recovered.

The influence of trauma and infection.—Tragic is the case of a young and shy girl who, after 6 days of pain and swelling, was driven to seek advice. An attempt was made to open the carbuncle by means of an incision, but pus was not found and the patient's condition rapidly worsened. When she was admitted to our research unit 24 hours later, the temperature was 97° F. and the pulse was thin, thready and uncountable; the patient was of an ashen bluish colour and sweat was beading the cold and clammy skin. Immediate resuscitative measures were undertaken and penicillin administration was begun, but in 8 hours the patient was dead. At necropsy the right facial vein was found to be thrombosed, there was early pericarditis with effusion and there were multiple very recent septic infarcts throughout the whole of both lungs, with an early fibrinous pleurisy. A coagulase-positive staphylococcus was cultured from the wound of the skin, from the blood stream and from the infarcts.

A carbuncle and metastatic lesions in the lungs.—A woman of 52 years of age was admitted with 2 weeks' history of a carbuncle of the right scapular region; the temperature was 102° F., the pulse was 130 and respirations were 28; the breathing was shallow and distressed on account of the pain in the right thorax. Sulphapyridine was given and in 24 hours the temperature had risen to 104° F. and the respirations to 40; diplopia had now occurred. The lumbar puncture was normal, the leucocyte count was 34,000, and from the blood a profuse growth of *Staph. aureus* was cultured; the skiagram showed widespread shadowing throughout both lungs and a small amount of fluid at the base of the right lung. Within a short time the patient was cyanosed and was in semi-coma; sulphapyridine was stopped and penicillin was begun. During the next 5 days there was a gradual improvement, and in 10 days the very large carbuncle was clean and free of sloughs and was healing; on the sixteenth day the general condition was remarkably improved, the leucocyte count had fallen to 8,000, but a low-grade toxaemia was present. A skiagram revealed a localized encysted empyema which on aspiration contained *Staph. aureus*. The empyema was treated by repeated aspiration and local instillation of penicillin; under this treatment the cavity became somewhat smaller, but it did not disappear and there was still evidence of mild toxaemia, although the pus was sterile. A second course of penicillin by the systemic route was given, aspiration was continued, the pus became thinner and the cavity gradually disappeared. The external rectus palsy was cured, and the patient regained her full health.

Quite often patients are admitted with the diagnosis of a fully developed metastatic lesion, correctly labelled, but, on account of the severity of the disease, the originating trivial lesion which is still present is overshadowed by the severity of the metastatic malady; alternatively, the originating focus has been healed for a week or two and has been forgotten by the patient and the relatives. The obvious continuity between a persistent minor lesion and the grave metastatic infection makes laboratory search entirely convincing.

A boy of 6 years old, who had had a boil over the left patella for a few days, was suddenly taken ill and was admitted in semi-delirium with an obvious osteomyelitis of the opposite left tibia. *Staph. aureus* was cultivated from the boil, the blood stream, and the soft tissues surrounding the tibia, and from beneath the periosteum and from the medulla of the bone itself. He made an excellent recovery under penicillin therapy.

Cellulitis and adenocellulitis

Of cellulitis and adenocellulitis 23 cases were encountered; in 16 of these the condition resolved without the necessity for surgery; in 7 pus formed and had to be evacuated through a ¼-inch incision with a temporary drain. On the average, pain was relieved in 2 days, the erythema had subsided in 3 and the lesion was healed in 7–10 days.

The concealed focus and spreading infection.—A spreading type of infection from a small concealed lesion is not uncommon; when it is present in the neck it is known as Ludwig's angina. A young airman of 18 years of age was admitted with a progressive cellulitis of the lower face and neck; the temperature was 100° F. and the pulse rate was 90. The patient was able to swallow only liquids and with effort, and he had considerable difficulty in opening his mouth. A few hours after admission there were the early signs of dyspnoea. The probable focus of infection was a small pocket behind the last molar tooth from which *Str. pyogenes* was isolated. Administration of penicillin was begun, and although in 6 hours there was an improvement in the patient's general condition, the oedema was progressing; in 24 hours, however, the dyspnoea was less and there was some improvement in swallowing. Thereafter progress was gradual and obvious; in 8 days there was complete resolution without the necessity for surgery, and the patient was discharged from hospital. Six weeks later, when he was perfectly well and had fully recovered, the last molar tooth was extracted after a 48-hour prophylactic systemic course of penicillin, and *Str. pyogenes* was again recovered from the tooth pocket.

Accidental trauma and fulminating infection.—Accidental trauma sometimes produces the most alarming symptoms due to a fulminating infection in a small abrasion. A boy of 11 dived into a swimming-pool and struck his head. Twenty-four hours later he was admitted in delirium, there was a small cut and an abrasion over the right eyebrow and the right eye was closed by a fiery red and very painful oedematous reaction; lumbar puncture showed no abnormality but the leucocyte count was 20,000; within the next few hours the inflammatory reaction had spread with increasing severity and had involved the left eye. Penicillin therapy was begun and within 2 days the patient was rational and quiet, and was taking food and fluids well; although the oedema was still present the signs of inflammation had disappeared and the swab from the wound—which previously had grown a coagulase-positive staphylococcus and a non-haemolytic streptotoccus—was sterile. In 10 days all inflammatory reaction had completely subsided and vision was normal. The small lesion had healed without loss of tissue and could not be detected.

Epithelium and endothelium as a complicating factor in infection

Inflammation of the breast.—The presence of epithelium is a complicating factor, and in inflammation of the breast the complicated structure of the tissue and the presence of epithelium—usually in a functioning state—adds to the difficulty of treatment. In the early stages penicillin can abort the inflammation. In many an abscess forms and this is best treated by a ¼-inch incision and temporary drainage. In only one of 22 patients with breast abscess who were admitted to the research clinic was there evidence of systemic involvement.

A woman of 37 years of age, who had given birth to a child 2 months previously, had been treated for 3 weeks by fomentations for a breast abscess. Three days prior to admission to hospital the abscess had been drained and had been packed with dry gauze. On admission the patient had pyrexia, a generalized dermatitis and a very swollen painful left breast; from the discharge was cultured a β-haemolytic streptococcus and a scanty growth of *Staph. aureus*. Sulphathiazole administration was begun, and although the condition improved the breast was still painful and swollen and was discharging pus; it was then found that the β-haemolytic streptococcus was sulphathiazole-resistant and therapy was stopped. Two days later the patient's temperature rose again and a course of penicillin was instituted; a collection of pus was localized and a ¼-inch incision was made; a temporary drain was put in position, and in 12 days the patient was discharged from hospital completely well.

Otitis media and mastoiditis.—The presence of epithelium in otitis media and in mastoiditis did not prevent successful therapy and in 31 of these cases under the care of my colleague, C. P. Wilson[12], there was response to penicillin. Surgical treatment was not necessary.

Pulmonary infections.—The response of pneumonia and bronchopneumonia infection due to penicillin-sensitive organisms was most satisfactory. Particularly so were those cases of mixed infection causing a postoperative complication; in 20 cases in which major surgical procedures had been satisfactory but were complicated either by early or established severe pulmonary infection, recovery was prompt and complete.

Subacute bacterial endocarditis.—The control and elimination of *Str. viridans* present in avascular infected tissue has proved the power of perfusion of penicillin, the necessity for adequate and prolonged dosage in certain types of infection and the low toxicity of commercial penicillin. To witness 14 of 18 patients making a full recovery, with the knowledge that the 4 who died did so from a mechanical cause and not because of the organism, was a culminating and gratifying experience. Whereas in gonorrhoea elimination of the gonococcus was successful within a few hours in the uncomplicated case, and within a day or two even when the organism complicated pregnancy or lay in the uterine tubes or peritoneum, in subacute bacterial endocarditis the majority of patients had to be under treatment for no less than one month before *Str. viridans* was completely eliminated.

The influence of bone

Osteomyelitis.—In osteomyelitis the results in the early stages of the disease were extremely satisfactory; they were satisfactory also in the later stages provided that correct ancillary surgery was employed. Of 37 cases treated, 13 responded to penicillin therapy only, and a further 5 to penicillin and stab drainage of the peri-osseous soft tissue abscess. In the other patients the site of the disease or the stage of the disease was such that radical surgery was necessary in addition. No other type of case demonstrates so well the success and future promise of early treatment and the difficulty experienced in the treatment of patients seen late in the course of the disease.

Septicaemia of unknown origin

Considerable difficulty may be experienced in determining the portal of entry and the cause of infection and particularly the feeding focus which is maintaining the organism in the blood stream.

A healthy girl of 20 years of age reported sick with a headache and pains in the limbs and in the back of the neck. There was not any evidence of abnormality in the ear or the throat, and lumbar puncture was normal, but on the fifth day of her illness blood culture showed a profuse growth of β-haemolytic streptococci. A course of sulphapyridine was begun and 2 days later there was swelling, redness and tenderness in the thenar eminence of the right hand and a lymphangitis of the forearm; the temperature was 104° F. The blood culture remained sterile and sulphonamide treatment was stopped at the end of 5 days after 82 grammes had been administered. Two days later the pyrexia was higher and the blood culture was again positive; the patient was given blood transfusions and another course of sulphonamide. After a further 56 grammes had been taken the leucocyte count was 15,000, the temperature was 105° F. and rigors were a daily occurrence. The patient was admitted to the research unit one month after the beginning of her illness, and on general examination no definite focus of infection could be discovered. A course of penicillin was begun and in 48 hours the patient's temperature was normal and the pulse rate was subsiding; for the first time, however, there was a complaint of pain in the left iliac fossa, and on physical examination it was found that there was tenderness over the symphysis pubis; x-ray examination showed an osteomyelitis of the symphysis pubis. Three weeks after treatment had been instituted, the signs and symptoms had disappeared and the patient was discharged. She was told to rest in bed at home and that she must not get up for a month. A return to work was made 3 months later and when she was seen in the follow-up, the patient had not any symptoms and was in excellent health, and function was normal. X-ray examination showed a healed osteomyelitis of the symphysis pubis.

In 7 similar cases it was found that the unexpected septicaemia was due to an undiscovered focus in bone. Had penicillin not saved the lives of these patients the focus would not have been discovered, for it was only during treatment and with repeated clinical examination and radiological assistance that the site of the feeding focus was discovered.

Septicaemia and multiple sites of infection

Puerperal sepsis, jaundice, osteomyelitis and empyema.—The physiological process of reproduction has its dangers. In a female of 34 years of age who had given birth to twins, the placenta had to be removed some 12 hours later. The uterus became infected and a septicaemia developed with *Staph. aureus* in the blood stream. The patient improved under intravenous sulphathiazole therapy and transfusions but rigors re-developed on the cessation of treatment. With a second course of sulphathiazole the patient became deeply jaundiced and the erythrocytes fell to 1,500,000; there was a complaint of fleeting pains in various joints, particularly in the left hip joint. The patient was admitted to hospital 7 weeks from the date of her illness; she was deeply jaundiced and there was gross enlargement of the liver and excruciating pain in the left half of the pelvis and in the left hip joint; the joint was fixed by spasm. The blood stream and the sputum contained *Staph. aureus*, x-ray examination showed marked osteoporosis and irregularity of the acetabulum, the upper end of the femur, the left hip bone and the sacro-iliac joint; the leucocytes were 27,000 but the erythrocytes were under 3,000,000. Penicillin therapy was begun and there was a rapid improvement, but on cessation of treatment there was still a low-grade toxaemia and the patient was increasingly troubled by an ineffectual cough. An x-ray picture showed an area of consolidation in the right lung and fluid in the right thorax. Aspiration of the chest was carried out and foul pus containing *Staph. aureus* was removed. Local aspiration and instillation of penicillin did not improve the condition and the patient was still considerably troubled by the pain in the left hip joint; her condition was such that immobilization by plaster was impossible and, as she was most intolerant of splinting with traction, even this means had to be abandoned. A second course of penicillin was given and the empyema was drained surgically. Recovery was rapid. The patient was discharged on crutches, and was told not to put weight on the affected limb, which had now recovered 80 per cent of its movements. Six months later the patient was in very good health with full movements of hip joint; the x-ray picture showed a healed lesion but there was narrowing of the joint space and a minor degree of arthritis. The patient has been walking well and has been in good health for the last 2 years.

The influence of the venous channels

It is commonly found that the spread of infection passes along the perivenous channels; as a result there may occur a perivenitis, a thrombosis containing organisms in the clot, or the actual production of intravenous pus. In either of these stages organisms may pour into the blood stream or clots may become detached to form emboli of the most dangerous character.

A man of 25 years of age suffered a gunshot wound of the right leg, which severed the sciatic nerve. At the time he was wounded he had been given penicillin. Some 7 months later while he was on leave in London he was admitted to hospital, acutely ill. He was found to be suffering from a complete lesion of the sciatic nerve and an anaesthetic and trophic ulcer on the ball of the great toe; from this coursed the scarlet lines of lymphangitis, the whole leg was oedematous and the superficial veins tender and firm, the inguinal glands were enlarged and very painful, and there was tenderness and pain on pressure over the right common iliac vein; from the ulcer *Staph. aureus* was cultivated.

Penicillin therapy was begun and complete resolution occurred; the patient was discharged after 10 days, and organisms could not be recovered from the persisting ulcer, which was soft and clean.

Periphlebitis.—In a man of 33 years of age who had had a major operation necessitating intravenous administration of saline, an infective thrombophlebitis of the arm developed. Sulphathiazole was administered and on several occasions localized collections of pus were incised in the forearm and the hand, but in spite of this his condition was deteriorating. On admission to hospital some 6 weeks after the onset of the illness he was exhausted, extremely ill and toxic, speech was hesitant and he was irrational at night; the whole arm was swollen and the incisions were discharging staphylococcal pus; in both lungs there were areas of consolidation which were the cause of an irritating and unproductive cough. Penicillin was begun and signs of recovery slowly became apparent. The original site of the infection healed first and the arm gradually regained full function, the cough became productive and quantities of foul sputum containing staphylococci were expectorated. The lung fields cleared but a persistent paravertebral empyema appeared and could not be reached with a needle. The chest was drained by a thoracic surgeon and from the pus *Staph. aureus* was recovered. The patient was later discharged from hospital with full function.

Infective venous thrombosis.—A girl of 19 years of age with a recurrent sinusitis was operated upon for nasal polypi and both maxillary sinuses were drained. Convalescence was not satisfactory, the patient began to run a temperature, and sulphathiazole was administered; the condition deteriorated and 14 days after operation she was admitted to the research unit. There was delirium with periods of cooperative attempts at lucidity, marked restlessness, swinging pyrexia and a pulse rate of 100. There was oedema of the whole face, both eyes were markedly proptosed and the lids were fixed by oedema, there was injection of the conjunctivae and papilloedema of both fundi, there was gross infection of the nose and the pus flowing from both maxillary sinuses contained *Staph. aureus*. On lumbar puncture the fluid was turbid, somewhat bloodstained, with a pressure of over 300 millimetres of water, but proved to be sterile; the leucocyte count was 11,000. A diagnosis of cavernous sinus thrombosis was made, penicillin was given and there was a rapid improvement of the general condition and a marked fall in pyrexia. On the fourth day the temperature rose again and all symptoms returned; the dose of penicillin was doubled and from then onwards a steady improvement occurred. First in the right orbit and then in the left a cold abscess appeared; these were opened by a fine tenotomy knife and pus was evacuated; from this pus a β-haemolytic streptococcus was cultured. Subsequent recovery was rapid and complete. When the patient was discharged from hospital there were not any residual ill effects or cosmetic impairment. It is noteworthy that the cultures from the nose constantly grew a culture of *Staph. aureus*, but the invasive causative organism proved to be the haemolytic streptococcus and was found on both occasions in the peri-ocular pus.

**Intravenous pus.*—Seven weeks prior to admission to hospital, a married woman of 41 years of age had had a swelling over the mastoid lanced; there was not any discharge and she continued to suffer severely with earache and headache for the next 6 weeks. Eventually she was admitted with a temperature of 106° F., rigors and severe pain down the right side of her neck; there was pain in the epigastrium, and an ineffectual cough. At times there was severe headache, nausea and retching, and loose motions were passed. The patient was drowsy and flushed and the tongue was brown and dry. There was a bloodstained discharge in the ear but there was not a perforation of the drum; a skiagram showed blurring and loss of outline of the right mastoid process, and consolidation of the left base and of the middle lobe of the right lung. There was moderate growth of β-haemolytic streptococcus in the blood stream, cellular granular casts in the urine, and a profuse growth of *Esch. coli*; the blood urea was 84 milligrams per 100 millilitres and the leucocytes were 57,000. A course of sulphathiazole was begun. The blood culture, however, was persistently positive with a profuse growth of haemolytic streptococci; vesicular lesions developed on the limbs; the pneumonic condition was resolving. The general condition now rapidly worsened and penicillin was given. In 6 days the condition had sufficiently improved to permit the jugular vein to be tied although the patient was stuporous and uncooperative. There was not any evidence of a cerebral abscess, but there was every evidence of a thrombosis of the lateral sinus. A few days later the mastoid process was exposed and pus was found in the cells; the lateral sinus was found to be thrombosed, so it was opened and pus was evacuated. The pus from the blood stream, the mastoid process and the lateral sinus was proved to be free of all organisms. Future progress was slow but satisfactory and the patient regained full health.

The constitution of the patient and the time necessary for repair of damaged tissues

The effect of a severe infection and the inevitable accompanying toxaemia, is obvious to the experienced clinician; it is not usual for him, however, to be able to give a specific reason for his "second sight", for his reason for anxiety during the early stages of the illness, and for his subsequent advice that convalescence should be adequate.

In certain cases of generalized infection—particularly in patients cured by penicillin of subacute bacterial endocarditis—the evidence of renal damage and the many weeks that elapse before all trace of this damage ceases to be evident is an indication of the severity of the strain thrown upon the tissues.

*The effect upon constitution can be illustrated by the case of a girl of 7 years old. During the week prior to admittance to hospital she had suffered from a fever and a sore throat and at times had complained of earache; it was noted that puffiness was developing round the eyes and that there was swelling of the feet. On admittance there was cyanosis and swelling of both eyelids and slight oedema of the legs, the blood pressure was 140/105, there were many erythrocytes and granular, hyaline and cellular casts in the urine and the blood urea was 25 milligrams per 100 millilitres. The right ear was discharging and culture gave a pure growth of β-haemolytic streptococci. Penicillin was begun; in 3 days the discharge was sterile and in 8 days it had ceased and the drum was healed. Recovery was uneventful, but it was 3 months before the urine was normal and free of erythrocytes.

SUMMARY AND CONCLUSIONS

Early diagnosis and early treatment mean economy in the use of penicillin and constitute prophylactic measures against complications. In generalized penicillin-sensitive infections the

* I am indebted to Mr. C. P. Wilson for the details of these cases.

successes obtained have been due to the maintenance of a bacteriostatic concentration in the tissues of sufficient strength and for a sufficient time to enable the patient to use to the full his natural defences. An apparent cure has been obtained when it has been possible to localize the infection so that the patient can absorb necrotic tissue, spontaneously extrude pus or dead tissue, or provide safe conditions for the surgeon to assist recovery by the removal of dead tissue.

The duration of treatment varies from one day to 28 days, depending upon the individual case and upon the necessity for the destruction of the organism in the remaining avascular tissue.

In the surgery of established infections, of the several methods tested two proved to be satisfactory. When administration of penicillin had converted the condition of an acute lesion to that of a chronic lesion, a small incision and temporary drainage was all that was necessary or advisable in the majority of cases, but in the minority, and for specific reasons, the radical removal of all visible infected material followed by primary suture and temporary drainage gave uniformly satisfactory results. No matter which of these two methods was employed it was found to be essential to continue penicillin for the length of time considered to be necessary for the purpose of controlling the residual infected tissue.

As an ancillary method, aspiration and local instillation of penicillin was of value in non-purulent effusions as opposed to purulent effusions. In all other infected lesions systemic therapy proved to be the most satisfactory, and the addition of penicillin applied locally was rendered unnecessary except in cases of meningitis and, possibly, empyemata.

BIBLIOGRAPHY AND REFERENCES

[1] Lourie, E. M., and Collier, H. O. J. (1943) *Ann. trop. Med. Parasit.*, **37**, 200.
[2] Heilman, F. R., and Herrell, W. E. (1944) *Proc. Mayo Clin.*, **19**, 257.
[3] Altemeier, W. A., Snyder, H., and Howe, Gertrude (1945) *J. Amer. med. Ass.*, **127**, 270.
[4] Kane, F. F. (1944) *Ulster med. J.*, **13**, 129.
[5] Robins, G. (1944) *Clinics*, **3**, 425.
[6] Wheeler, W. E. (1945) *Amer. J. Dis. Child.*, **69**, 215.
[7] Weber, R. A., and Favour, C. B. (1945) *Johns Hopk. Hosp. Bull.*, **77**, 132.
[8] Alston, J. M., and Broom, J. C. (1944) *Brit. med. J.*, **2**, 718.
[9] Hart, V. L. (1944) *Brit. med. J.*, **2**, 720.
[10] Cross, R. M. (1945) *Lancet*, **1**, 211.
[11] Jones, T. R. L., Maitland, F. G., and Allen, S. J. (1945) *Lancet*, **1**, 368.
[12] Wilson, C. P. (1946) *Proc. R. Soc. Med.* (in press).
Hudson, R. V., McIntosh, J., Meanock, R. I., and Selbie, F. R. (1946) *Lancet*, **1**, 409.
Hudson, R. V. (1946) *Proc. R. Soc. Med.* (in press).
Hudson, R. V. (1944) *Proc. R. Soc. Med.*, **37**, 109, 503.
Selbie, F. R., Simon, Rosemary D., and McIntosh, J. (1945) *J. Path. Bact.*, **57**, 47.
Ward, G. E. S., Meanock, R. I., Selbie, F. R., and Simon, R. D. (1946) *Brit. med. J.*, **1**, 383.

BACTERIAL ENDOCARDITIS

By Ronald V. Christie, M.D., D.Sc., F.R.C.P.
Professor of Medicine, University of London; Director, Medical Professorial Clinic and Physician, St. Bartholomew's Hospital, London

SUBACUTE BACTERIAL ENDOCARDITIS

Subacute bacterial endocarditis is a unique disease in many respects, not least in its resistance to treatment although the infecting organism may be sensitive to a variety of chemotherapeutic agents. Sulphonamides proved a failure, and at first it seemed likely that penicillin would be equally ineffective. Florey and Florey[1], Herrell[2], and others showed that the blood could be sterilized, and transient clinical improvement obtained, by comparatively small doses of penicillin but, as with the sulphonamides, relapse was the rule when treatment was stopped. Penicillin differs, however, from the sulphonamides in that it is devoid of toxicity, and there is therefore no theoretical limit to the amount which may be given, and this suggested that a more ambitious system of dosage should be tried. Further progress at that time was hindered by limitation of supplies and by demands for the treatment of diseases more susceptible to penicillin. Dawson and Hobby[3] reported one patient cured out of 10 treated with amounts of penicillin which at the time seemed large, although small according to present standards. The results obtained by Loewe and his collaborators[4] using both penicillin and heparin, were much more encouraging. Seven patients were treated, some receiving as much as 7,800,000 units, and in all of them sterilization of the blood and relief of clinical manifestations were obtained, although the period of follow-up was quite insufficient to justify conclusions on the efficacy of treatment. In the following year, Loewe[5] reported a larger series of 54 patients treated with heparin and penicillin, and the results were less spectacular than those previously described. Heparin was given by subcutaneous deposition, a coagulation time of between 30 and 60 minutes being the objective. The daily dose of penicillin varied from 40,000 units to 1,000,000 units and the total amount given from 0·87 mega-units to 48·9 mega-units, administered over a period of 2 weeks or more. Treatment failed to control the infection in 14 patients, it was effective in 40, of whom 3 died, leaving 37 out of 54, or 68 per cent, who remained well for periods of from 2 to 15 months, during which time they were under observation. The bearing of these results on the value of heparin in the treatment of this disease is discussed later.

Results as good as those of Loewe and his colleagues[4] were obtained without the use of heparin. Bloomfield and Halpern[6] treated 18 patients with about 200,000 units daily given continuously for 2 months. All were apparently cured, but the significance of these results is uncertain since the patients formed a selected group, one criterion being that the strain of streptococcus should be sensitive to penicillin in a dilution of at the most 0·1 unit per millilitre.

Flippin and his collaborators[7] describe 22 patients treated with 300,000 units of penicillin daily for 14 days; 10 died, 4 relapsed, and 12, or 55 per cent, remained well for periods of a year or more during which they were under observation.

During the past 2 years the treatment with penicillin of several hundred patients suffering from subacute bacterial endocarditis has been described in American literature, and still it is not possible to draw any definite conclusions as to the method of treatment which should be recommended. Many investigators have not used a standard system of dosage, others have selected patients because of physical fitness, or on the basis of sensitivity of the organism to penicillin, and others have combined the use of penicillin and heparin. In contrast, the use of penicillin in Great Britain for the treatment of subacute bacterial endocarditis has been for the most part confined to 14 research centres appointed by the Penicillin Clinical Trials Committee of the Medical Research Council, and working according to a carefully prepared plan. The centres were established in February 1945, and within 7 months 147 patients had been treated. The recommendations made here are for the most part based on a report on these patients (Christie[8, 9]), and to a lesser extent on my own experience in the treatment with penicillin of more than 30 patients. This emphasis on results obtained in Great Britain is not due to insularity, or to any lack of appreciation of the pioneer work on the treatment of this disease in the United States of America. It rather illustrates an advantage of poverty. It was scarcity of penicillin that led to the formation of special centres for the coordinated treatment of a rare but fatal disease, in which the only hope of cure lay in the administration of an expensive drug still in short supply.

Daily dose and duration of treatment

There is not any uniformity of opinion on the system of dosage which should be used in the treatment of this disease. As the purity of penicillin increases, and its price diminishes, it is probable that amounts which now appear astronomical will be used, and the duration of treatment may be reduced. The system of dosage now recommended is 500,000 units daily for 28 days but, since this is unlikely to be the last word on the subject, the steps which have led to this provisional recommendation, and the evidence on which it is based, will be described in some detail.

The relative importance of duration of treatment and the total amount of penicillin given had first to be determined. The 14 research centres referred to were divided into 3 groups; all gave their patients a total of 5 mega-units of penicillin, but over

TABLE 1. PATIENTS RECEIVING A TOTAL OF 5 MEGA-UNITS OF PENICILLIN GIVEN IN COURSES LASTING 5, 10, AND 20 DAYS

Dose	Died	Relapsed	"Cured"	Average follow-up
1 mega-unit for 5 days	6 (30%)	14 (70%)	0	—
500,000 units for 10 days ..	2 (17%)	7 (58%)	3 (25%)	217 days
250,000 units for 20 days ..	4 (29%)	3 (21%)	7 (50%)	249 days

different periods of time. One group gave a mega-unit daily for 5 days, another half a mega-unit daily for 10 days and the third group a quarter of a mega-unit daily for 20 days. The results of this experiment clearly showed that, within these limits of dosage, the duration of treatment was of much greater importance than the total amount of penicillin given (see Table 1).

The next step in this investigation was to vary the total amount of penicillin given over a constant period of time. The duration of treatment was established at 28 days; one group of patients

TABLE 2. PATIENTS TREATED FOR 28 DAYS WITH A DAILY DOSE OF 0·1, 0·25, AND 0·5 MEGA-UNITS

Dose	Died	Relapsed	"Cured"	Average follow-up
100,000 units a day	3 (21%)	5 (36%)	6 (43%)	198 days
250,000 units a day	13 (38%)	4 (12%)	17 (50%)	117 days
500,000 units a day	7 (39%)	0	11 (61%)	114 days

received 100,000 units daily, another 250,000 units a day and the third 500,000 units daily (see Table 2). The results indicated that a daily dose of 100,000 units of penicillin was insufficient and that 250,000 units daily was not quite so effective as 500,000 units daily. Eighteen patients received 500,000 units of penicillin daily for 28 days and none relapsed; 7 died, but these deaths cannot be ascribed to failure of penicillin therapy. It should be remembered that no matter how effective penicillin may prove to be in the treatment of this disease a significant death rate will remain from causes such as heart failure, uraemia and major emboli. When this is borne in mind, the results obtained by giving 500,000 units daily to previously untreated patients are all the more remarkable. None of the 18 patients relapsed and in only one of the 7 deaths was there any evidence that penicillin had failed to control the infection.

Experience in Great Britain subsequent to the publication of this report supports the policy that provided the patient has not relapsed after a previous course of treatment and provided the organism is not more than 10 times as resistant to penicillin as the Oxford staphylococcus, 500,000 units daily should be given for 28 days.

Significance of *in vitro* sensitivity tests

The infecting organism is almost always a streptococcus not more than 5 times as resistant as the standard test staphylococcus. Only when the organism is more than 10 times as resistant, and this occurred in only 4 of the 147 patients described, can this measurement be said to have definite prognostic or therapeutic importance. With this degree of resistance failure to respond to treatment is common, and evidence on the system of dosage which should be adopted is meagre. Our own policy is to continue the administration of 500,000 units daily for 6 weeks or more, although it is possible that a larger daily dose should be adopted.

Importance of early and adequate treatment

Delay in treatment undoubtedly diminishes the chances of survival, not because the infection is less readily controlled, but because structural damage in this disease is both progressive and dangerous. Inadequate treatment not only means delay and exposure of the patient to the many complications of the disease. It is also possible that resistance to treatment with penicillin may develop. Evidence on the last point is not yet conclusive, but it is clearly safer to assume that inadequate treatment is prejudicial to later success. Early diagnosis of the disease has become of great therapeutic importance.

Methods of administration and general care

Many of the centres involved in this investigation have found that most patients prefer continuous intramuscular infusion, while other centres have found intermittent intramuscular injections more satisfactory. No difference has been shown in the therapeutic results obtained by these two methods and it is generally agreed that both should be available if the treatment of subacute bacterial endocarditis is to be undertaken. In the United States of America many have preferred the intravenous drip, but in Great Britain the high incidence of venous thrombosis, possibly due to impurities, has prevented the general use of this method.

For obvious reasons the patient should be confined to bed and the general principles involved in the treatment of any prolonged febrile illness should be applied. Anaemia should be given treatment appropriate to its severity.

Response to treatment

The blood culture becomes sterile within a few days of the commencement of treatment, but not infrequently fever persists longer, although it usually falls within a week. The temperature chart can be very misleading, and I have seen several patients who remained febrile throughout while penicillin was being given, and yet had an uninterrupted and afebrile convalescence. Alternatively, some patients who remain afebrile during the last few weeks of treatment have subsequently relapsed because dosage was inadequate. Neither the cause nor the prognostic significance of this fever which may persist during treatment is known, but it is presumably not due to septicaemia or to impurities in penicillin.

The dangers of infarction and other embolic phenomena remain throughout treatment and convalescence, but probably in lessening degree. The spleen diminishes in size, often quite rapidly. In contrast haematuria persists long into convalescence and may remain months after the patient has returned to an active life. The erythrocyte sedimentation rate also remains high during treatment but falls slowly during convalescence.

The rate of general improvement in health is very variable, and is usually associated with increase in the haemoglobin percentage and gain in weight. Many patients show subjective improvement within a few days of the commencement of treatment and it may be difficult to restrain activity during early convalescence. In the absence of complications such as heart failure or major emboli it has been our custom, 2 weeks after cessation of treatment, to allow patients to sit in a chair and then to encourage an increase in activity according to the patient's capacity.

Relapses

Although none of the 18 patients relapsed following the system of dosage now recommended, 500,000 units for 28 days (see Table 2), one patient who had failed to respond to treatment died. As more patients are treated with this dosage, occasional relapses are likely to be observed. These should, however, become apparent soon after treatment has been completed, since of 54 relapses, after courses of penicillin which must be considered inadequate according to present standards, 49, or 91 per cent, occurred within 30 days (Christie [8, 9]). The treatment of relapses, and the treatment of patients in whom the daily administration of 500,000 units of penicillin fails to sterilize the blood after 7-10 days, present special and difficult problems. If penicillin were in ample supply a larger dose over a longer period of time would probably be recommended. At present 500,000 units daily for 6 or 8 weeks is being used and in the few patients to whom this has been given, results have been satisfactory.

Heparin

The results already described, in which penicillin alone was given, compare favourably with those obtained from a combination of penicillin and heparin (Loewe[5]). The hazards of heparin are well known and its use appears to be contra-indicated unless a controlled investigation on the treatment of penicillin-insensitive cases is being undertaken. Heparin must add the additional hazard of severe haemorrhage from a vascular lesion which might otherwise have been trivial if used in cases in which penicillin alone would be effective.

Prophylaxis

Dental extraction and removal of other foci of infection other than in the mouth have long been considered as precipitating factors in this disease. In patients with rheumatic endocarditis, or congenital heart disease, a prophylactic course of penicillin for these minor operations has been recommended by several investigators. Ward and his colleagues[10] suggest administration of 500,000 units daily for 3 days.

Prognosis

An analysis of the results of treatment in the different types of rheumatic and congenital heart disease is not yet possible, but it is our impression that severe aortic regurgitation is a bad prognostic feature, and that the results in congenital heart disease are slightly better than those in rheumatic heart disease. This does not suggest any difference in the action of penicillin in these various types of heart disease but probably only reflects the incidence of heart failure. It is not surprising that even moderate heart failure should be a bad prognostic sign and that few patients with severe heart failure survive even if the infection is easily controlled.

Another important factor in prognosis is the sensitivity of the infecting organism. If this is more than 10 times as resistant as the standard test staphylococcus, the chance of a favourable response to penicillin is inversely proportional to the resistance of the organism.

ACUTE BACTERIAL ENDOCARDITIS

Acute bacterial endocarditis, often only diagnosed by the pathologist, is a complication of septicaemia, the treatment of which is described elsewhere. When the diagnosis is made clinically in patients with septicaemia the chances of recovery are uncertain, but the outlook is by no means so hopeless as it has been supposed to be. Even when treated with the moderate doses required in uncomplicated septicaemia, about one-third of these patients recover (Dolphin and Cruickshank[11], Meads, Harris and Finland[12]). This recovery rate is, however, very unsatisfactory, and it is obvious that a more ambitious system of dosage should be tried. Although acute bacterial endocarditis differs in many fundamental respects from the subacute variety, it seems reasonable to recommend that the same principles of treatment should be adopted, and that 500,000 units daily for 28 days should be given.

REFERENCES

[1] Florey, M. E., and Florey, H. W. (1943) *Lancet*, **1**, 387.
[2] Herrell, W. E. (1943) *Proc. Mayo Clin.*, **18**, 65.
[3] Dawson, M. H., and Hobby, Gladys L. (1944) *J. Amer. med. Ass.*, **124**, 611.
[4] Loewe, L., Rosenblatt, P., Greene, H. J., and Russell, M. (1944) *J. Amer. med. Ass.*, **124**, 144.
[5] Loewe, L. (1945) *Bull. N.Y. Acad. Med.*, **21**, 59.
[6] Bloomfield, A. L., and Halpern, R. M. (1945) *J. Amer. med. Ass.*, **129**, 1135.
[7] Flippin, H. F., Mayock, R. L., Murphy, F. D., and Wolferth, C. C. (1945) *J. Amer. med. Ass.*, **129**, 841.
[8] Christie, R. V. (1946) *Brit. med. J.*, **1**, 381.
[9] Christie, R. V. (1946) *Lancet*, **1**, 369.
[10] Ward, G. E. S., Meanock, R. I., Selbie, F. R., and Simon, R. D. (1946) *Brit. med. J.*, **1**, 383.
[11] Dolphin, A., and Cruickshank, R. (1945) *Brit. med. J.*, **1**, 897.
[12] Meads, M., Harris, H. W., and Finland, M. (1945) *New Engl. J. Med.*, **232**, 463.

CHEST INFECTIONS

By A. Hope Gosse, M.D., F.R.C.P.
Physician, St. Mary's Hospital; Physician, Brompton Hospital, London;
Consulting Physician, King Edward VII Sanatorium, Midhurst

INTRODUCTION

Common infections of the respiratory system are due to the presence of *D. pneumoniae*, of streptococci, of staphylococci and of *D. catarrhalis*. All these organisms are very sensitive to penicillin and their elimination is now often possible and is of great value.

Pfeiffer's bacillus (*H. influenzae*) and Friedländer's bacillus (*K. pneumoniae*) are sometimes sensitive to the very high rates of concentration which can be obtained by local treatment. The tubercle bacillus is insensitive, and tuberculosis therefore is not benefited at all by the drug.

The medical practitioner must not expect, as yet, dogmatic directions for his employment of penicillin in the treatment of respiratory infections, for the various techniques already employed are constantly undergoing change with the introduction of new and improved methods. There is, however, an over-riding principle in this therapy which applies to any of the techniques of its administration: that when penicillin can be brought in close enough contact with a penicillin-sensitive organism—and the closer the better—it can be confidently expected to eliminate that organism. The decision will always have to be made whether it would be more beneficial to the patient for the penicillin to be given intramuscularly, as in pneumonia, locally, as into an empyema, or by inhalation, as in bronchitis. Further, a decision may be required concerning the employment of these methods separately or in combination. When the principle described above is borne in mind the choice is relatively easy and almost automatic.

The introduction of this new therapy will surely increase the tendency to consider the morbid conditions of the chest in terms of bacteriology rather than of morbid anatomy. The clinician's questions will now be concerned with the type of organism which is producing the disease rather than with the morbid changes which have been, or are being, produced.

To determine whether or not the respiratory infection is being caused by a penicillin-sensitive organism it is essential to have a specimen of sputum or pus bacteriologically examined. The report can be expected to be returned from a good laboratory within 24 hours. In acute infections of the chest when the patient is seriously ill, it is desirable to start penicillin treatment without bacteriological confirmation and it should be continued only when the report indicates penicillin-sensitive infection.

The selection of cases for treatment largely depends at present on the severity of the disease, the availability of trained nurses, and the supply of penicillin in the required form. These three factors taken together were adequate reasons for issuing penicillin almost exclusively to hospitals when it was in short supply. In the future, because of the rapid increase in the quantity manufactured, it will rapidly become available to every registered medical practitioner for use in the treatment of his patients.

The practitioner may well ask for guidance regarding the relative values of sulphonamides and penicillin in respiratory infections. They will be discussed under the headings of the separate infections. Alternative treatment with a sulphonamide will often be expedient and, in some cases—especially of pneumonia—it will be adequate, whereas in empyema of the pleural cavity, penicillin is likely to stand alone in medical, as contrasted with surgical, therapy.

It is expected that increasing numbers of cocci causing infection of the respiratory tract and at present sensitive to sulphonamides, will be found to be sulphonamide-resistant in spite of having retained their morphological and cultural characteristics. This disquieting change in character is attributed to prolonged and inadequate dosage of the sulphonamides in the same or in an intermediate host. Such cases, although still rare, will necessitate the choice of penicillin should danger threaten.

Sometimes the response to penicillin treatment in infections of the lung is as dramatic and immediate as in other systems affected by penicillin-sensitive organisms, such as infection of the meninges by the meningococcus and the urethra by the gonococcus, and in any system by the staphylococcus when the causative and curative agents contact each other. In many cases it may be found to be of use only as a temporary sterilizing agent, as in bronchiectasis, without elimination of the insensitive organisms, which retain their activity unimpaired.

It is desirable to state here categorically that penicillin has no place in the treatment of any disease caused entirely by the tubercle bacillus. It is too early to say whether or not it is ever to be considered as contra-indicated in a mixed infection partly caused by the tubercle bacillus, but there must be few, if any, clinicians who would withhold its use to eliminate a penicillin-sensitive organism which added to the severity of the tuberculous disease.

In making a diagnosis of pneumonia it is now of little but academic interest whether the case is one of lobar pneumonia or of bronchopneumonia, although it is important to estimate the probable severity of the disease. The mode of onset helps this estimation: the acute onset with a rigor and a temperature of 104° F. in a few hours is of much graver import than is the insidious onset in which pyrexia is present for 2 or 3 days before the diagnosis is established. The essential feature in the diagnosis of any of the pneumonias is causation. What is the organism? Is it penicillin-sensitive? If sputum is available it is surely the first duty of the clinician to see that its bacteriology is determined without delay. If assumption is necessary it may be assumed that whenever the prevailing organism in the sputum of the pneumonia patient is a pneumococcus, a staphylococcus, or a streptococcus (with certain exceptions), then it is penicillin-sensitive and the patient can be expected to react favourably to treatment.

Any patient with pneumonia who responds favourably to the sulphonamides would improve as much, and often more, on penicillin. The oral administration of 2 tablets of a sulphonamide 4-hourly is, however, less wearying to the patient than are 3-hourly injections of penicillin day and night for some 3–5 days.

If sputum is not available or if the causative organism cannot be determined, the clinical diagnosis of pneumonia is in itself an indication for a choice of one of these specific remedies and for its immediate administration.

Penicillin treatment of pneumonia is carried out by the intramuscular injection of 15,000 units of penicillin in sterile solution 3-hourly day and night for 5 days. There are many alternative methods. Sometimes the drip method is preferred to the intramuscular route by the scientific clinician but seldom is it preferred by the patient. The dosage is varied and 15,000 units is probably a minimal dose for an adult with pneumonia. A dose of 30,000 units is preferred by some physicians and larger doses in a suspension have been found to maintain a fairly constant level of penicillin in the blood, even when given only twice daily. The establishment of this method, if it is found to be as satisfactory as the 3-hourly method, will be the greatest boon to the general practitioner and to the patient.

Apart from the fact that penicillin administration is more wearisome to the patient than is the oral administration of a sulphonamide, the question now almost always arises concerning the relative merits of the two in every case diagnosed as pneumonia. The well established specificity of the sulphonamides will often be found adequate to control the toxaemia and reduce the temperature to a normal level within 2 or 3 days. In this connexion it may be recommended that Sulphamezathine (sulphadimethyl-pyrimidine) is to be preferred to any of the earlier introduced sulphonamides because relatively, it causes little nausea and other toxic symptoms. Sulphamezathine, or sulphadiazine, will do all that, or even more than, the previously introduced sulphonamides did and with far less toxic effect than sulphanilamide and its immediate successors. In such cases the need for penicillin therapy either concurrently or alone does not seem to be insistent. When, however, the toxaemia and the pyrexia do not respond well in 2–3 days and the patient's condition is becoming more disquieting, administration of penicillin is clearly indicated. Further, in every case of pneumonia in which the prognosis seems dangerous both the sulphonamide and the penicillin treatments may, and perhaps should, be given. As an injury to a limb calls for the rites of radiological diagnosis, in a case of pneumonia, from a medico-legal point of view, so a dangerously ill pneumonia case may call for the rites of penicillin in therapy.

In the case of average severity therefore the increased difficulty of administration and the greater efficacy of penicillin, as balanced against sulphonamide, treatment, does not leave much to choose between these two specific treatments for pneumonia. In the severest cases, marked by later decade of life, delirium, cyanosis, low blood pressure, rapid pulse and, above all, a positive blood culture, both methods of therapy should be employed. Contra-indications for the use of sulphonamides are leucopenia, severe nausea or vomiting, and excessive headache. The only known scientific contra-indication to the use of penicillin in pneumonia is a sure knowledge that the causative organism is not penicillin-sensitive.

In favourable cases fall in temperature, by lysis, and subsidence of toxaemic symptoms can be expected in 1–2 days. In some cases this improvement is only partial; the temperature may fall from a level of 104° F. to 101° F. in 36 hours but no further immediate drop may take place although the treatment is continued. It would appear that the pyrexia in these cases is due to more than one micro-organism. The penicillin-sensitive organism is eliminated but the non-sensitive organisms induce some degree of pyrexia until the natural processes of the inflamed areas produce their antibodies. In the absence of any complication the temperature may not become normal until 3 weeks after the onset of the pneumonia. Should the pyrexia last longer than 21 days some complication should be sought, and, if it has not already been done, tuberculosis should be excluded. It would occasionally save some humiliation to the practitioner if he were to make a rule of having the sputum examined for acid-fast bacilli quite early in every case of penumonia in an adult.

EMPYEMA

Penicillin is altering materially the treatment of empyema thoracis even while the principles of treatment are being evolved. In penicillin-sensitive infections of the pleura causing empyemata, the essential treatment is the injection of 30,000–50,000 units of penicillin in 30–50 millilitres of solution into the pleural space after fluid has been withdrawn and with the position of the needle unchanged so as to ensure that the penicillin is injected into the pus or fluid of the empyema. This process should be repeated in from 24 to 48 hours when it is desirable to aspirate as much fluid as possible before injecting another dose of penicillin. Every 2 or 3 days this procedure may require repetition until the fluid is sterile and shows signs of absorption, or until surgical intervention is required to obtain the quickest return to good health and activity.

The most favourable results can be expected when good fortune has enabled the clinician to make the diagnosis early, when the fluid is only turbid although containing numerous pus cells but is not yet frankly purulent. Complete resolution may take place and a skiagram of the chest taken some weeks later may show hardly any evidence of the former purulent pleurisy. In every case the clinical and radiological signs should be checked throughout the convalescence to guard against a relapse of the empyema going unrecognized and therefore untreated.

Pneumonia treated by penicillin may be accompanied or followed by a small pleural effusion which remains sterile suggesting that a septic effusion has been avoided by this specific therapy.

By systemic treatment alone little penicillin can be expected to appear in the empyema. Systemic treatment does, however, affect the adjacent inflamed lung with its bountiful blood supply. This, materially at times, improves the condition of the patient for later surgical drainage.

Satisfactory as are the results of treatment of empyemata by penicillin when an early diagnosis has been made, it is all too true that often an empyema is diagnosed only after it has been frankly purulent for days and perhaps weeks, even in specialist hands. In these established cases the empyema should be sterilized by sufficient penicillin injections and then surgical drainage should be established with, or perhaps without, resection of a rib. Otherwise the fibrinous exudate and debris will cause a thickened pleura and be liable to reinfection before organization of the scar tissue is complete. For the further consideration of this problem see elsewhere.

TRAUMATIC HAEMOTHORAX

The presence of blood in the pleural cavity following trauma, such as crush injuries of the chest or the fractured end of a rib perforating the pleura and lung, is a potentially dangerous source of infection by pyogenic organisms. While it is important to aspirate the blood as far as possible as soon as the patient has completely recovered from the shock of the accident, and in any case within 48 hours, penicillin, 50,000 units, should be introduced prophylactically into the pleural space after aspiration. With each aspiration further penicillin should be introduced as in the treatment of incipient empyema.

TUBERCULOUS PYOTHORAX

The same treatment can be employed in a case of secondary infection of a tuberculous pyothorax by a penicillin-sensitive organism. This occurs, although rarely, in some cases of artificial pneumothorax treatment in every large pneumothorax clinic. Whereas formerly it was almost imperative to drain the secondarily infected tuberculous empyema with the certainty of a permanent tuberculous sinus, it can now be treated with penicillin and without surgical drainage. When the pus is freed from any pathogenic organisms, apart from the tubercle bacillus, then thoracoplasty or the more conservative treatments of the tuberculous pyothorax can be employed, and a permanent sinus perhaps avoided. The prognosis is thereby materially improved.

ABSCESS OF THE LUNG

The treatment of abscess of the lung by penicillin is still in the experimental stage and it is difficult to indicate with accuracy the result likely to be achieved in any given case. In some cases it is dramatic; in others it is disappointing even to the extent of failing to prevent a fatal termination.

There can, however, be no doubt that penicillin has an important place in the future therapy of the lung abscess, single or multiple. The examination of the offensive purulent sputum bacteriologically for penicillin-sensitive organisms is a prerequisite to its use. The present indication is that the staphylococcal abscess will give good results, as may also be obtained in a mixed infection, whereas in streptococcal abscesses of the lung variable results, some curative, others ineffective, will be encountered.

In the classification of lung abscesses on the basis of response to penicillin therapy by intramuscular injection of 15,000–30,000 units 3-hourly there are grounds for division into the following groups.

Type	*Response*
(1) Multiple staphylococcal lung abscesses associated with staphylococcal septicaemia	Very good
(2) Bronchiectatic lung abscess	Poor
(3) Acute single lung abscess	Often good
(4) Chronic single lung abscess:	
(a) with adequate bronchial drainage	Good
(b) with inadequate bronchial drainage	Poor
(5) Mixed infection lung abscess	Variable

The best results are obtained with early and adequate therapy. If necessary the penicillin treatment should be maintained for weeks, even months.

The method of administration mostly employed up to the present has been systematic intramuscular injection 3-hourly of 15,000 units. Inhalation therapy is being employed and has been regarded as beneficial in a few cases.

If the course of this disease is complicated by an empyema or bronchiectasis the treatment described for these conditions should be employed.

Encouraging reports have been received on the treatment of abscess of the lung by the injection of about 50,000 units of penicillin direct into the abscess cavity by a hollow needle introduced through an intercostal space. It would seem that radiological control would be necessary to ensure that the point of the needle is in the abscess cavity. It may well prove that by a combination of systemic treatment with direct injection into the abscess cavity the best result will be obtained. The former objection to exploring an abscess cavity at all was based on the danger of infecting the pleural cavity and on the striking increase in the severity of the prognosis if this occurred. Should such infection be caused by a penicillin-sensitive organism and be recognized early the danger now can be largely, if not entirely, eliminated. The improved prognosis, yet to be established, of direct cavity injection is to be set against any potential danger.

BRONCHIECTASIS

Progress in radiological technique has led to the increasing recognition of this condition which is one of the common causes of chronic disease of the lungs. The onset is often insidious as the bronchi may remain apparently dry for years with perhaps an occasional haemoptysis, the cause of which demands diagnosis. This is effected by a bronchogram, in which the pathological condition of the bronchi is shown. At any stage of its development from a few days to even years septic infection of the bronchiectatic wall may occur and it is then that penicillin is first to be considered in the treatment of this disease. If the patient has pyrexia due to the septic organisms invading the parenchyma of the lung and if the organisms in the pus are penicillin-sensitive, then systemic penicillin, 15,000 units by intramuscular injection, can be expected to reduce the pyrexia quite rapidly; only 3-hourly injections for a period up to 5 days is required in most cases.

When, however, the thick green nummular sputum, sometimes offensive in odour and to taste, becomes chronic and lasts continuously, sometimes for months, then the purulent bronchiectasis should be treated with penicillin by the inhalation method. Oxygen under pressure is bubbled through glycerin for a few minutes into a rubber bag and thence to a B.L.B. nasal mask which must be accurately and as comfortably as possible adjusted to the patient's face. He breathes in through his nose and breathes out through his mouth. When he is accustomed to the method the switch is turned to make the oxygen bubble through the penicillin; this method should be continued for half an hour or so, by which time 100,000 units of penicillin dissolved in 3 millilitres of physiological saline may be vaporized and inhaled. Deep breaths are desirable so that the penicillin-concentrated atmosphere of oxygen mixing with air can be sucked into the smallest bronchi and alveoli.

It is early yet to speak of the ultimate value of penicillin in chronic septic bronchiectasis but early experience shows that, although the penicillin-sensitive organisms in the bronchiectatic pus can be reduced for a time, the sputum usually remains purulent and in a short time, even a few days, the organisms may be present again in all their former vigour and quantity.

BRONCHITIS

When penicillin first became available for therapeutic trial it was in such short supply that its use was largely restricted to the dangerous or at least more severe infections and it is difficult to indicate with confidence the probable value of its use in bronchitis. On general principles, but with as yet inadequate experience, it would seem that its use is more likely to be of greater benefit in recent and acute bronchitis than in established chronic bronchitis. It may well prove to be true that when there have been chronic tissue changes of a fibrotic nature its use may be limited to the temporary elimination of penicillin-sensitive organisms. In acute bronchitis treated early by inhalation of from 100,000 to 200,000 units a day in 2 or more inhalations, there is promise of the early termination of the bronchitis. The clinical condition is so variable in its severity and duration, that it is no easy matter to judge results. There is not any doubt, however, that the penicillin-sensitive organisms rapidly disappear from the sputum.

When chronic bronchitis and bronchial asthma have coexisted in a patient, the results clinically appear to be at times encouraging but what new treatment for bronchial asthma has not won commendation from the unfortunate sufferer? Experience shows that only a few, if any, patients obtain a real measure of control over the asthmatic paroxysms.

The best results obtained in bronchitis would therefore appear to be in the acute attack in a patient with previously "dry" bronchial tubes, when the organism is penicillin-sensitive and the infection is single and not multiple.

It may not be out of place to raise here the question how far the possible indiscriminate or prolonged inadequate use of penicillin for all minor infections may be to the disadvantage of the patient's, and even to public, health. Will such use of it lead to the sensitive organisms developing into an insensitive strain? The answer must be left to the future. For the present the value of penicillin has been proved and its use should be emphasized in full doses in every severe infection by a penicillin-sensitive organism.

CHEST SURGERY

By T. Holmes Sellors, D.M., M.Ch., F.R.C.S.
Surgeon, London Chest Hospital

INTRODUCTION

There are two main headings under which the use of penicillin can be considered in chest surgery. First there is its role in the active treatment of lung and of pleural infections, and secondly there is its value as a prophylactic agent in minimizing the infective complications of surgery.

The chief importance of penicillin in the active treatment of surgical chest conditions must centre around empyema, which is discussed in detail. Pulmonary conditions which do not require surgical treatment are considered elsewhere.

The prophylactic value of penicillin in actual operative work is well established, since many procedures are liable to infective complications and any reduction in their incidence will be of great advantage. The improvement in the results of chest surgery can be attributed in part to penicillin but it must not be overlooked that there also has been a considerable advance in technical developments in the same period.

There must not be, however, any impression that the basic principles of surgery can be relaxed or that the accepted rigid aseptic technique can in any way be modified. The importance of the drug lies in the fact that it can eliminate certain infections or, at least, can minimize their severity.

METHODS OF ADMINISTRATION

The principal methods of administration are discussed elsewhere and there are only minor comments which need to be made in connexion with chest surgery. Systemic penicillin in acute chest infections is usually adequate in a dosage of from 1,000,000 to 2,000,000 units over a period of 10–14 days. There is some doubt with regard to the extent to which penicillin, given systemically, can reach the pleural cavity, but it is probable that a limited concentration can be achieved by this method.

Local injection of penicillin into the pleura should aim at covering all infected surfaces and a dose which maintains an adequate concentration is usually in the neighbourhood of 20,000–40,000 units. The drug disappears from the pleura in about 24 hours and must therefore be repeated daily or as often as the concentration falls. In the case of an empyema cavity with thick fibrous walls, however, penicillin does not disappear at anything like this speed and it can be identified in an adequate concentration even after several days.

It has been suggested[1] that much larger doses of penicillin injected into the pleura will be absorbed into the circulation and maintain an adequate penicillin blood level, so that a dose given locally will produce a general systemic effect; 120,000 units of penicillin injected into the pleural cavity passes out into the blood stream at a fairly steady rate and the blood level is adequately maintained for about 24 hours; there is usually just enough left in the pleural sac to be effective locally. Doubling the dose (up to 240,000 units) maintains sufficient penicillin in the blood for 48 hours.

Inhalation and instillation of penicillin into the bronchi is a method which will probably increase in popularity since a reasonable blood concentration can be obtained in this way. Ten thousand units administered in a vaporized form gives a good blood concentration in addition to the local action on the bronchi and lung tissues. The Collinson inhaler which uses oxygen to atomize the penicillin solution or a Rybar inhaler with a hand pump have been found to be effective in producing penicillin in a spray fine enough to reach the lung tissue.

Penicillin and sulphathiazole powder, and pastes and jellies containing these substances can be used on raw areas, but it will be realized that the exudate which forms on these surfaces will inevitably carry the substances away from the point at which they were applied. Dusting of operative incisions with the powder is effective but when there is a granulating surface the substance is usually swept away from its point of application or fails to penetrate the crevices sufficiently well to be entirely effective.

CLINICAL APPLICATIONS

Empyema

General considerations.—Pleural empyema is the most important condition which has to be treated in chest surgery and is one in which penicillin can play an important part. The infecting organisms are usually penicillin-sensitive and the contents of the pleural cavity can often be sterilized with surprising rapidity. A definite warning must be given in this connexion: the sterilization of pus does not necessarily mean the healing of the empyema. Closure of the cavity is just as important a feature; it is of little value to eliminate infection from the pleural cavity and leave a chronic dead space which produces considerable incapacity, since a dead space may be reinfected at some future date. Enthusiasm for chemotherapy, therefore, must be coupled with strict attention to the obliteration of the actual cavity and the restoration of the underlying lung function.

The experience of thoracic surgeons in empyema suggests that, on the whole, treatment of this condition is most unsatisfactory. Late recognition, lack of coordination in the management and indifferent handling result in an unnecessarily high proportion of chronic empyemata with consequent severe disability. These comments still apply to many cases treated with penicillin and it is important therefore to consider the principles of treatment in some detail.

Principles of treatment.—Pleural infection almost always follows some underlying pulmonary inflammation. The pleura reacts by producing a thin effusion, loaded with organisms, which becomes turbid and steadily increases in thickness until frank pus is recognized. In the early stages there is no localization of the infection and the whole pleural cavity is potentially involved. As the process develops and the pus becomes thick, localization occurs and an abscess with relatively firm walls is produced; at this stage there is less fear of the development of a total empyema. In addition to the formation of pus, the result of pneumococcal or staphylococcal infection is to produce masses of fibrin which lie in strips on the walls and float loose in the base of the cavity. This fibrin may prevent adequate aspiration of pus by blocking the needle and there is no point in sterilizing the contents of an empyema cavity and leaving a fibrin mass behind, since this will act only as dead tissue and become a possible source of infection.

An untreated empyema, if left alone, rapidly develops a thick wall which is more noticeable on the parietal than on the visceral pleural surface. The underlying lung tissue is immobilized and the chest wall is rendered rigid and contracted. Very considerable efforts on the part of surgery and physiotherapy are required to overcome this disability.

In the literature which has been published on the use of penicillin in pleural infections, there is a possibility that confusion may arise unless it is clearly understood at which stage the treatment advocated is used. The use of penicillin in the early stages is far more likely to bring about resolution than its use in a well established and chronic abscess cavity which shows little tendency to obliterate.

Complete and repeated aspiration helps to obliterate the empyema cavity so long as the pleural layers are thin and re-expansion is unimpeded. When fibrin flakes are present and there is fibrosis over the lung surface, aspiration will fail and must be replaced by a more effective form of drainage. An intercostal tube provides a better channel for emptying thick pus and fibrin, but this cannot compare in efficiency with a wide-bore tube such as that used after rib resection.

The introduction of chemotherapy has slightly increased the incidence of empyema owing to the fact that patients with severe pulmonary inflammation who previously might have died, now survive, and thus add to the number of cases in which empyema may develop. It has been suggested that the use of sulphonamides and penicillin has increased the incidence of pleural infection in pneumonic conditions, but there is little evidence to support the suggestion.

The bacteriology of empyemata in relation to penicillin therapy is important. The majority of cases are caused by sensitive organisms such as pneumococci, streptococci and staphylococci, but other bacteria which are insensitive may be encountered, and in consequence of this the causative organisms must be established as soon as possible, namely, at the time of the first diagnostic aspiration. Penicillin can produce sterility in pneumococcal and streptococcal infections in 2–4 days, although with staphylococcal organisms the period of time is a little longer. The response is slower when thick pus and fibrin are present. The effect of penicillin on the actual formation of pus is to convert thin turbid effusions into frank pus several days earlier than would be the case without its use.

A disadvantage of prolonged open drainage of an empyema is that secondary invading organisms sooner or later gain access to the cavity. Organisms commonly encountered are *B. proteus*, *Ps. aeruginosa* and coliform bacilli insensitive to penicillin. This secondary infection cannot be effectively dealt with by chemotherapy and is responsible for delay in healing.

This point should be borne in mind when any empyema is approached, and the advantages of the closed chemotherapy form of treatment are obvious if the cavity can be obliterated at the same time; it is useless to try the method when the walls of the cavity are so thick that they will mechanically interfere with healing. It is safer to use efficient surgical drainage when there is any doubt concerning the final healing: slight prolongation of the convalescent period is of less disadvantage than is a persistent dead space.

Treatment of early pleural infection

The line of treatment recommended by Fatti and his colleagues[2] seems to be eminently satisfactory for the early type of case;

compared with cases in which ordinary methods of treatment were used the time of healing was more than halved. As soon as fluid has been recognized, the aspirating needle is used and if there be any suggestion of pus, penicillin is injected at the same time. The frequency with which penicillin-sensitive causative organisms are found is so great that the bacteriological report can be anticipated on these occasions. Once the organism has been identified, however, aspiration is again performed and this time as much fluid is withdrawn as is possible. Penicillin (120,000 units or more in 10 millilitres of physiological saline) is injected. This procedure is repeated, daily if necessary, as the pus develops and thickens; when the pus is too thick to pass through the aspirating needle, an intercostal tube is inserted. The tube is probably best placed at a point some distance above the lowest limit of the empyema pocket. It is not necessarily placed at the lowest and most dependent point, because in a rapidly healing empyema obliteration is more or less concentric. This must be contrasted with more orthodox drainage in which the tube is placed at the lowest point.

The outline of the cavity can be gauged by the injection of a few millilitres of Lipiodol or radio-opaque oil (Oleum Iodisatum B.P. Add. I, Oleum Iodatum U.S.P. XII) and the taking of X-ray films from the anteroposterior and lateral aspects. With the intercostal tube in place, the cavity contents are drained off once or twice a day, and penicillin is instilled along the tube, which is then closed with a spigot. In favourable cases, the lung steadily re-expands and when the cavity is estimated to have closed, the intercostal tube is removed and the wound is covered with a sterile dressing and is left untouched.

Assessment of the obliteration of the cavity is not entirely simple. Drainage will have ceased, but there will still be a considerable amount of dullness over the empyema area and some diffuse radiological opacity. If injection of radio-opaque oil shows that the empyema has been reduced to a simple tube track, healing clearly has been obtained.

The constitutional improvement of the patient as the empyema is rendered sterile, is marked, and from the earliest stages lung function should be encouraged by use of special breathing exercises which aim at re-expansion. These breathing exercises and general active movement of the patient are essential to recovery. If the infection is not controlled the closed method of treatment should be abandoned and more definitive drainage established.

This type of treatment requires meticulous control and rigid asepsis even in the performance of simple procedures such as aspiration. The admission of secondary insensitive organisms will vitiate the effect of penicillin. The treatment, moreover, cannot be undertaken without the full cooperation of an experienced bacteriologist. Such treatment has considerable scope in the management of empyemata in children and also in that of bilateral cases in which the risks of bilateral and simultaneous drainage are considerable.

Treatment of late pleural infection

The majority of empyemata are recognized only when they are well established and localized. In these cases there is much fibrin present and re-expansion of the collapsed lung is likely to be slow. Drainage should therefore be considered in preference to aspiration and penicillin therapy. When empyema is first recognized it is reasonable to use aspiration and penicillin for a few days, but when aspiration becomes difficult or ineffective drainage should be instituted. An intercostal tube is rarely adequate on account of the comparative narrowness of its lumen and if it be used for the relief of pressure in large and comparatively early effusions it should be replaced by rib resection and insertion of a wide tube within a week or 10 days; the only exception to the use of this measure is the rare case in which rapid re-expansion occurs. The most satisfactory procedure is to perform deliberate rib resection at the site of election—the lowest and most posterior point of the cavity. The contents of the cavity are sucked out under open vision and the walls are cleared of fibrin masses. If the empyema has been effectively sterilized by penicillin, suture of the wound followed by aspiration is feasible[3,4], but it has been found to be more satisfactory to use wide-tube drainage and to control the closure of the cavity in the ordinary way. Breathing exercises and effective drainage ensure ultimate healing.

As has been stated, secondary infection develops sooner or later with an open tube and a careful watch should be kept on the bacteriology of the material removed so that local or systemic penicillin can be used should occasion arise. A cream of phenoxetol (β-phenoxylethyl-alcohol) 2 per cent with penicillin has a good effect in some mixed infections. A further point to be borne in mind is based on the observation that young bacteriological cells are particularly susceptible to the action of penicillin[5]. The effect of drainage is to allow rapid cell multiplication; therefore at this point penicillin used in full doses may be of value.

Note on aspiration.—There are minor points about the technique of aspiration which should be stressed, particularly when the needle is inserted into the pleural cavity in the early (unlocalized) stages. A fine needle and a local anaesthetic should be used for diagnostic aspiration and in the event of a dry tap, the needle point should not be advanced carelessly in case infective lung is punctured. In no circumstances should the needle be disconnected from its syringe lest air be sucked into the pleural cavity. An air bubble introduced in this way will rise, and in the absence of pleural adhesions may ascend to the apex. An apical empyema is much more difficult to manage than is a basal empyema.

The aspiration of thick pus requires a wider needle and it is useful to use a 2-way tap between the needle and syringe so that the syringe can be emptied without disconnecting the apparatus. The holding steady of a syringe for a prolonged period is not easy when many ounces of pus have to be evacuated. Coughing, tightness and distress are indications of too rapid a removal of fluid, and when this occurs, a pause of several minutes should be made before the operation is continued. The removal of a pint or more of pus may well take a quarter of an hour or 20 minutes and it is important that both patient and operator should be comfortable for this period. When a wide needle is used the anaesthetized skin should be nicked in order to avoid the carrying in of a plug of skin with the needle point. Recognition of the lowest point of the cavity is judged by injection of a small amount of Lipiodol and the taking of 2-plane skiagrams.

Aspiration is an operation usually carried out with the patient in bed and is one in which aseptic precautions are easily relaxed. If it is to be effective there must be complete asepsis and attention to detail on every occasion.

Chronic empyema

Chronic empyema is a most disabling condition and one that often could be avoided. It is usually the result of improper management and lack of control in the acute stages. Often, the tube has been removed too early, or too small a tube is provided so that drainage is inadequate and infection is maintained. The condition may also be caused by other factors such as retained foreign body, unrecognized tuberculous infection and new growth.

The most common example of empyema as referred to the chest surgeon, consists in a case which has been drained and, because drainage of pus has stopped or because the tube has not been replaced, is left with a small sinus which intermittently drains a large intrapleural pocket with thickened rigid walls. The chest is contracted and there is gross interference with expansion of the underlying lung. Secondary infection of the cavity is usual and the discharge is often profuse and has a foul odour. Bacteriology should be studied at the earliest opportunity so that the possible use of chemotherapy can be considered.

Treatment usually involves re-drainage of the space; an

adequate opening is made into the cavity at the most dependent point and the inside of the space is inspected for a foreign body such as a drainage tube or piece of bone, before a large size tube is inserted. The tube should remain in position and should be altered only when the size and shape of the cavity make change desirable; the tube is not removed until the empyema is reduced to a simple tube track. The process, however, can be properly controlled only by the taking of pleurograms at regular intervals.

In the majority of cases the organisms found are not penicillin-sensitive and there is little indication for the use of the drug locally or generally. It has been found in a number of cases that the organisms encountered are so profuse as to cover the presence of some underlying penicillin-sensitive organisms. This is noticeable in the case of *B. proteus* and *Ps. aeruginosa*, which, however, can be eliminated through culture by the use of selective media such as sodium azide 0·05 per cent or by covering the culture with a layer of melted agar as suggested by Fry. In a number of cases an underlying sensitive organism which responds to penicillin is found. It may be noted that in these cases local applications are unsuccessful and a systemic course of penicillin has to be used. In nearly all cases, empyema treated by adequate drainage ultimately heals, although it may take weeks and even months to obtain final closure. Occasionally some subsidiary operation which involves further resection of rib and the use of pleural or muscle flaps to obliterate the cavity, is used. In these cases penicillin is a valuable pre-operative prophylactic and the use of penicillin powder has been found to be effective in achieving a lower rate of infection and improved healing.

Haemothorax.—Particularly when occasioned by penetrating wounds, haemothorax is treated by aspiration with simultaneous prophylactic injections of penicillin. The incidence of infection in the recent war was much less than it was formerly and, even allowing for the varying circumstances, penicillin undoubtedly contributed to the continued sterility and early healing in a great many of these cases.

Tuberculous empyema.—In pure tuberculous empyema penicillin has not a place but when mixed infection occurs and sensitive organisms are encountered, intrapleural injection may be considered so that the empyema can be converted into a sterile tuberculous condition. This result is not always achieved, but when the method is successful external drainage of the empyema is avoided.

The problem of empyema treatment is rarely studied in adequate detail and much greater use should be made of bacteriology in order to discover how much help can be obtained from chemotherapy.

Bronchiectasis

In bronchiectasis, examination of the sputum usually shows a mixed flora; if penicillin-sensitive organisms are present the drug should certainly be used. Systemic courses improve the amount and character of the sputum and inhalations cause the sputum to become more fluid; in the case of foetid pus, the odour is lessened.

It is probable that inhalations will prove to be of considerable value as a prophylactic in cases which are not considered to be suitable for surgery[6]. Penicillin, however, cannot be regarded as having any place in replacing surgery in cases considered to be suitable for lobectomy, or as being a substitute for postural drainage, which is the only effective way of removing secretions.

In lobectomy cases pre-operative treatment should consist of prolonged postural drainage and intermittent penicillin inhalations. A systemic course started 2 or 3 days before operation and continued through the postoperative period has been found to be valuable. At operation itself penicillin powder is used over the bronchial stump and raw hilar area, and enclosure of a tablet of penicillin (7,000 units) in the bronchial stump helps to prevent infection in that area and assists primary healing. The importance of infection in relation to bronchial healing is discussed below in more detail.

After operation, aspiration of the pleural cavity is performed as often as fluid collects, and on each occasion 20,000–40,000 units of penicillin should be injected. Drainage will be required only when secondary infection cannot be controlled by aspiration and penicillin. The use of intrapleural penicillin during the period of expansion of the residual lung tissue undoubtedly reduces infection; even should a fistula develop, the pleural contents may remain sterile.

Lung abscess

The use of penicillin in the treatment of lung abscess is not as important as it might be thought to be. The infection is essentially an acute one resulting from obstruction of a segmental bronchus by infected material. Fusiform bacilli and anaerobic organisms predominate and these, plus necrosis of lung tissue, account for the foetor of the condition. The response to systemic penicillin is not usually marked, and the same observation applies to inhalations. It is difficult to see how the actual penicillin can reach the infected area as long as there is bronchial obstruction. If the abscess does not rupture into a bronchus and be coughed up within a week or so, surgical drainage should be considered, particularly if the cavity increases in size.

Early formation of pleural adhesions is now recognized as

being constant over the surface of the abscess and drainage in one or two stages should be made through these adhesions after careful localization. The prophylactic use of penicillin after the operation period may be considered but injections of penicillin directly into the cavity is not a procedure that should be accepted for routine use, although good results have been reported[7].

It is essential that drainage should be established through firmly adherent pleural layers, since the escape of pus into a free pleural cavity will lead to the formation of a fulminating empyema. Should this happen, the use of penicillin in large doses may prevent the condition becoming disastrous, and in the initial stages of the lung abscess drainage, penicillin powder has considerable value in eliminating certain organisms from the raw surfaces.

There are certain suppurative conditions of the lung which may be considered as coming within the province of surgery and in which an extensive trial of penicillin has been made. The results here are variable, but because of the severity of the condition penicillin should be given a trial since unexpected improvement may result.

A specific form of abscess which produces large distension cavities may be due to staphylococcal infection. Surgery is not indicated in these cases and the extensive use of systemic penicillin should be considered.

PENICILLIN IN MAJOR THORACIC SURGERY

As a prophylactic agent in major forms of thoracic surgery penicillin has a definite place. The drug can be used systemically or locally when operation is being done on cases in which infection already exists; an example is the infection which occurs behind a bronchial carcinoma when pneumonectomy is contemplated. Infective complications are undoubtedly reduced and in pneumonectomy, for example, primary healing may be obtained. In this event convalescence is complete in a period of weeks, whereas if the dead space becomes infected the resulting empyema may require months of treatment.

The most important aspect of lung excision is the healing of the bronchus. The tendency of this structure to break down after suture is considerable and when this occurs organisms from the air tubes reach the hitherto clean pleura and may produce an empyema.

Many methods of bronchus closure have been tried but prevention of a secondary infection is undoubtedly the most important feature; here penicillin plays a valuable part. The incidence of fistula formation has diminished considerably since its introduction[8]. At operation the practice is to apply penicillin and sulphathiazole powder over all the raw areas, which include the incision through the chest wall. Postoperative aspirations of any fluid should be followed by injection of penicillin into the pleura.

In other types of operation which involve much trauma of tissue, application of penicillin-sulphathiazole powder to the wounds may be considered, although it is doubtful whether it should be employed as a routine. In an operation such as thoracoplasty a great deal of muscle is divided, and as the incision is made through skin which is frequently a source of minor infections, the value of prophylactic penicillin is obvious. After thoracoplasty a dead space is left under the scapula and in this, fluid may collect. In addition the lung will probably have been stripped from its apical attachments (apicolysis or Semb type of operation) and infected lymphatic vessels may have been divided. Infection of this dead space is therefore occasionally encountered and it produces considerable distress. The extensive use of penicillin may allow the next stage of the operation to be proceeded with and primary union to be obtained in the wound. Hitherto, such cases would have had to be drained and, as the dead space is almost mechanically incapable of closure, a more or less permanent track would have been produced.

Heart

Suppurative pericarditis is usually of staphylococcal origin and often occurs as part of a general metastatic infection. Here the treatment to be adopted is essentially one of aspiration in order to avoid the effects of a cardiac tamponade, and at the same time penicillin can be injected. A systemic course would usually have been given and some penicillin will reach the pericardium from the blood stream[9,10]. There is not enough evidence to determine whether or not administration of penicillin and aspirations will produce sufficiently good results to enable drainage of the pericardium in this condition to be avoided, nor is it known whether or not the thickening of the pericardium which follows the inflammation produces constrictive pericarditis in later years.

In operations on the heart for such conditions as foreign body or for constrictive pericarditis, the use of local penicillin for the dusting of raw areas should be considered.

The rôle of penicillin in the treatment of acute and infective endocarditis is discussed elsewhere. In cases which are associated with patent ductus arteriosus its value pre-operatively is obvious, but even if the infection be controlled the patent ductus should still be obliterated surgically; if this is undertaken a course of penicillin should be given during the operative period.

Mediastinitis

Mediastinitis, although not often encountered, is a very dangerous condition. It may arise from a retained foreign body in the oesophagus or from perforation as a result of instrumentation. It can also occur with new growth formation. The main hope in these cases is to establish adequate drainage in the loose cellular tissues of the mediastinum and to insert fine tubes along which penicillin can be instilled. If early treatment be undertaken, some successful results may be achieved.

REFERENCES

[1] Florey, M. E., and Heatley, N. G. (1945) *Lancet*, **1**, 748.
[2] Fatti, L., Florey, M. E., Joules, H., Humphrey, J. H., and Sakula, J. (1946) *Lancet*, **1**, 257, 295.
[3] Roberts, J. E. H., Tubbs, O. S., and Bates, M. (1945) *Lancet*, **1**, 39.
[4] Butler, E. C. B., Perry, K. M. A., and Valentine, F. C. O. (1944) *Brit. med. J.*, **2**, 171.
[5] Knox, R. (1945) *Lancet*, **1**, 559.
[6] May, H. B., and Floyer, M. A. (1945) *Brit. med. J.*, **1**, 907.
[7] Pickering, D., and Grenville-Mathers, R. (1945) *Lancet*, **1**, 530.
[8] White, W. L., Burnett, W. E., Bailey, C. P., Rosemond, G. P., Norris, C. W., Favorite, G. O., Spaulding, E. H., Bondi, A., Jun., and Fowler, R. H. (1944) *J. Amer. med. Ass.*, **126**, 1016.
[9] McAdam, I. W. J., Challinor, S. W., Duguid, J. P., and McCall, A. (1945) *Lancet*, **2**, 843.
[10] Norman, H. B., and Ainsworth, R. M. (1945) *Brit. med. J.*, **1**, 806.

WOUNDS AND GAS GANGRENE

By A. E. Porritt, C.B.E., M.Ch., F.R.C.S.
Surgeon, H.M. Household; Surgeon to Out-patients and Assistant Director of the Surgical Unit, St. Mary's Hospital, London

and

G. A. G. Mitchell, O.B.E., M.B., Ch.M.
Late Adviser in Penicillin and Chemotherapy, 21 Army Group; Professor (Elect) of Anatomy, Manchester University

The pioneer work performed by Florey and Cairns[1] and by Pulvertaft[2] in Africa, aroused hopes that the use of penicillin might transform the treatment of war wounds, and results in later campaigns confirmed these expectations. As we were closely associated with the clinical application and assessment of penicillin throughout the North-West European campaign, we had unequalled opportunities for studying the effects of penicillin in war wounds, and the observations recorded here mainly deal with experiences in the 21st Army Group (the combined British and Canadian Armies constituting the British Liberation Army). These experiences were very extensive. Between D-day and VE-day (6th June 1944 and 8th May 1945, respectively) there were approximately 406,000 admissions to the 21st Army Group Medical units, including about 182,000 battle casualties. Of these, 100,000 patients at least received penicillin treatment, the majority being wounded men.

THERAPEUTIC APPLICATIONS OF PENICILLIN IN WAR WOUNDS

These are discussed in general terms because wounds of particular regions, such as those of the head and chest, are dealt with separately.

We have shown (see p. 106) that the widespread use of penicillin in prophylaxis effected a marked improvement in the condition of war wounds, and that in the British Liberation Army at least 9 out of 10 wounds were clinically clean when they were first examined at base hospital level. In consequence secondary closures became the most commonly performed operations, and this procedure was not confined entirely to apparently clean wounds. It was also carried out regularly, and with impunity, in many wounds which in pre-penicillin days would have been considered quite unsuitable for suture. This was one of the most notable therapeutic advances achieved during World War II and brought untold benefit in the prevention of pain, in providing better functional and cosmetic results, in avoiding prolonged suppuration with consequent visceral damage, and in shortening convalescence. This one advance alone must have saved many limbs and even lives. The success led to one curious result. Men who thought they had "blighty" wounds found themselves instead in convalescent depots with completely healed wounds within 3–4 weeks of being hit, and, although the physical result was excellent, the psychological response was poor. This problem assumed such importance that the Director of Medical Services of the 21st Army Group, had to introduce a rule that any man who had been in a hospital and convalescent depot for a month after he had been wounded should invariably be granted a week's sick leave in the United Kingdom. Even then they returned to duty more rapidly than in pre-penicillin days because so much time had been saved by quicker healing of wounds and recovery of function. "The results achieved led to a saving of manpower, a reduction in wound-complications and an economy in hospitalisation, in supplies of drugs and equipment, in surgeons' and nurses' time which it is quite impossible either to compute or to appreciate fully."[3]

Closure of wounds

Before results are discussed the methods in general use are here summarized. These are applicable to any wound suitable for closure, although modifications were necessary in special cases, for example, open bone and joint wounds.

In the 21st Army Group guide to penicillin therapy, medical officers were advised as follows.

> "When patients can be held for the requisite 4–5 days the possibility of closing wounds and covering raw surfaces by suture or grafting should be constantly explored, and if prophylaxis and forward treatment have been adequate most wounds can be closed on the first occasion they are examined in hospital. In some cases closure is mechanically impossible because of extensive tissue loss. In these skin grafting or plastic procedures should be considered and employed if possible; they are especially desirable if bones, tendons, main vessels or nerves are exposed. . . . Even a partial closure is better than none at all and may lead to reduction in oedema, thus facilitating further closure at a subsequent date. The decision to allow healing by granulations should be regarded as an unfortunate necessity and should not be made until more satisfactory alternatives have been considered."

Definition of sutures.—In order to obtain uniformity in records certain common terms were defined precisely: (1) Primary suture—any suture performed during the first day; (2) Delayed primary suture—any suture performed in the first week, that is between the first and seventh days; (3) Secondary suture—any suture performed after the first week, irrespective of whether or not any former attempt at suture has been made.

Even with the potent aid of penicillin the scope for primary suture in war wounds was small; it was confined mainly to men with penetrating abdominal or sucking chest wounds. Experience taught that suture of wounds should never be performed unless the patient could be kept in hospital for 4–5 days, and breaches of this elementary rule of war surgery by inexperienced or over-confident operators produced some of the relatively few serious wound infections seen during the course of the British Liberation Army campaign. The transportable casualties seldom reached a hospital on the first day, so that any sutures performed were mainly of the delayed primary or secondary variety. The results detailed in subsequent tables refer to closures of this type.

Surgical methods of treatment.—The surgeon who first examined the wound in hospital normally decided then and there upon the best course of treatment.

(1) Superficial, clean, or mildly infected wounds were sutured at once after a single dusting with penicillin powder.

(2) Larger and deeper wounds without evidence of serious or spreading infection were also closed at once, but small tubes were often left in the wound through which penicillin solution was injected for 4–5 days.

(3) More heavily infected wounds of any size were treated for 2–3 days with penicillin before suture was attempted, and wound swabs were taken and cultured. If the pathogens were penicillin-sensitive, improvement, usually rapid, followed combined local and parenteral therapy and the wound was then treated as under (2).

Surgeons learned quickly that a transient initial increase in the amount of discharge sometimes occurred after applications of penicillin to a wound. This soon diminished or ceased unless penicillin-insensitive organisms were present or subsequently gained access during the course of treatment, but these were never highly pathogenic and rarely delayed healing to an appreciable extent.*

In a typical operation, after the usual preliminary gentle cleansing, the surgeon removed from the wound any debris, devitalized tissue or any foreign material which remained. The wound edges were freshened by the removal of minimal amounts of skin, and in older wounds granulation tissue was excised; it was recognized that undercutting for the purpose of mobilizing the skin edges and of eliminating tension was permissible to the limits imposed by anatomical considerations. Haemostasis was

* According to an article published recently by Harley, Baty and Bowie (*Brit. Med. J.*, **1**, 639) this was not so in the Eastern theatres of war. There penicillin-insensitive Gram negative bacilli proved a common cause of prolonged low-grade infection and occasionally produced severe spreading infection.

then secured, the wound was dried, and all the surfaces were insufflated with penicillin powder (5,000 units of penicillin in 1 gramme of a sulphonamide or of dried plasma). Small drains were inserted if any pocket or dead space could not be eliminated. In deep or irregular wounds 1–3 fine rubber tubes were often inserted through small stab incisions in the flaps, and through these 1–2 millilitres of penicillin solution (500 units in 1 millilitre of isotonic saline solution) were injected twice daily for 4–5 days after preliminary aspiration, on each occasion, of any pus or exudate. This was done very gently in order to minimize any disruptive effect, and full aseptic precautions were employed in order to avoid the possibility of introducing penicillin-insensitive pathogens. These tubes were brought out through the inner dressings which were not disturbed during the injections, and between instillations the tube ends were stoppered with small sterile rods and were covered with sterile wool. Most surgeons preferred interrupted silkworm gut sutures for the actual closure of the wound and when there was any tension they did not remove the stitches for 10–12 days.

In all the more severe and contaminated wounds parenteral penicillin was given for 3–4 days after operation, and sometimes for a day prior to operation. Some surgeons exploited the knowledge that the wound exudates are bacteriostatic when there is an adequate level of penicillin in the blood. They gave only parenteral penicillin[4], and local applications other than the penicillin powder applied at the time of operation were not used. This obviated local disturbance of the wound and possible infection with penicillin-insensitive organisms. The results were excellent, but the method was less economical. Other surgeons obtained very good results by intensive therapy[5]; by the injection of penicillin solution locally through a syringe and needle instead of through indwelling tubes; or by local applications of penicillin in a slow-release vehicle. These variations in detail need not be described separately.

There were only two serious complications after the many thousands of sutures performed—both cases of localized gas gangrene which responded favourably to treatment—although many closures were performed in frankly infected wounds or in those requiring extensive excisions of devitalized tissues or foreign materials.

Scheme to investigate relative value of penicillin

Several agents were being recommended as adjuvants to good surgery in 1943–1944 when the Normandy invasion was being planned and when penicillin was known to most surgeons only by repute. Preliminary reports about penicillin were very encouraging, but many surgeons were of the opinion that the original casualties treated with penicillin had received preferential care by being held at forward base hospitals for a much longer period than was usual. Some surgeons claimed that this alone was sufficient to explain the improved results, and most of them were not prepared, without further evidence, to accept the claim that penicillin was better than were all other agents. Here was a problem of both practical and academic importance and it was decided to investigate the relative value of different preparations in the control or the elimination of infection in order to enable early suture or skin grafting to be carried out. For this purpose we instigated a special investigation in August 1944. Surgeons were asked to treat alternate cases: (a) with penicillin and (b) with a contrast agent—each surgeon to select the agent which he regarded to be the best alternative to penicillin. It was stipulated that, apart from the chemotherapeutic agents employed, every other controllable factor such as surgery, rest, nursing, diet and so forth, should be of the same standard in all cases, without preferential treatment for any one group. In order to avoid confusion of the issue it was suggested that wounds uncomplicated by visceral or skeletal damage should be selected, and therefore the cases studied were consecutive unselected wounds of the soft tissues. Records were kept on special forms and the following assessment was employed.

Grade I. Success. Wound healed and completely dry at the end of 14 days (this interval was selected because stitches were commonly left until the eleventh or twelfth day when suture had been performed under some degree of tension—as was not uncommon).

Grade II. Partial success. Wound incompletely healed at the end of 14 days (some moisture or gaping at areas along suture line, mild stitch suppuration and so forth), but healed and completely dry at the end of 21 days.

Grade III. Failure. Wound incompletely healed at the end of 21 days.

RESULTS OF INVESTIGATION

By March 1945, when the investigation was terminated, reports on almost 5,000 wounds had been received from more than 20 hospitals. The great majority of these reports were suitable for analysis and they provided a representative cross section of war wounds treated by many surgeons—an important point, since published reports often deal with relatively small groups of patients who received preferential treatment or who were operated upon by someone above the average in surgical skill.

The results are summarized in Tables I and II.

TABLE I RESULTS OF WOUND SUTURES IN 4,432 CASES, USING VARIOUS AGENTS

Agents used	Total cases	Grade I		Grade II		Grade III		Percentage Grades I and II
		Number	Per cent	Number	Per cent	Number	Per cent	
Penicillin—local applications only	2,359	1,881	79·73	348	14·75	130	5·52	94·48
Penicillin—local and parenteral ..	1,485	1,221	82·22	185	12·46	79	5·32	94·68
Penicillin—parenteral only ..	107	92	85·98	12	11·21	3	2·81	97·19
Nuflav—local applications ..	137	80	58·39	33	24·09	24	17·52	82·48
Sulphonamides—local & systemic	141	88	62·41	30	21·27	23	16·32	83·68
Sulphathiazole and 1 per cent proflavine—local	46	19	41·30	18	39·13	9	19·57	80·43
Nil	157	114	72·61	25	15·92	18	11·47	88·53

The results may be shown more simply by contrasting the penicillin cases with all the others.

TABLE II SUMMARY OF RESULTS

Agents used	Total cases	Grade I		Grade II		Grade III		Percentage Grades I and II
		Number	Per cent	Number	Per cent	Number	Per cent	
Penicillin	3,951	3,194	80·84	545	13·79	212	5·37	94·63
Others	481	301	62·57	106	22·04	74	15·39	84·61

Theoretically, the two groups should be about equal. In fact, the penicillin cases outnumber the others by about 8 to 1 because many surgeons became convinced at a relatively early stage of the superiority of penicillin, and abandoned the use of contrast agents. Although in Table I some of the groups are so small that the range of possible statistical error is great, the problem under investigation was clearly answered in both Tables I and II—in this large series of wounds operated upon by many different surgeons those treated with penicillin definitely did better than did the others. This is more evident if the highest standard (Grade I) is adopted as the criterion of success; and it is interesting to observe that, by lowering the standard and including both Grades I and II, the differences become less evident.

The results in the group of men who did not receive local or general therapy will attract attention, but they cannot be compared strictly with the others as this group does not contain any major cases. It represents what can be accomplished by unaided surgery in small clean wounds, and it must be remembered that the majority of these patients had had prophylactic penicillin or sulphonamides before admission to the hospital where suture was performed.

On the other hand the penicillin groups—and particularly those receiving parenteral penicillin—contained almost all the major wounds, yet these show the highest degree of success whatever standard is adopted. Viewed in the light of this knowledge the penicillin results appear to be still better.

It has been emphasized that all controllable factors were standardized as far as is possible in a clinical investigation, and in large series such as this one, wounds of every part, type, duration, severity and degree of contamination were represented, so that the effects of variables were minimized or equalized. In fact certain of these factors were analysed separately and it was found that they did not produce any significant difference in the results. One of these additional analyses may be quoted as an example, and in support of the statement that penicillin proved to be superior to other agents. The next tables (III and IV) show the effect on the chances of success, of increasing time intervals between the receipt of the wound and the closure of the wound.

TABLE III PENICILLIN CASES: EFFECT OF INCREASING TIME INTERVALS

Days between receipt of wound and suture	Total cases	Grades I & II		Grade III	
		Number	Per cent	Number	Per cent
1–7 days	1,290	1,236	95·81	54	4·19
8–14 days	667	627	94·01	40	5·99
15–21 days	148	133	89·86	15	10·14

The next table deals with wounds treated with Nuflav. The number of cases is much smaller, but it was the largest amongst the contrast groups for which accurate time intervals were available.

TABLE IV NUFLAV CASES: EFFECT OF INCREASING TIME INTERVALS

Days between receipt of wound and suture	Total cases	Grades I & II		Grade III	
		Number	Per cent	Number	Per cent
1–7 days	39	36	92·31	3	7·69
8–14 days	42	33	78·57	9	21·43
15–21 days	19	11	57·89	8	42·11

These tables support the view that increasing time intervals diminish the chances of successful suture and, even allowing for possible error owing to the relatively small numbers of Nuflav cases, it is interesting to observe that better results were obtained with penicillin at all intervals after the receipt of wounds. The relatively steep fall in the percentage success in the Nuflav cases was additional evidence suggestive of the superiority of penicillin, but was not conclusive because of the small numbers.

Wounds which in prepenicillin days would have been considered to be quite unsuitable for suture were closed regularly and with impunity, and the results were good, as is shown in the table which follows.

TABLE V RESULTS RELATED TO CONDITION OF WOUND BEFORE SUTURE

Condition of wound	Total cases	Grade I		Grade II		Grade III		Percentage Grades I and II
		Number	Per cent	Number	Per cent	Number	Per cent	
Clean ..	760	612	80·53	107	14·08	41	5·39	94·61
Dirty ..	117	80	68·38	24	20·51	13	11·11	88·89

The term, clean, is employed in the clinical sense. It was applied to wounds which showed only mild evidence of inflammation inseparable from any injury, and with minimal discharge and contamination, but which were not necessarily sterile. Many, in fact, contained pathogenic organisms and these were doubtless held in check and finally eliminated by the combined effects of the normal body defences and penicillin. The dirty wounds were frankly purulent, often with tags of devitalized tissue and well formed granulations, and sometimes were contaminated with foreign material.

The difference in the results is significant, especially if Grade I healing be regarded as the standard. It is remarkable that 9 out of 10 unclean wounds were completely healed within 21 days after suture. Only a few years ago any sensible surgeon would not have considered it wise to close them.

Failures.—The failures were instructive. Of 3,951 wounds closed with the aid of penicillin, 212 (5·4 per cent) were regarded as complete failures because they were incompletely healed at the end of 21 days. The principal causes were as follows, but often two or more factors shared responsibility.

(1) Infection was noted as the chief, or as a contributory, cause in at least 47 cases. Coliform bacilli (23) and staphylococci (21) were implicated most frequently, and the latter were not all penicillin-insensitive. *Ps. aeruginosa* was implicated in 9 cases. A number of failures were due to infection in underlying structures such as bone, fascia and tendons.

(2) Tension was the reputed chief cause of failure in 28 cases and was a contributory cause in others.

(3) An unfavourable site was the third most common cause of failure and was implicated 27 times: buttock (7), back (4), over scapula (3), axilla (2), over tibia (4), dorsum of foot (2), dorsum of hand (2), perineum (1), dorsum of finger (1), over vertebral spinous process (1). In the back and buttock areas mechanical and physical factors played a part—pressure, movement, lack of ventilation and so forth.

(4) Type of wound. In 9 cases failure was attributed to the gross size of the wound and the extensive degree of tissue damage. In 5 cases cruciate or T-shaped wounds broke down slightly at the centre, and in 3 cases a bridge of undermined skin between two wounds sloughed owing to interference with its blood supply.

(5) Time. The effects of increasing time intervals in predisposing to failure have been demonstrated in Table III.

(6) Foreign material was regarded as the chief cause of failure in 15 cases: cloth (7), phosphorus (4), catgut (1), metal (3). The irritant or dangerous nature of the materials most frequently implicated is noteworthy.

Various other factors such as inadequate general or local rest, inexpert or excessive primary surgery, badly designed flaps, incomplete haemostasis, tentage, pocketing, voluminous oily dressings and so forth were all blamed on occasion; but the most common causes of failure were those cited at the beginning —infection, undue tension, an unfavourable site, gross tissue damage, irritant foreign material, or a lengthy time interval between the receipt of wounds and closure.

WOUNDS COMPLICATED BY VISCERAL OR SKELETAL DAMAGE

Diseases and injuries of special regions are discussed in other chapters and in order to avoid reduplication they are not considered here.

SUMMARY AND APPLICATION TO CIVIL PRACTICE

From the results recorded in the foregoing pages it seems to be obvious that in future it will be routine practice to suture or to apply a skin graft to almost all wounds at the first surgical opportunity. The probability of efficient prophylaxis, the likelihood of early and uninterrupted surgical attention, and the absence of the time-distance factor so important in war wounds, should all tend to facilitate and to render safe this ideal procedure. It should hardly be necessary to re-emphasize the benefits which may result from early suture or from the application of a skin graft, or the urgency of covering exposed bones, tendons, main vessels and nerves, if need be with the aid of plastic procedures. A surgeon will now have to adduce very particular reasons for not closing a wound at an early date.

Application of war methods to civil practice.—The methods used in the closure of war wounds have been summarized above, and with minor modifications they could be used in treating any wounds. In general, minor wounds should require only local applications of penicillin powder, but more severe, complicated, or obviously contaminated wounds should receive both local and parenteral penicillin. The dosage and methods of administration employed in therapy should resemble those already described in the section on prophylaxis, namely 15,000–20,000 Oxford units injected intramuscularly every 3 hours, or 100,000–120,000 units daily if continuous injection methods of administration are used. Parenteral treatment should seldom be necessary for more than 3–4 days and may be discontinued after 48 hours if the wound is "quiet" and painless, and the patient is afebrile. On the other hand, in grossly lacerated or contaminated wounds, and in those which are sutured under tension, the administration of penicillin should be continued for 4–5 days and the stitches should be left *in situ* for 11–12 days. When there is any suggestion of anaerobic infection the dosage of penicillin could be doubled with advantage. Let it be repeated again: penicillin therapy without sound surgery will produce many failures. Only by a judicious combination of the two can this great advance in traumatic surgery be consolidated.

ANAEROBIC MYOSITIS

The high rate of incidence of gas gangrene in World War I, in the short, bitter struggle of 1940, and in the Italian campaign, gave rise to inevitable fears of a similar high rate in the invasion of North-West Europe planned for 1944. The possible opportunity to investigate this dreaded complication was not to be missed and the Medical Research Council, with the willing cooperation of the 21st Army Group and of the Emergency Medical Services authorities, devised an elaborate scheme for detailed studies at all levels from the front to the base. Any estimates had to be purely conjectural, but it was confidently anticipated that the special investigation team would collect an adequate number—probably 400–500 cases—in the first 6–8 weeks. In fact the total for the entire 11 months of the campaign was 384 cases (251 Allied and 133 prisoners of war). This figure is approximately correct but, for various reasons, it was not possible to verify all cases reported during the last 2 months of the campaign. The figures given in Table VI are those for the first 9 months (June 1944–February 1945 inclusive) and they are based on corrected figures supplied by Major J. D. MacLennan, R.A.M.C., who was engaged on special duties connected with anaerobic myositis, and who investigated not only those cases reported on the official forms, but also others discovered by us during routine tours.

TABLE VI TOTAL ANAEROBIC CASES TREATED IN BRITISH LIBERATION ARMY MEDICAL UNITS FOR 9 MONTHS

Categories	Total cases	Deaths	Percentage recovery
Allied troops	238	52	78·1
Prisoners	118	57	51·7
Totals	356	109	69·4

The incidence and mortality rates were constantly more favourable in Allied than in enemy troops and, as will be shown later, they were lower in this campaign than in any previous campaign. It would be very interesting to discover why this was so, but the solution of any problem with many variable factors is never easy, and the difficulties are increased by the absence of official records for many cases and by omissions and ambiguities in the records of others. This was not always the result of carelessness. Certain officers had never heard of Army Form I. 1241—the special form for reporting cases of gas gangrene—or believed that it had not to be rendered in prisoner of war cases; others found it impossible to obtain details about times and dates of the receipt of wounds, primary treatment, serotherapy, chemotherapy and so forth, from confused patients or incomplete entries in field cards. Of 156 official records available only 78 were sufficiently complete to justify detailed analysis (59 Allied cases with 8 deaths and 19 enemy cases with 4 deaths), and even then it was not possible to obtain information about every point. Definite conclusions cannot be based on such small groups, but certain suggestive evidence can be extracted about various points.

The importance of surgery

The meticulous excision of all dead and devitalized tissues, the removal of obvious foreign material, the relief of tension, the abolition of pockets, the provision of adequate drainage, the protection of the blood and nerve supplies and various other measures taken by the competent surgeon, are of prime importance in prophylaxis. Should clostridial myositis actually develop, the extirpation of all infected muscle is absolutely essential. Penicillin and the sulphonamides provide powerful support in both prophylaxis and therapy but can affect only the fringe of devitalized or devascularized tissues—an elementary fact which is not always appreciated. It cannot be overemphasized that surgery is still the main prophylactic bulwark; this is borne out in Table VII, which summarizes the primary operative treatment in 78 men in whom gas gangrene developed.

TABLE VII PRIMARY SURGERY

Categories	Adequate primary surgery	Inadequate primary surgery	No primary surgery	Total cases
Allied troops	35	12	5	52
Prisoners	10	5	4	19
Paratroops	3	1	3	7

A higher proportion of Allied troops received adequate primary surgery and they had a lower incidence of gas gangrene than had enemy wounded.

It is generally agreed that the time interval between the receipt of wounds and primary surgery is important and this interval could be determined exactly in 48 of the above 78 cases: in 35 Allied cases it averaged 17·2 hours; in 10 prisoner of war cases it averaged 26·1 hours; in 3 Allied paratroops it averaged 52 hours.

Paratroops could not always have treatment as early as could ground troops, and in order to avoid giving erroneous impressions of average time intervals they are shown separately.

It will be noted that Allied cases received primary surgery on an average about 9 hours earlier than did prisoners. Of the total 48 cases, in 18 the interval exceeded 20 hours, and in at least 15 patients the clostridial infection was established before they were admitted to a surgical unit; 3 of these men died, one before operation was possible and 2 who were operated upon at some unknown interval after the onset.

The quality of the surgery after diagnosis cannot be assessed from records, but from personal observations we know that in the great majority of cases it was prompt and efficient. There were 43 primary amputations in the series and 2 secondary amputations after traumatic amputations by a missile. The remainder were treated by excision of the affected muscles. Table XI shows that 38 of these amputations were performed in men with major vascular injuries.

Serum and drugs in prophylaxis

Opinions vary about the exact values of drugs and serum, but most surgeons believe that they help in the prevention or the control of infection.

TABLE VIII ADMINISTRATION OF PROPHYLACTIC AGENTS

Categories	Total cases	Penicillin			Gas gangrene antitoxin			Sulphonamides		
		Given	Doubtful	None	Given	Doubtful	None	Given	Doubtful	None
Allied troops	59	32	3	24	31	1	27	31	2	26
Prisoners	19	1	—	18	5	1	13	12	1	6

It is evident that a much smaller proportion of prisoners received penicillin and gas gangrene antitoxin and a higher percentage received sulphonamides. Naturally, while penicillin was in short supply, prisoners were given sulphonamides in routine prophylaxis. Normally, sulphonamides were also used for routine prophylaxis in our own troops, but for a considerable part of the period under review they were deliberately withheld if penicillin was being administered, in order to test the relative value of penicillin and sulphonamides in prophylaxis; the results of this investigation are recorded elsewhere (see p. 112).

Unless all other relevant factors are considered, erroneous deductions may be drawn from the above table. It is known that the incidence of gas gangrene was higher amongst prisoners, and it might be assumed that penicillin is a better prophylactic agent than is a sulphonamide. Or it might be argued that neither was any good, unless one remembered that in many cases with vascular injuries the agent never reached the affected parts in adequate concentration, and that other factors such as time intervals, primary surgery, and state of nutrition, also played a part.

Serum and drugs in therapy

The next table gives a summary of the use of penicillin, gas gangrene antitoxin, and sulphonamides after the diagnosis of anaerobic myositis was made. The first column records those who apparently received adequate doses and the last those who did not receive any at all. The "doubtful" column includes those who had inadequate doses, or cases in which the records were too indefinite for the facts to be certain. Thus, men who received less than 150,000 units of parenteral penicillin, 50,000 units of gas gangrene antitoxin, and 12 grammes of sulphonamides are included in this column. Possibly these limits are set too low, but in fact, when the agents were given, the doses were usually adequate or even excessive; for example, one man received 2,100,000 units of penicillin and another 437,500 units of gas gangrene antitoxin. The maximum oral dosage of a sulphonamide substance noted was 45 grammes of sulphathiazole.

TABLE IX ADMINISTRATION OF THERAPEUTIC AGENTS

Categories	Total cases	Penicillin			Gas gangrene antitoxin			Sulphonamides		
		Given	Doubtful	None	Given	Doubtful	None	Given	Doubtful	None
Allied troops	59	53	6	—	49	8	2	37	14	8
Prisoners	19	10	2	7	17	—	2	16	2	1

The table shows that a higher proportion of Allied troops than of prisoners received penicillin; in the case of the sulphonamides the position was reversed.

Analysis of the chemotherapy and serotherapy in the fatal cases provided the following information.

TABLE X CHEMOTHERAPY AND SEROTHERAPY IN FATAL CASES

Administration and dosage	Penicillin	Gas gangrene antitoxin	Sulphonamides
No prophylactic measures: adequate therapeutic measures	4	8	4
Adequate prophylactic and therapeutic measures	3	2	6
None at all: or inadequate doses ..	5	2	2
Totals	12	12	12

The conclusion is evident. Drugs and sera, even in adequate dosage, will not save every patient; a number will always arrive too late, and others will die from the severity of the injuries or from renal or other complications. Amongst the 12 deaths, one was due to an associated abdominal wound, one man was moribund before a surgeon saw him, another died on the table, in 3 the infections were fulminating, and 4 had high arm or thigh amputations.

Parts affected and types of wound

The sites of origin were: leg (45), thigh (18), arm (6), buttock (4), shoulder (2), foot (2) and back (1).

The high rate of incidence of wounds in the lower limb was associated with a large proportion of vascular injuries. Of the 45 leg cases, 30 involved the posterior group, 12 the anterior group, and 3 were generalized and involved muscles in both groups. In 15 cases the posterior tibial artery was certainly injured and in 2 others it was possibly damaged. In 35 patients there were associated open bone or joint injuries. In 31 cases the degree of muscle damage was recorded as slight to moderate, and in 47 it was said to be very extensive.

Curiously enough the official form does not ask for information about the degree of contamination or the presence of foreign material, so that reliable figures cannot be supplied concerning this point.

The reputed causes were: shell wounds (39), gun-shot wounds (12), mortar-bomb wounds (11), mine wounds (7), missile uncertain (6) and accidental injuries—vehicles (3).

Predisposing causes

Certain figures relating to predisposing causes such as lengthy time intervals, absent or inadequate primary surgery, insufficient chemotherapy, and extensive muscle damage have already been given.

In 5 cases a tourniquet had been applied and in another patient one probably had been used; one tourniquet had been in position for 10 hours. In 2 cases it was noted that tension had not been prevented or relieved by splitting of the deep fascia at the primary operation; tension in the deeper compartment of the calf is not relieved by incision of the more superficial layer of deep fascia alone. In 2 other cases the patients had tight, unsplit plasters around the affected part.

In this series of 78 cases, however, vascular injuries were undoubtedly the chief predisposing factors. Their distribution is set out in the final table, and the last column shows the number of limbs amputated: in many cases the injuries in themselves were so severe that amputation would have been necessary in any case.

Needless to say, most vascular injuries were not complicated by gas gangrene. In the 9 months under review at least 900 men in the 21st Army Group had severe wounds complicated by main vessel injuries.

TABLE XI ASSOCIATED VASCULAR INJURIES

Vessel injured	Certainly Injured	Probably injured	Limb amputated
Post. tibial artery ..	15	2	12
Popliteal artery ..	7	1	8
Ant. tibial artery ..	6	—	4
Femoral artery ..	5	—	4
Both tibial arteries ..	4	1	5
Brachial artery ..	2	—	2
Sup. gluteal artery ..	2	—	—
Plantar arteries ..	1	—	1
Axillary vein	1	—	1
Popliteal vein	1	—	1
Totals ..	44	4	38

Bacteriology

Many cases occurred in field units without any pathologist or laboratory facilities and therefore it is not surprising that information concerning this point was incomplete. In 33 cases *Cl. welchii* was clearly identified; in one case *Cl. oedematiens* was implicated; in 20 cases clostridia were found, but the exact types were not specified; in 24 cases bacteriological examinations were not made, but clinically there was not any doubt about the diagnosis. The infections were often mixed, and in a few cultures other clostridia (*sporogenes*, *tetani*, *bifermentans*, *tertium*) were detected.

An interesting observation was made by Major J. D. MacLennan (personal communication). He obtained smears from a number of severe wounds sustained in France and Belgium, and isolated *Cl. welchii* in about 80 per cent. In similar wounds investigated by the same observer in the Desert, *Cl. welchii* were found in 28–30 per cent.

Incidence and mortality rates

According to MacLennan[6] the incidence of gas gangrene was 3·4 per 1,000 in the Middle East and 6·7 per 1,000 in Tunisia; Jeffrey and Thomson[7] estimated that the figure in Italy would be "not less than 10 per 1,000". The incidence in Allied troops in the British Liberation Army was 1·5 per 1,000, but in prisoners it was 20–30 per 1,000 cases which were treated in British or

Canadian medical units. The British Liberation Army calculations are based on "split" figures kindly supplied by the Statistical Department, 21st Army Group, and although the figures for Allied troops are accurate within narrow limits, they are less accurate than are those for prisoners. Obviously, without further information concerning the figures for other campaigns, direct comparison is not legitimate; but Major MacLennan, who had had experience in the Middle East Forces, the Central Mediterranean Force and the British Liberation Army, informed us verbally before he left the British Liberation Army in February 1945, that the rate of incidence of gas gangrene had been lower in North-West Europe than in any other theatre of war.

The rate of incidence was much higher amongst prisoners, and our impression is, that during the period under review the proportion of severe wounds was greater amongst enemy prisoners than amongst our own troops and that their state of nutrition and bodily cleanliness were on a lower level. A retreating army may secure its lightly wounded, but may be forced to leave the more serious and helpless cases behind. This was one possible reason for the higher rate of incidence amongst prisoners. There were others. The average time interval between the receipt of wounds and primary operation was distinctly greater amongst prisoners and a higher percentage had not had any primary surgery. These factors alone were sufficient to explain a disproportionate incidence, and largely invalidated attempts to evaluate other factors such as chemotherapy. Nevertheless it should be observed that Allied troops received much more prophylactic penicillin and that prisoners had more prophylactic sulphonamides. In regard to the therapeutic use of these drugs the same thing occurred, although the disparity was less pronounced.

Writing in 1944, MacLennan and Macfarlane[8] stated that "the case fatality rate of gas gangrene in the present war has been approximately 50%". The rates have fluctuated at various times and places from approximately 70 per cent in Sicily in 1943 to 30 per cent in Italy in December 1943. In the previous three months in Italy, however, the mortality rate was 70 per cent; Jeffrey and Thomson[9] record that Colonel Churchill, the American Consulting Surgeon in Italy, informed them that "in over 100 cases of undoubted gas gangrene the mortality was 54%". In a series of 33 cases in Italy in the spring of 1944, the mortality was 36·4 per cent (Jeffrey and Thomson). In the British Liberation Army, in a series of 356 consecutive cases (Allied and prisoner of war) which occurred between June 1944 and February 1945, the overall mortality was 30·6 per cent. Comparatively, this was a good figure, but if the figures were "split" the result was still better: of the total 356 cases 238 occurred in Allied troops with 52 deaths, representing a mortality rate of 21·8 per cent. This figure is very interesting when compared with a prediction made by Jeffrey and Thomson[9]: "Given fair conditions, and with penicillin, we may hope to see the mortality from gas gangrene in the Field reduced to the region of 20%". With the more favourable conditions prevailing in civil life even better results should be achieved, although a certain number of fulminating cases will always be too late for treatment and other patients will die from associated injuries or renal and other complications.

Factors influencing the occurrence of infection and the results have already been discussed on p. 106, so we only repeat that the one new factor in the British Liberation Army scheme of prophylaxis and treatment was the widespread use of both parenteral and local penicillin at all levels, including the most forward surgical units. We cannot escape the conclusion that this potent agent must be accorded a good deal of the credit for the diminished incidence and improved results.

It is obvious therefore that in civil practice parenteral and local administration of penicillin—in larger than normal doses—must be added to both the prophylactic and therapeutic armamentarium of the surgeon in dealing with either the threat or the fact of this dire infection.

REFERENCES

[1] Florey, H. W., and Cairns, H. (1943) *Investigation of War Wounds. Penicillin. A Preliminary Report to the War Office and the Medical Research Council on Investigations concerning the Use of Penicillin in War Wounds.* War Office A.M.D. 7/90D/43. London.
[2] Pulvertaft, R. J. V. (1943) *Lancet*, **2**, 341.
[3] Porritt, A. E., Debenham, R. K., and Ross, C. C. (1946) *Brit. med. J.*, **2**, 377.
[4] Young, D. H., Evans, R. W., and Hughes, K. E. A. (1945) "Delayed Suture of Soft Tissue Wounds using Parenteral Penicillin". *Penicillin Therapy and Control in* 21 *Army Group*, p. 135.
[5] Heatley, S. (1945) "Intensive Intravenous Penicillin Therapy: A Report on 100 Consecutive Cases Treated by this Method". *Penicillin Therapy and Control in* 21 *Army Group*, p. 157.
[6] MacLennan, J. D. (1944) *Lancet*, **1**, 203.
[7] Jeffrey, J. S., and Thomson, S. (1944) *Brit. J. Surg.*, **32**, 159.
[8] MacLennan, J. D., and Macfarlane, M. G. (1944) *Brit. med. J.*, **1**, 683.
[9] Jeffrey, J. S., and Thomson, S. (1944) *Brit. J. Surg.*, **32**, 159.

BURNS AND PLASTIC SURGERY

By Rainsford Mowlem, F.R.C.S.

Surgeon in Charge, Plastic Department, Middlesex Hospital, London; Surgeon in Charge, Plastic Unit, Hill End (E.M.S.) Hospital, St. Albans

GENERAL CONSIDERATIONS

In all operations upon the superficial soft tissues, bacterial contamination is an ever present risk. In the ordinary course of events the normal defensive mechanisms are so effective that there is little danger that infection will occur or, should it do so, that it will cause any serious tissue destruction. When the defence breaks down it does so either because of the grossness and overwhelming virulence of the organism responsible for the infection, or because of inadequacy of local tissue response to the contamination.

In reconstructive surgery both of these conditions are commonly encountered. The great majority of granulating wounds are grossly infected and surgical procedures upon them may expose the deeper tissues to an overwhelming contamination which will result in cellulitis[1]. In many phases of the transference of pedicles or flaps from one part of the body to another, their blood supply may be reduced to a level which is sufficient to maintain viability but at which a normal inflammatory response cannot be produced. In these conditions even minimal bacterial contamination may cause serious tissue loss and so invalidate the whole plan of operation. It is in such circumstances that bacterial control is of particular importance and for this purpose penicillin is one of the most effective substances at our disposal. Its use must always be dependent upon an accurate knowledge of the bacteriology of the affected area, and its efficacy is determined by the choice of an appropriate method for its application. It is not a substitute for surgery or an excuse for indifferent technique; provided that it is applied intelligently it can permit of safe and early surgical intervention.

THERAPEUTIC METHODS

Systemic route

Before deciding upon the method of administration, it must be certain that the area which requires treatment is, in fact, accessible *via* the blood stream. In many cases the area cannot be reached by this systemic route and a more effective approach should be chosen.

Penicillin is given systemically by (1) continuous injection (intravenous or intramuscular)[2] and (2) repeated intramuscular injection. The technique and dosage for both these methods has been described elsewhere.

Local application

Most local methods presuppose intermittent application. The frequency of such applications should be determined by periodic testing of the area for the presence of penicillin[3]. For example, if it is decided to apply penicillin to a raw surface at, say, 12-hourly intervals, a first application should be made and, immediately before the second is due, serum from the surface should be assayed for the continued presence of penicillin. If it is recovered in adequate amounts the period between dressings can be longer, and its absence is an indication that applications must be more frequent. Such control is desirable in all cases in which local application is indicated. (It should be noted that, in this chapter, when a time period between dressings is given, this is only approximate.)

Penicillin is used locally as follows.

(1) Penicillin solution in physiological saline (100 units per millilitre). (a) As a surface spray for raw areas such as burns. An even film is easily produced and may be allowed to dry before it is covered with the usual dressings. In some stages of healing such an application may cause severe burning pain which persists for about an hour and which is so unaffected by sedatives that the application must be abandoned. The calcium salt appears to be a little more unpleasant in use than does the sodium salt.

(b) The solution may be injected into relatively avascular deeper areas through a fine rubber tube in order to produce a high rate of local concentration of the drug. The arrangements for either intermittent or continuous application are easily made.

(2) Penicillin powder (500 units per gramme). This is particularly useful for insufflation into wounds or on to raw surfaces.

(3) Penicillin cream (Lanette wax SX base, 500 units per gramme). The water-soluble wax base ensures an adequate supply of the drug over a longer period of time than is possible when either the solution or the powder is used. In addition, the dressing is non-adherent and it is therefore very suitable for some burns and for wounds in which frequent change of dressings is undesirable.

(4) Penicillin pastilles (gelatin base, 500 units per pastille). There is an increasing amount of evidence that in such a base a constant supply of penicillin can be maintained for the purpose of controlling oral and pharyngeal infection[4].

SPECIAL APPLICATIONS

Wounds

Most lacerations are contaminated; the amount of infection which will result is more usually an indication of inadequate debridement or of vascular insufficiency than it is of the initial virulence of the organism causing the infection. In the face, the blood supply is so good that there is seldom need to rely on anything other than the inherent bactericidal action of living tissue. One exception to this is the extensive graze which results in loss of the superficial layers of the skin. In these cases infection may cause destruction of the remaining deep layers of the skin so that, instead of epithelialization occurring simultaneously over the whole area, it can occur only from the margins. Careful cleansing, followed by closed dressings of penicillin cream will, in most instances, avoid such a complication.

Another type of wound which justifies the use of penicillin is the ragged laceration which penetrates the mucous membrane of the mouth. A watertight closure of the mucosa is difficult to obtain and the torn and bruised condition of the cheek tissues seriously diminishes their resistance to normal infection. Such injuries were seen commonly as the result of the detonation of high explosives but they are less often encountered in civil practice. Good results were obtained by careful surgical closure and by the injection of penicillin through one or more tubes at the rate of 4,000–10,000 units daily. It is probable that systemic treatment would produce the same result, but the local application gives a high degree of concentration which deals with any infection tending to spread back from the infected oral cavity.

In the limbs the problem is different. The blood supply of the skin and the subcutaneous tissue is much less generous than it is in the face, and any laceration may interfere with the vascularity of a large area. Ordinary recent lacerations seldom require more than careful surgical management together with a local dusting of penicillin powder and perhaps a short course of penicillin by systemic injection[5].

Skin losses and skin grafts

The partial avulsion of large flaps of skin and subcutaneous tissue is often encountered as the result of road accidents. In this type of case loss of blood supply of the flap is the important factor. Bacteriological sterility is of no value in the presence of dead tissue. It is essential to trim back the avulsed flaps until there is free bleeding from their edges. An extensive skin defect will thereby be created, but this defect will be much less than that caused by the infection which is inevitable if all non-viable tissue is not removed. When it is at all probable that even small areas of devitalized tissue have been left behind, it is wise to dust the surface with penicillin powder before the skin flap is sutured into its correct position and a skin graft to cover the residual defect is applied. In addition, it is wise to institute systemic penicillin immediately before operation and to continue it for about 4 days after operation.

Treatment of granulating areas.—The regimen outlined above should obviate the occurrence of large raw surfaces in traumatic cases but there still will be many instances in which they may arise. The essential aim in all these cases is to produce epithelialization—spontaneous or surgical—at the earliest moment, for if these wounds are untreated they will ultimately become avascular and fibrotic. In that state, neither spontaneous healing nor grafting is possible. Every effort should therefore be directed to the creation of the requisite state for early and successful grafting. Slough removal can be hastened by the use of Eusol (Liquor Calcis Chlorinatae cum Acido Borico B.P.C.) or of 5 per cent solution of trypsin, or by employment of the knife; the aim is to produce a granulating area which is relatively dry, smooth and not exuberant. An important factor in the creation of such a bed is the elimination of infection. Insufflation of penicillin provides an easy method of even distribution of the drug but will not necessarily ensure the application of a sufficient quantity of penicillin to ensure bacteriostasis without frequent extensive dressings. It may therefore be preferable to use penicillin cream every 24 hours. Split-skin grafts are indicated for the primary repair of the majority of such areas and the operation for their application does not usually entail any disturbance of the granulating surface. Should it do so, however, a dusting of penicillin powder immediately before the application of the skin graft is all that is necessary.

It may be impossible or undesirable to wait until optimal conditions have been produced in the raw surface. It may be essential to produce skin cover at the earliest moment and to consider achieving this before slough separation is complete. It is practicable in many cases to remove such sloughs immediately prior to grafting. It might also be that, for reasons outside the surgeon's control, the granulating area is so old that its base is fibrotic and that excision will be necessary prior to grafting. In both these instances there will be active surgical intervention immediately before the graft is applied and this intervention will have to take place in an infected area. The chances therefore of spreading infection and of causing cellulitis are much greater than they are in those instances in which the skin graft is to be applied over undisturbed granulations. In such circumstances it is desirable to commence systemic penicillin prior to operation and to continue using it for about 4 days after operation, and it is desirable to apply penicillin locally at the time of operation when it is considered that slough excision has not been complete.

Such treatment will provide general protection against bacterial invasion for a time long enough to allow the normal defences of the tissues to react and it will also eliminate the surface infection which would tend to cause failure of the graft.

Full-thickness flaps.—These are used when it is desirable to transfer skin and subcutaneous tissue from one part of the body to another. The flaps often have their blood supply reduced to a point just above the limit of viability; they are therefore incapable of the normal tissue resistance even to minimal infection and once infection has occurred intravascular stasis and thrombosis may cause necrosis of large areas. It is occasionally necessary, for example, to transpose a flap of skin and subcutaneous tissue from the calf of one leg to the anterior aspect of the other leg in order to protect the tibia. This may have to be undertaken in the presence of a low-grade infection in the recipient area. In this type of case systemic penicillin should precede and should follow operation but because the blood supply in the flap itself is small it may be as well to supplement the amount of penicillin reaching the flap by the instillation underneath the flap and through a capillary tube, every 12 hours at least, of a few millilitres of penicillin solution (1,000 units per millilitre).

Bone grafts

The transference of bone from one area to another means that it must be completely detached from its blood supply. In such a state bone cannot tolerate any infection but, in spite of this, it has been found to be possible to transfer it into an infected area provided that the organism concerned is sensitive to penicillin and provided that an adequate vascular cover for the graft can be supplied[6]. For example, in the reconstruction of frontal contour after radical exenteration of the frontal sinuses, it may be unnecessary to wait until the wound has completely healed. If the organism is penicillin-sensitive and there are not any remnants of mucosa, excision of the granulating area and building up of the frontal bone together with apposition of the cranial aponeurosis can be carried out in one stage. A capillary tube is left in the depths of the wound beneath the bone graft and through this from 2,000 to 5,000 units of penicillin a day are instilled. It is preferable to ensure a constant titre of penicillin by giving small doses frequently rather than larger doses at longer intervals. Systemic penicillin cannot be expected to reach all parts of the bone graft which, although it is enclosed in the patient's tissues, is, at first, outside the reach of his circulation. A similar technique can be applied if by mischance the oral cavity should be opened in the insertion of a mandibular graft. The defect in the mucosa must be accurately closed and a capillary tube inserted down to that region. It is known that the great majority of mouth organisms are penicillin-sensitive, and provided that 5,000–10,000 units daily are injected for 5–7 days, no ill effects are likely to result.

Intra-oral operations

Apart from the usual operations associated with dental abnormalities, there are many indications for operation within the mouth and in all of them infection is a potential danger. Such danger is, fortunately, more theoretical than practical since the results of these operations are usually good, but there appears to be little doubt that, in many instances, infection slows the healing processes and increases postoperative discomfort. Almost all the organisms commonly encountered in the mouth are sensitive to penicillin. If therefore a constant supply of penicillin can be made available for the first 5 days, infection can be controlled. There is considerable evidence that pastilles made with a gelatin base and each containing 500 units, are effective in rendering the mouth sterile for from 4 to 5 days. At the same time their prolonged use may lead to the appearance of extraneous organisms which are not penicillin-sensitive and the presence of which is more disastrous than is that of the normal flora of the mouth.

Actinomycosis

The causal organism may be recovered often from the normal mouth and it is therefore not unexpected that sometimes it may obtain access to the soft tissues, presumably through a tooth socket. The infection is seldom found primarily in the bone but is confined to the soft tissues superficial to it. Two main types of infection are seen, as follows.

(1) A small chronic abscess, usually at some distance from the site of the tooth. The condition proceeds very slowly to perforation and then there is a discharge of pus for a considerable time; ultimately it may heal. The contents of such an abscess are almost invariably said to be sterile but under careful cultural conditions the mycelium often can be recovered.

(2) The better known cervicofacial actinomycosis, which ends in multiple abscesses and multiple fistulae. These tend to sclerose and, after destruction of most of the subcutaneous fat in the area, and many months of treatment, the condition becomes quiescent.

The sensitivity of the causative organism of actinomycosis is variable, some strains being quite as sensitive as is the standard Oxford staphylococcus, whereas others are from 8 to 16 times more resistant. In most cases, however, good results have been obtained by the use of penicillin provided that the concentration is high and that its use is continued for considerably longer than is necessary in dealing with ordinary penicillin-sensitive organisms[7,8]. The small localized abscess may be treated by the insertion of a capillary tube into its centre, preferably from a distance (as in the aspiration of a tuberculous gland). Through this tube the contents of the abscess are withdrawn and are replaced by not less than 1,000 units of penicillin; this is done every 8 hours. It may be necessary to continue the process for as long as 3 weeks.

The more generalized type of lesion may be treated either by systemic penicillin or by "rafting" the whole of the affected area with many capillary tubes. All of these are finally brought together at a single point, and either continuous irrigations or intermittent injections of up to 20,000 units of penicillin solution a day are carried out. Local application appears to offer a method of producing a degree of tissue saturation which is greater than systemic injection normally can effect, and it must be appreciated clearly that both concentration and duration of treatment are important. Actinomycosis elsewhere would, it is presumed, respond to the same type of treatment, although in many areas access can be obtained only through the blood stream.

Osteomyelitis

Acute osteomyelitis of the mandible in adults is most often associated with the removal of a tooth. It is probable that the determining factor is a vascular rather than a bacterial one. Through the root socket, a large area of dead bone is exposed to infection from within the mouth, and in my experience—up to the present time—it has not been found that the institution of systemic penicillin controls the disease. This is not inexplicable if the vascular theory of causation is accepted. Once the disease is established, then here, as elsewhere in the body, bone destruction is irreversible and penicillin is not of any value. About the end of the second or third week, when the extent of the damage becomes obvious in X-ray examination, it is possible, however, to cut short the development of the condition. This is done by the removal of the lower margin and outer plate of the affected bone together with extraction of all teeth in that area. Any defect in the mucous membrane is closed by accurate suture. Capillary tubes are inserted and the surface wound is closed. Provided that the surgical procedure has been adequate and that only living bone is left behind, the injection of from 5,000 to 10,000 units of penicillin daily will result in primary healing. Treatment is continued for 5–7 days only and at the end of this time there is seldom any evidence of residual infection; if it is still present it is an indication not of the inefficacy of penicillin but of the insufficiency of the surgery[9].

Burns

When the extent of the burn does not jeopardize the patient's life the problem resolves itself into the production of the earliest possible healing with minimal scarring and retention of maximal function. First degree or second degree burns expose the depths of the skin and from this region local regeneration very readily occurs. When, however, there is gross superadded infection, the remaining skin elements may be destroyed and thus a full-thickness loss is caused. Healing will then occur only from the periphery and therefore may be indefinitely delayed. In the face, the potentiality of infection from one or other orifice is very great and here in particular penicillin has its advantages. A generous application of penicillin in Lanette wax SX cream will usually be found to be effective for about 24 hours; in some instances it may be desirable to lengthen this time to 48 hours. It is comparatively simple to ascertain, at the end of a given period, whether any active penicillin remains and thus to determine the frequency with which dressings need to be changed.

When the burn itself causes full-thickness destruction of skin, adequate bacterial control usually can be obtained by similar dressings. By the end of about one week a leucocytic barrier will have been erected round the affected area and the danger of tissue invasion will have decreased. The continuation of penicillin may then have one of two results.

(1) It may result in complete and continued sterility of the surface, and in these circumstances the separation of slough appears unduly prolonged[10]. When surgical removal and skin grafting is contemplated the conditions are optimal, but if it is desired to wait until a clean granulating surface has been produced, there will be unnecessary delay.

(2) Penicillin-insensitive organisms may make their appearance. *B. proteus*, *Ps. aeruginosa* and *Esch. coli* are all too often seen and when they do occur the difficulties of obtaining a satisfactory graft are considerably increased.

On the whole, therefore, it may be wise to continue penicillin only until the patient is safe from active invasion of tissue by bacteria and then to revert to the older methods of treatment until the time for skin grafting is imminent. The treatment is as described in the section on granulating areas (see p. 183).

In a very extensive burn the local problem is identical with that outlined above but the extent of the burn will make it difficult to ensure that all areas are satisfactorily protected by penicillin dressings throughout the whole of the 24 hours. It is often desirable to reinforce local treatment with systemic treatment and to continue this until there has been time for the creation of a leucocytic barrier beneath the affected areas which will protect the patient against cellulitic invasion. With the added safeguard of systemic treatment the frequency of change of local dressings can be safely reduced and this will contribute to the patient's comfort and, perhaps, to his recovery.

REFERENCES

[1] Rank, B. K. (1940) *Brit. med. J.*, **1**, 846.
[2] Morgan, H. V., Christie, R. V., and Roxburgh, I. A. (1944) *Brit. med. J.*, **1**, 515.
[3] Garrod, L. P. (1944) *Brit. med. J.*, **1**, 528.
[4] MacGregor, A. B., and Long, D. A. (1944) *Brit. med. J.*, **2**, 686.
[5] Jeffrey, J. S. (1943) Investigation of War Wounds. Penicillin. Preliminary Report to the War Office and the Medical Research Council. War Office (A.M.D.7), p. 47.
[6] Mowlem, A. R. (1945) *Proc. R. Soc. Med.*, **38**, 171.
[7] MacGregor, A. B. (1945) *Proc. R. Soc. Med.*, **38**, 639.
[8] MacGregor, A. B. (1945) *ibid.*, **38**, 201.
[9] Mowlem, R. (1944) *Brit. med. J.*, **1**, 517.
[10] Barron, J. N., and Mansfield, O. T. (1944) *Brit. med. J.*, **1**, 521.

ORTHOPAEDIC SURGERY AND FRACTURES

By V. H. Ellis, F.R.C.S.
Orthopaedic Surgeon, St. Mary's Hospital, London

GENERAL CONSIDERATIONS

The use of penicillin in orthopaedic surgery ensures freedom from the complication of generalized or local spread of infection from the affected area, and consequently the long interval which had to be allowed between the healing of infected wounds, particularly those involving bone, and reconstructive operations has been greatly shortened. Although this has been most noticeable in the case of infected fractures, it is equally true, and with an even higher degree of security, in the case of soft tissue injuries. This time saving sometimes effects a considerable improvement in the ultimate result by reducing fibrosis, contractures or stiff joints. For example, the repair of nerves by suture may be completely ruined by the recurrence of sepsis, yet delay in repair adds still more to the necessarily long time of recovery and entails prolonged and careful treatment to prevent stiffness of joints and to maintain the integrity of the affected muscles' condition. As some of the sulphonamide group of drugs have an unfavourable action on nerves, penicillin is useful both as a local application and as penicillin-plasma or penicillin-sulphanilamide powder.

Similar considerations arise in the repair of tendons, in the treatment of which early restoration of movements of joints, particularly of the fingers, is of great importance. Wounds of flexor tendons of the hand or suppuration in a tendon sheath are common in civil practice, particularly in industry, and although the greatest usefulness of penicillin lies undoubtedly in the prevention of infection in these cases, yet tendon grafts and sutures can be carried out earlier and more safely under the protection of the drug.

PENICILLIN IN FRACTURE TREATMENT

The object of fracture treatment is the restoration of normal function as quickly and completely as possible. One of the chief causes of failure is infection, which doubles the average time of healing of fractures and can be prevented almost entirely by good surgery with the help of penicillin.

The only common cause of infection in closed fractures is surgical intervention, which, therefore, should never be carried out unless the full requirements for aseptic surgery are available.

Open fractures may become contaminated with organisms at

the time of injury or by their subsequent introduction. Infection of compound fractures with haemolytic streptococci is usually secondary and is preventable.

The change from contamination to infection is chiefly a question of time. Its prevention by adequate early surgery is of prime importance and is achieved by careful wound toilet followed by closure of the wound immediately, or after an interval. The old rule that compound fractures receiving adequate treatment within 6 hours of injury might be immediately sutured, was generally satisfactory.

The parenteral use of penicillin soon after injury increases the margin of safety, but does not supplant early surgery as the prime requirement. Early penicillin treatment will minimize the likelihood of infection of fractures with pyogenic organisms, of which staphylococci are the most significant, provided that the exposed and contaminated tissues have an adequate blood supply by which the circulating penicillin can reach them. It is therefore advisable that all patients with compound fractures be immediately treated with parenteral penicillin (15,000 units 3-hourly), followed as soon as possible by surgical wound toilet. If these conditions can be fully satisfied, and if continuous supervision of the patient is possible, primary closure of the wound is permissible. If there is delay, heavy contamination of the wound, or necessity for transfer of the patient, the wound should be left open under a sterile dressing of tulle gras, with adequate immobilization of the fractured limb.

Delayed primary suture from 3 to 5 days after injury can be effected with a very high percentage of success by good primary surgery and a course of penicillin, which should be continued from the time of wounding until after suture, reduction, and immobilization of the fracture have been performed. Whatever the nature of the organisms present may be, if the wound does not appear inflamed or grossly oedematous, suture will result in nearly 100 per cent primary healing.

Parenteral penicillin is preferable to the local application of the powder, and probably makes the latter superfluous in uninfected fractures where the local blood supply is good. Penicillin-sulphanilamide powder—5,000 units per gramme—is, however, effective in preventing secondary contamination of the fracture, and is of value if parenteral penicillin cannot be given or if there is avascular tissue in the wound, such as loose bone fragments. Such fragments should not be removed at the primary surgical treatment as avoidance of sepsis will allow them to play the part of grafts and help union without the formation of gaps or cavities.

The local instillation of penicillin through tubes into the wound tends to delay healing, even when inserted through separate stab wounds, and may encourage infection by penicillin-resistant organisms. It is, therefore, a less satisfactory method of treatment for uninfected compound fractures. In the very few cases where the correct early treatment fails, or where it is not initiated, an infected fracture usually results.

Even then, if early parenteral penicillin is given, it will prevent a secondary osteomyelitis or septicaemia. In a series of 192 septic wounds involving long bones severe osteomyelitis did not occur in patients receiving penicillin within 24 hours.

INFECTED FRACTURES

Within a few days the infected area becomes walled off from the surrounding tissues by granulation tissue, which is a barrier to the spread of organisms. This barrier, however, may be easily broken down by movement at the fracture, or even of the soft parts. Manipulation of an infected fracture should, therefore, be preceded by at least one single injection of 50,000 units of penicillin given intramuscularly. This single injection will prevent the extension or generalization of the infection, and should be repeated as often as required for changing plasters, re-reduction of fractures, or for any operation, such as sequestrectomy, on an infected fracture.

Rapid healing will not occur in infected fractures where there is more than nominal skin loss, or where a bone cavity or gap persists. In such cases a course of penicillin of 3-5 days will avert danger while a skin graft and cancellous chips are applied. Under this protection, cancellous chips may be successfully inserted even into a septic bone cavity, provided there is no dead infected bone present and the skin is sutured over the grafts. In this way many chronic sinuses can be avoided or healed.

The treatment of infected ununited fractures, bone gaps or cavities has been made very much easier by the use of grafts of purely cancellous bone and penicillin. The grafts have great osteogenic power, considerable resistance to infection, and rapidly become revascularized. Grafts of cortical bone such as those taken from the tibia are likely to sequestrate in the presence of any infection and, probably owing to their dense nature, penicillin does not prevent this occurrence, at least not without a very prolonged course of the drug. The complete revascularization of a cortical graft requires months as compared with a few weeks for cancellous bone, which if it succumbs to infection is completely absorbed and is seldom sequestrated. The use of cancellous bone almost eliminates the necessity of wide saucerization of cavities, the introduction of pedunculated muscle grafts and various other procedures.

The cancellous bone chips are usually taken from the iliac crest, and as this inevitably leads to the formation of a haematoma between the cortical tables of the ilium, blood-borne infection of this haematoma may occur in the presence of bone infection elsewhere. It is safer, therefore, to prepare the infected bone cavity at a preliminary operation and follow after an interval by the taking and placing of the grafts. On both occasions penicillin protection is used. For the first operation a single dose is often sufficient, but a course of several days should be employed after the grafting. This two-stage technique is unnecessary unless there is chronic infection of the recipient bone.

The simultaneous application of whole skin, such as cross-leg or abdominal flaps, with the insertion of cancellous chips, is a formidable procedure, and it needs the cooperation of a plastic and an orthopaedic surgeon. The correct planning of multiple operations, often proceeding simultaneously with changes in the patient's position, is necessary.

In these circumstances even the most careful aseptic technique is liable to fail, but the concurrent protection of penicillin given systemically renders the procedure safe in skilled hands.

Long operations do increase the liability to secondary contamination of the wound; insufflation of penicillin powder provides security, but should not allow any relaxation of vigilant aseptic technique.

The routine use of penicillin—sulphanilamide or penicillin-sulphathiazole powder—from a Royal Air Force type insufflator is advisable at the conclusion of operations on infected fractures. It produces a greater concentration of penicillin locally, economizes the amount of systemic requirement and allows the drug to reach comparatively avascular tissues. In addition, the sulphonamide has an effect on the penicillin-resistant organisms which are frequently present in chronic bone infection, and which in some cases interfere with healing, or, by producing penicillinase, decrease the efficacy of the drug.

WOUNDS OF JOINTS

Penicillin does not easily pass the barriers of normal serous membranes, and consequently the synovial fluid of a normal joint will contain much less penicillin than the blood in patients receiving intramuscular injection. This statement is less true of the fluid in injured or inflamed joints, and in fresh haemathroses the joint penicillin level may reach that of the blood.

As parenteral penicillin dosage has to be high to reach a good level in a joint, it is much more economical to inject the drug directly into the joint. Forty-eight hours after injection of 100,000 units into a knee joint the fluid showed a good bacteriostatic level.

Wounds of large joints are particularly prone to infection. The wound may be either direct, or caused by involvement of the joint in a nearby compound fracture.

Direct wounds

In direct wounds of joints the primary surgery is of great importance. The wound should be excised together with the removal of any foreign body and damaged tissue from the joint. The synovial membrane should be closed with interrupted sutures, and the remainder of the wound left open under Vaseline gauze after dusting with penicillin powder. Where the synovial membrane cannot be closed, and where continuous supervision is certain, it is justifiable to close the skin at once, or this should be done between the third and the fifth day provided that the wound is quiet.

One reason for making every effort to close off the joint is to retain the injection of 50,000 or 100,000 units of penicillin, which should be injected through sound tissues.

The joint should be aspirated at intervals of 48 hours subsequently and further injections of penicillin made. Two or three aspirations only are required, generally. Immobilization should be absolute, and continued after operation until the joint is healed—usually in from 2 to 3 weeks.

Compound fractures involving joints

If a compound fracture extends into a joint it is obvious that infection may easily spread from the former to the latter which may be inadequately protected by systemic penicillin. A feeble barrier of blood clot soon walls off the joint, but any movement of the bone fragments may disrupt it. All efforts previously described should be made to prevent infection of the fracture, but immobilization is of even greater importance where an infected fracture involves a joint. The joint itself should be protected by a direct injection of penicillin, particularly if any manipulation of the fracture must be performed. In such cases both systemic and local penicillin must be given, and this should also be carried out with direct wounds when there is much soft tissue damage.

In considering the direct injection of penicillin into a joint the necessity for the sterility of the solution cannot be too much emphasized. Sometimes prepared solutions of penicillin have been contaminated, usually by *Ps. aeruginosa,* while sterility of the syringe and needle has not always been achieved.

It is not yet certain what is the best dosage and concentration of penicillin for injection into the joints. Impurities may have a cumulative inhibitory effect with concentration, so that 50,000 may be preferable to 100,000 units. The volume of fluid also may be important and it should be sufficient to reach all recesses of the joint without causing painful distension. Much will depend on the capacity of the joint and the amount of fluid aspirated before injection. Penicillin disappears more rapidly from joints in which absorption of fluid is occurring, but in these circumstances maintenance of a high level is not so important.

The after-treatment of infected wounds of joints presents some difficulties. Although the joint is soundly healed and quiet, movement may lead to pain and swelling of the joint, particularly when intra-articular adhesions are present.

Suppuration rarely recurs but the joint becomes "irritable" and further efforts at movement are likely to decrease rather than increase the active range.

A short course of penicillin causes some of these irritable joints to subside, proving that there is an underlying infective process. If such an irritable joint is anticipated, the first attempts at movement should be made only after an injection of penicillin into the joint. Active and not passive movements alone are allowed, and, if in spite of this irritability of the joint occurs, immobilization must be prolonged.

OSTEOMYELITIS

Penicillin is of great value in bone infection by staphylococci and streptococci, which together cause more than 90 per cent of pyogenic osteomyelitis, of which proportion three-quarters are staphylococcal infections. With only occasional exceptions all these organisms are penicillin-sensitive.

Haematogenous osteomyelitis must be preceded by a bacteriaemia, and this can always be overcome by sufficiently early treatment with systemic penicillin if the organism is vulnerable. Unfortunately, diagnosis is difficult, and only a few hours may elapse before there is a definite bone focus.

There is now considerable evidence to show that acute osteomyelitis can be cured by early surgical and penicillin treatment. If the process is not arrested early, necrosis of the bone will occur, due to cutting off its blood supply by thrombosis of the intraosseous capillaries, or separation of the periosteum. As soon as the blood supply fails the circulating penicillin will be unable to reach the infecting organisms except by slow diffusion. All organisms in contact with penicillin may be destroyed, so that all signs and symptoms of infection may be abolished, yet live staphylococci may remain walled up in the bone to recommence their spread as soon as the penicillin in the surrounding tissues falls below the bacteriostatic level. It is, therefore, evident that in osteomyelitis prolonged treatment with penicillin is necessary, and that in chronic osteomyelitis, where there may be large areas of sclerosed and comparatively avascular tissue, penicillin alone will not produce a cure within reasonable time.

Theoretically, chronic osteomyelitis could be cured by removal of all infected bone, at the same time protecting the body and the uninfected bone by maintaining an adequate level of penicillin in the serum. In some cases, for example in Brodie's abscess, this can be done, and where the infected bone is localized and accessible.

Where massive bones are extensively involved—for example, the upper or lower ends of the femur or the pelvis—it is evident that the technical difficulties of adequate surgery become overwhelming unless extremely mutilating procedures are undertaken.

The three indications for operation in chronic osteomyelitis taught in former days—complete removal of diseased bone, removal of sequestra and evacuation of abscess—therefore, still hold, but their scope has been widened and execution made much less hazardous by the introduction of penicillin.

One of the most persistent features of chronic pyogenic osteomyelitis is its tendency to repeated flares with acute local inflammation, toxaemia, and a liability to the formation of new metastatic foci. These flares can be rapidly aborted or controlled by a short course (3-5 days) of intramuscular penicillin therapy, and the morbidity and mortality of this very serious disease can be greatly reduced.

Brodie's abscess with a definite wall not grossly sclerosed has been successfully treated by the direct introduction of 50,000 units of penicillin. After localization by skiagram, the affected portion of bone is exposed and a small drill hole made into the abscess. The penicillin is then injected into the cavity and the wound sutured.

All operations on osteomyelitis should be done under the protection of penicillin, but there are certain dangers attached to this form of treatment which must be borne in mind.

DANGERS OF PENICILLIN TREATMENT

As adequate dosage of penicillin will inhibit all sensitive organisms within its reach, a local bone lesion may not be discoverable in cases already under systemic treatment. All redness, tenderness and pain may rapidly disappear, and if an abscess forms or is already present it will become "cold", and being detectable only by the presence of swelling and fluctuation may easily be missed, or the identity of affected bone mistaken.

A child aged 4 years was admitted to hospital with what appeared to be a very early osteomyelitis of the tibia. Continuous intramuscular penicillin was immediately begun and the periosteum over the upper end of the tibia was incised and the bone drilled. Pus was not found and the wound was closed. The child's condition immediately improved, the temperature became flat, and continued so during a 2 weeks' course of penicillin. On withholding the penicillin, however, the condition rapidly deteriorated and the child died in spite of another course of the drug. At necropsy osteomyelitis of the fibula was found with a large subperiosteal abscess. There was pus in the pericardium caused by a penicillin-sensitive staphylococcus.

Staphylococci in a large abscess cannot be reached by systemic penicillin, although the signs are marked. Abscesses must always be aspirated or drained.

In cases of pyaemia treated by penicillin a most thorough examination of the whole patient must be made without delay, otherwise metastatic abscesses will remain undiscovered.

Inadequate dosage of penicillin may also give a false sense of security, and it is essential that a bacteriostatic level in the blood be continued uninterruptedly as long as necessary. This requires continuous intramuscular instillation, or 3-hourly injections of at least 15,000 units night and day; an unpleasant treatment for adults, and even more severe for sick children.

Some preparations of penicillin contain impurities which themselves cause a rise of temperature. With increasing purity of the supplies this becomes less common, but the rise in temperature may deceive the surgeon with regard to the sensitivity of the organism and the progress of the case. Such rises of temperature are more common where continuous intramuscular drip is maintained for a long time, and may lead to redness of the area even though the injection site remains sterile.

PYOGENIC ARTHRITIS

Pyogenic infection of joints due to penetrating wounds has already been considered. In civil practice pyogenic arthritis is more commonly blood-borne.

The lesion may occur apparently as a primary manifestation or as secondary to a single focus, such as otitis media, a boil, or in the course of a general blood stream infection, causing the pyaemic joint; it may also spread from osteomyelitis in a contiguous bone.

Gonococcal infections are not considered here as they are seldom intra-articular infections, and are best dealt with as a complication of the general disease.

Suppurative arthritis may occur at any age and is a well defined condition in infants, but the commonest age incidence is from 4 to 14 years, and it is 3 times commoner in males than in females. The joints most often involved in haemotogenous infection are the hip, knee, elbow and wrist, in descending order. Suppuration in the hip of children often occurs as a complication of otitis media and may have an insidious onset.

This form of arthritis was a fairly common complication of scarlet fever, but with the decreasing virulence of the disease it has become less frequent.

About 50 per cent of joint infections are due to staphylococci and 25 per cent to streptococci. The remainder are mixed infections, or are due to pneumococci, *Ps. aeruginosa,* the typhoid group and others.

Diagnosis in the more superficial joints is usually easy, the signs being a rapid onset with an effusion which becomes painful, high temperature, loss of function, and some spasm (though this may be an early sign). In joints such as the hip, surrounded by much muscle, the effusion may not be easily detectable, and diagnosis is consequently difficult.

Diagnostic aspiration is essential and should be done with scrupulous aseptic precautions, and great care should be taken to ensure that the infection is not extra-articular before the needle is inserted into the joint. The aspirated fluid may be turbid and in the early stages a positive smear may be obtained from the centrifuged deposit, but cultures may be sterile, the organisms having been killed by the bactericidal action of the synovial fluid.

The first stage in pyogenic arthritis is an acute inflammation of the synovial membrane, and is only later associated with destruction of the articular cartilage by tryptic ferments. Much later the suppuration extends outside the synovia and capsule, and oedema around the joint becomes obvious.

It is most important that penicillin be given before irretrievable damage has been done to joint structures. This damage may occur within a few hours, and consequently treatment should not be delayed pending a report on the culture of the aspirated fluid.

Aspiration in itself is a therapeutic measure and the pouring out of more fluid which occurs has some action against the infection. The aspirated fluid should be replaced by a sterile solution of penicillin, about 50,000 units dissolved in an equivalent amount of fluid to that aspirated is satisfactory.

If the joint becomes distended, aspiration may be repeated as often as necessary, but as penicillin will probably persist in a bacteriostatic concentration for 48 hours, this will be the normal interval between aspirations at which further injections of penicillin should be administered.

If the treatment is begun at an early stage, two or three injections may suffice, but they should be continued until the general and local conditions have returned to normal. During treatment the joint should be continuously and adequately immobilized. Unless some other focus of infection requires it, systemic penicillin is unnecessary in early cases of suppurative arthritis, but where there is any danger of the infection spreading beyond the confines of the joint cavity it is essential, but should be additional to local treatment.

Early and adequate treatment by penicillin will abort the majority of joint infections caused by sensitive organisms. If this is done before the articular cartilage has been damaged a normally functioning joint should result. Drainage of the joint or surrounding soft parts should not be required unless treatment is late or inadequate.

If penicillin treatment is undertaken at a later stage in the disease, when the articular cartilage has been destroyed, the general and local condition of the patient will be much improved, but the joint cannot be restored to normal. It is important to note that gross distention of the joint may lead to pathological dislocation which may occur without marked symptoms if the patient is under penicillin treatment. It is important, therefore, that repeated aspiration and examination of these cases are carefully carried out.

The usual result of an acute suppurative arthritis, except in infants, is a bony ankylosis following subsidence of the infection. With penicillin treatment the inflammatory process which leads to this result is cut short, so that ankylosis does not occur and a restricted range of movement persists. If the articular cartilage has been severely damaged the joint will rapidly show an osteoarthritic type of change, producing a painful movable joint, more disabling to its owner than a sound bony ankylosis. The subsequent treatment of such a joint may have to be by operative fixation, and this cannot be immediately undertaken for fear of a flare-up of the infection. With penicillin protection, however, it is unnecessary to wait as long as 6 months, which period was formerly considered a minimum. There should be one or two months' delay, and operation should be done during a 5-day course of penicillin. It is well to start the course 24 hours before operation to allow a bacteriostatic level to be reached by diffusion in the more sclerosed and less vascular areas involved in the operation.

PENICILLIN IN SURGICAL TUBERCULOSIS

Although penicillin has no effective action on the tubercle bacillus, it is a very useful drug in the treatment of bone and joint tuberculosis. It has been stated that whereas the overall mortality of spinal caries is about 25 per cent, that from similar cases with secondary pyogenic infection is about 75 per cent.

Every effort is made to prevent the formation of sinuses in surgical tuberculosis by aspiration and other means, but if such sinuses occur the greatest care is taken to prevent secondary pyogenic infection. This prevention is rendered very much easier by penicillin. The discoloured area of skin, or the sinus, is dusted with penicillin-sulphathiazole powder, and covered with an occlusive dressing, thereby effectively preventing the ingress of the more common pyogenic organisms. Even longstanding sinuses not clinically secondarily infected have been known to heal rapidly with this treatment, and it is a procedure worthy of further trial. Whether or not frankly infected tuberculous lesions can be benefited by systemic penicillin is not known, and all the difficulties encountered in the treatment of chronic pyogenic osteomyelitis are met in an aggravated form.

REFERENCES

Jones, G. B. (1945) "The Local Use of Penicillin in War Wounds of the Knee Joint". *Penicillin Therapy and Control in* 21 *Army Group*, p. 167.

OSTEOMYELITIS

By Ian Aird, Ch.M., F.R.C.S.Ed.

Lecturer in Surgery, University of Edinburgh.

ACUTE HAEMATOGENOUS OSTEOMYELITIS OF LONG BONES

Sir Howard and Lady Florey[1], reporting in 1943 the first therapeutic trial of penicillin in osteomyelitis, prophesied that a time would come when that disease, treated early and intensively with penicillin, would not require surgical intervention. This prophecy has proved extremely accurate, and it is now true to say that penicillin, administered in acute haematogenous osteomyelitis, will control septicaemia, prevent the development of metastatic foci, and induce the resolution of the initial bone lesion in three or four weeks provided that (1) the infecting organism is penicillin-sensitive (as it is in more than 90 per cent of cases), (2) administration is begun early, (3) dosage is adequate, (4) treatment is continued over a sufficient period and (5) local periosteal abscesses and metastatic abscesses, present when treatment is begun, are evacuated.

Preliminary investigation

Although treatment should always begin promptly and should never be delayed until laboratory data are available, the suitability of a case of osteomyelitis for penicillin treatment, the prognosis, and the final assessment of results depend upon exact clinical and bacteriological diagnosis, and not only all possible clinical data, but also all available bacteriological material should be collected when the patient is first seen. This preliminary investigation need not occupy more than a few minutes. Chemotherapy has increased rather than lessened the surgeon's responsibility for precise diagnosis.

The site of osteomyelitis is seldom in doubt. Even if the patient is comatose, and the evidence of local inflammation slight, pressure over an infected metaphysis will disturb him. The discovery of an overt bone lesion does not absolve the clinician, however, from the duty of performing a complete general examination, with particular attention to the other parts of the skeleton, to the pericardium, and to the respiratory tract; distant metastatic abscesses may be already present when the patient is first seen.

When a provisional clinical diagnosis has been established,

material should be obtained if possible for bacteriological examination. A carefully collected specimen of venous blood yields a culture of the causative organism in approximately 50 per cent of all cases. In others, pus aspirated or evacuated from a subperiosteal abscess is available for bacteriological examination. Material can also be obtained suitably and safely by the insertion of a sternal puncture needle into the suspected metaphysis, under local or general anaesthesia[2]. If the metaphysis is infected, the fluid withdrawn by way of this needle, whether it be pus or blood or a mixture of the two, provides the responsible organism.

Commencement of treatment

Penicillin administration should begin as soon as the clinical diagnosis of osteomyelitis is made, and should not await bacteriological reports. In a fulminant infection an hour's delay may have fatal consequences. Since the introduction of penicillin and the proof of its efficacy, acute osteomyelitis has become an urgent surgical emergency. In exceptional cases, where symptoms of septicaemia precede the signs of a bone focus, it is possible to begin treatment and to control the infection before the bone inflammation develops, if the general signs of staphylococcal septicaemia are promptly recognized.

Method of administration

The systemic administration of penicillin into the muscle of an unaffected limb by repeated injection or by continuous drip appears to control adequately not only the systemic infection, but also, provided abscesses are evacuated, the bone lesion and its metastases. The local administration of penicillin, by continuous drip through a sternal puncture needle inserted into the infected metaphysis[2], gives a high local concentration of penicillin and an adequate blood level. It has, however, no advantage over the standard intramuscular methods, except perhaps in the case of osteomyelitis of the upper end of the femur complicated by suppurative arthritis of the hip. (See p. 198.)

Dosage

McAdam[3] used a standard daily dose of 100,000 units successfully in a series of 40 cases. The tendency today, however, is to give larger doses. Vaughan Hudson[4] advises the administration of 60,000 units 3-hourly, and Trueta[5] recommends a total dose of 400,000 units on the first day, 200,000 on the second, and 100,000 on subsequent days.

There is a strong case, as Bodian[6] has shown, for grading the dose to suit the body weight. At the Hospital for Sick Children,

London, a daily dose of 1,000 units per pound of body weight has been found adequate. In young children the repeated injection of penicillin into muscles of small volume may produce sterile abscesses, and it is therefore desirable to reduce as far as possible the volume of injected fluid—to prevent tension necrosis of muscle fibres—and its concentration of penicillin—to lessen the risk of chemical irritation by impurities.

Duration of treatment

It has been shown[3] by the repeated aspiration of infected marrow that neither the temperature chart nor the leucocyte count is a reliable criterion of the time of sterilization of infected bone, and that organisms may linger in a metaphysis for more than a fortnight. It is wise therefore to continue penicillin administration for 3 weeks. In the case of bone infection, shortening of the duration of treatment cannot be fully compensated by an increase in dosage. Early mild infections certainly respond to large doses of penicillin in a fortnight or less, but no rules are yet available to permit the grading of the course of treatment to suit the severity of the infection.

The scope of operative intervention

In prepenicillin days the danger of dislodging septic emboli by radical operations upon infected bone was well recognized, and a relatively conservative management of osteomyelitis was increasing in popularity; there was a growing tendency to limit operation to the drainage of subperiosteal abscesses. Penicillin now affords such certain control of the systemic infection, and such reliable assurance against the development of metastatic foci, that it may seem to invite a return to radical surgical intervention. Available statistical evidence shows clearly that any tendency to adopt guttering, saucerization, or trephining of bone as a standard part of the management of acute osteomyelitis should be resisted. In McAdam's series of 40 cases, wide sequestration requiring sequestrectomy occurred only twice, in 2 of 5 patients—these were not the most severely affected—who had been treated by open marrow drainage. Altemeier and Helmsworth[7] similarly were disappointed in the progress of patients treated by radical operation.

On the other hand, surgery cannot with impunity be discarded completely. Once an abscess has formed, it cannot be sterilized by the general administration of penicillin, and all authors are agreed that a fluctuating subperiosteal abscess should be emptied. McAdam has found that subperiosteal abscesses resolve if evacuated by aspiration, but the practice now is to open them by incision. Trueta advises, in addition, that the bone be drilled, and others have practised aspiration[2] and continuous drainage[3] of the marrow by way of a sternal puncture needle, but there is no convincing evidence that even such a limited intervention on the bone is necessary or desirable, and there is abundant evidence that evacuation of the abscess is a sufficient operative supplement for penicillin administration.

Even the evacuation of a subperiosteal abscess may be followed by the appearance of metastatic foci unless septicaemia is controlled and the patient is protected against septic embolism by a high blood penicillin level. Operation, even the evacuation of a fluctuating abscess, should be performed only after at least 24 hours of penicillin administration.

The abscess may be evacuated equally well by aspiration or by incision. The advantage of aspiration is the security it affords against secondary infection. Evacuation by incision provides a wound through which, particularly in young children, penicillin-resistant organisms may effect an entry to the bone. If an open wound is made, its value as a portal of entry should be reduced by immediate suture, which can be performed with safety under the penicillin umbrella.

In the later stages of the disease, sequestrectomy is rarely necessary. In McAdam's series of 40 cases it was required only twice, on both occasions in patients who had been submitted to radical operation early in the course of penicillin treatment. I also have performed sequestrectomy twice: in patients whose course of penicillin had been discontinued after only 14 days, and who are now considered to have been treated for an inadequate period; staphylococci were obtained from the fluid evacuated from the bone at the time of sequestrectomy.

Immobilization

In the early stage of the disease the limb is immobilized in accordance with the general principles of the treatment of inflammation, but with the more particular intention of affording the patient comfort and of reducing the risk of septic embolism. Later, immobilization is continued to avoid pathological fracture when the bone becomes progressively decalcified, as it so often does.

Provided the joints immediately proximal and distal to the inflamed bone are completely immobilized, it is of no great consequence which method of splinting is used. Complete plaster of Paris encasement should be avoided during the first few days of treatment lest it conceal the development of a subperiosteal abscess or the signs of suppurative arthritis in an adjacent joint; initially a plaster gutter or a Thomas splint is preferable. When an abscess has resolved after aspiration or incision, or when, at the end of the first week of treatment, the risk of abscess has passed, a complete plaster case may safely be applied. Plaster immobilization should be continued until radiological examination shows the stage of decalcification to be ended and the stage of recondensation to be well advanced.

Infants suffering from osteomyelitis in a lower extremity can be conveniently immobilized in a gallows splint.

The treatment of associated arthritis

There is evidence that penicillin administered at a distant site may penetrate to the cavity of an inflamed, if not of a healthy, joint, but an effective concentration of penicillin in a joint the seat of suppurative arthritis cannot be guaranteed by systemic administration alone. A joint coincidentally infected is probably best treated on alternate days by aspiration of as much fluid as possible, and its replacement by 30,000 units of penicillin in a volume of 3 millilitres. The hip joint offers a special difficulty in this connexion. If the joint has not been greatly distended by pus, one cannot be certain that injected penicillin is reaching the joint cavity. The uncertainty is even greater at the second injection, when the pyarthrosis is beginning to resolve, than at the first. Osteomyelitis of the upper end of the femur, complicated by suppurative arthritis of the hip, is consequently the chief, or perhaps the only, specific indication for the use of the continuous intramedullary drip. A sternal puncture needle can be readily introduced so that its point lies in the metaphyseal abscess of the neck of the femur. The needle, inserted below the greater trochanter, can be made to follow the axis of the neck at an angle determined by study of a skiagram taken previously. The procedure is particularly simple in a young child, the position of whose femoral head, palpated from the femoral triangle, offers an easy target. The required daily dose of penicillin, introduced by continuous drip through the needle, not only maintains an adequate blood level, as McAdam has shown, but ensures a high concentration in the adjacent joint, for the metaphyseal abscess cavity usually communicates directly with the hip joint.

Suppurative staphylococcal arthritis of infants.—In young infants the epiphyseal cartilages afford less resistance to the passage of infection than they do in older children, and suppurative arthritis is in the first 2 years of life a common complication of osteomyelitis. Indeed, the first sign of disease at this age is usually a swollen joint, or several joints concurrently or successively inflamed.

In this form of osteomyelitis resolution can be expected with general administration of penicillin by intramuscular drip, without local penicillin administration and without surgical intervention. A movable joint can usually be obtained. The success of systemic penicillin administration in this form of suppurative arthritis probably depends upon (1) the relatively high dosage of penicillin these infants receive in proportion to their body weight, and (2) the loss of integrity of the joint space; the sinus established from bone to joint through the fragile epiphyseal cartilage persists as a channel for the passage of inflammatory exudate, rich in penicillin, from metaphyseal abscess to joint cavity.

Management of metastatic lesions

Metastatic foci seldom arise after penicillin administration has begun, but those which are already present at the start of treatment may not subside without surgical intervention. A close watch should be kept therefore for signs of metastatic infection arising unobtrusively, particularly during the first few days of treatment. A distant subperiosteal abscess may require evacuation, or suppurative arthritis in a distant joint may demand aspiration and penicillin injection. Pericarditis, which before the introduction of penicillin occurred in 50 per cent of the fatal cases, may still cause death[8] unless promptly recognized and suitably treated by aspiration and penicillin injection. The treatment of metastatic foci in the pericardium, lungs, serous cavities, central nervous system and kidneys follows the lines described elsewhere for suppuration in these organs.

Systemic response to penicillin treatment

The response of septicaemia in osteomyelitis to penicillin is neither immediate nor dramatic. Improvement in general well-being and lessening of the depth of coma, if present, are slowly progressive from the time when treatment starts, but the patient remains seriously ill, usually for some days. If the patient has septicaemia when first seen, pyrexia usually continues for from 7 to 14 days, resolving finally by lysis. A transient fall of temperature to normal on the second or third day of treatment is not unusual. The blood culture, if positive initially, becomes sterile after a few days. The leucocyte count may rise progressively during the early days of treatment and falls again to normal only after 2 or 3 weeks.

The mortality rate of acute osteomyelitis is extremely difficult to interpret, as the severity of the disease varies so much from place to place and from time to time, but in general it may be said that the percentage of positive blood cultures in any series of cases is a fair guide to the proportion of serious illness. Of McAdam's, and Altemeier and Helmsworth's patients, more than 50 per cent afforded a positive blood culture. Only one of McAdam's 40 patients died, and from an infection by a partially penicillin-resistant staphylococcus. Altemeier and Helmsworth in 34 cases had also one fatality: a patient with severe haematogenous osteomyelitis of the tibia neglected for 14 days, who died 17 hours after admission to hospital. Trueta has treated a series of 30 successive patients with acute osteomyelitis, not one of whom died. The present mortality rate of acute osteomyelitis may thus be assumed to be in the region of 2 per cent, and the mortality rate of the septicaemic form of the disease to be rather more than 3 per cent.

Local response of the bone lesion to penicillin treatment

McAdam has shown by repeated marrow aspiration that, provided secondary infection is excluded, penicillin-sensitive organisms disappear from the bone lesion after an average period of 14 days. Pain is relieved almost at once if penicillin treatment is effective and if mobilization is complete. Swelling due to soft tissue oedema subsides in from 5 to 7 days; swelling of longer duration should raise the suspicion of a persistent subperiosteal abscess requiring drainage. A full recovery of function may be expected in the affected limb if there is no joint involvement, the organism is penicillin-sensitive, the treatment is adequate, and subperiosteal abscesses are punctually drained. In cases complicated by suppurative arthritis in a joint contiguous to the infected bone, there is fair prospect of recovery of full function if the joint lesion is detected early and properly treated, but figures are not yet available to express this prospect mathematically. It is safe to say that there is more than an even chance of full recovery.

Massive sequestrum formation and the persistence of sinuses appear to be nearly always due to a penicillin-resistant organism, inadequate dosage or insufficient duration of treatment, delay in evacuating subperiosteal abscesses, or over-elaborate operative intervention in the early stages of the disease.

Radiological appearances

The pathological course of the local lesion in osteomyelitis treated with penicillin, as illustrated by radiological appearances, differs substantially from the pathological course of unmodified osteomyelitis. The initial radiological appearance is the same whether or not penicillin has been given. In from 7-10 days after the onset of the disease a localized translucent patch of decalcification in the metaphysis indicates the site of the primary focus. At the same time, or a little later, a thin line of subperiosteal new bone may be visible along the surface of the shaft. In a case treated by penicillin, however, the osteoblastic reaction is never extensive, and it may be long delayed or entirely absent; a thick involucrum is exceptional. The most striking change is a decalcification which is progressive during treatment and for some time after treatment ends. Decalcification may increase for as long as 18 weeks after infection has been eradicated from the bone and subperiosteal space. The trabeculations lose their density, definition and regularity, and then regain these attributes to re-form the original bone pattern very exactly. So exact indeed is the resemblance of the new bone shadow to the old, and so rapid may be the recovery in density, that the process must in some cases at least be a decalcification followed by recalcification, rather than bone destruction followed by bone synthesis. The stage of decalcification is of some practical importance, for the risk of pathological fracture during it is a real one, and free movement should not be allowed until recondensation is complete.

The pathological process which underlies the radiological sequence is not yet fully understood. It is probable that the same decalcification occurs in unmodified osteomyelitis, but its radiological translucency is obscured by the thickness of the sequestrum jacket through which the bone shadow is seen. The decalcification is at all events a sequel of the original infection, which incites a process that is progressive after the infection disappears. Whether the decalcification is due to the initial effect of bacterial toxins, or to the pressure of granulation tissue, or to the increased vascularity of inflammation, is still uncertain. Decalcification may be slight if penicillin treatment is begun early enough, and it may be so transient that it is missed, if radiological examination is infrequent. It is less obvious in cases treated by radical operation; the more extensive subperiosteal deposit of new bone which operation excites destroys the effect of translucency.

Small sequestra can sometimes be detected in the cortex of the affected bone after sterilization is complete. These may be completely and quite rapidly absorbed, by the same mechanism as sterile bone chips transplanted to repair a defect. Even quite large surface sequestra have sometimes been absorbed[3, 7]. Exploration of areas suspected of sequestrum formation should not be precipitate. In osteomyelitis of the femoral neck, complicated by arthritis of the hip, the capital epiphysis may undergo a condensation strongly suggestive of necrosis, to recover in due course its normal density if not its normal outline.

Streptococcal osteomyelitis

A streptococcus is isolated from pus withdrawn from the marrow cavity in approximately 5 per cent of cases of acute osteomyelitis. In none of the cases so far reported has the streptococcus of osteomyelitis proved resistant to penicillin. Indeed, in those cases which have been reported, the local and systemic effects of inflammation have yielded to penicillin treatment more rapidly than is the rule in staphylococcal osteomyelitis.

Osteomyelitis of the short bones and flat bones

Osteomyelitis in parts of the skeleton other than the limb bones is treated on the same general lines as have been detailed above. Cranial or vertebral osteomyelitis may require early operation, with wide removal of infected bone, to drain adequately an extradural abscess ; in such cases operation should be done only under a penicillin umbrella.

Osteomyelitis complicating compound fracture

Traumatic osteomyelitis is a separate problem, and is dealt with elsewhere.

CHRONIC OSTEOMYELITIS

Penicillin has little value in eradicating chronic infection from a bone which is the seat of longstanding osteomyelitis, with sequestra, sinuses, and recurrent abscess formation, even if the responsible organism is penicillin-sensitive. While in acute osteomyelitis surgery is the handmaiden of penicillin, in chronic suppurative osteomyelitis penicillin is the handmaiden of surgery. The scope of penicillin treatment in chronic cases is restricted to the control of systemic disturbance and the prevention of metastases during flares and after operations for the drainage of abscesses and the removal of sequestra. Any operation for the treatment of chronic osteomyelitis should be preceded by 3 days and followed by 5 days of full dosage penicillin administration.

Brodie's circumscribed abscess of bone

Penicillin has a special function in the treatment of this condition. Under its umbrella protection the skin may be closed safely by primary suture after the content of the abscess has been evacuated and its sclerosed bony wall has been chiselled away to leave a shallow depression in the affected bone. Penicillin protection may also be employed to prevent the resurrection of latent infection when a chronic osteomyelitis cavity is filled with a muscle graft, or when the deformity of an old osteomyelitis is corrected by open operation.

Only one form of chronic osteomyelitis, the rare non-suppurative sclerosing osteomyelitis of Garré, appears to respond well to penicillin treatment. A 3-week course of intensive penicillin administration may afford long-continued relief of pain and of pyrexia when these are features of the disease. The condition is so rare and so slowly progressive that a final assessment of the value of penicillin in its treatment is not yet possible.

OSTEOMYELITIS DUE TO PENICILLIN-RESISTANT ORGANISMS

Most of the failures of the intensive penicillin treatment of osteomyelitis can be ascribed to penicillin-resistance of the responsible organism. It has already been stipulated that the start of penicillin treatment in a case of osteomyelitis should not await precise bacteriological diagnosis. It is important, however, to obtain material for bacteriological examination in all cases where that can be done, since the bacteriologist's report, which is rendered usually 24 hours after the commencement of treatment, permits exact prognosis. The staphylococci of osteomyelitis vary in their sensitivity to penicillin, and in most cases when penicillin-resistance of the organism is reported, it is advantageous to increase substantially the daily dose of penicillin, and to continue treatment with a dose of from 60,000 to 100,000 units 3-hourly. Sulphathiazole, too, should be administered in full doses, though it is seldom that sulphathiazole has a therapeutic effect when penicillin fails. After a few days there is clinical as well as bacteriological evidence of the inefficacy of penicillin treatment if the organism's resistance to penicillin is high. The coma persists or deepens, and tenderness and swelling in the affected limb appear. Metastatic foci, too, develop and the occurrence of a new metastatic focus 3 days or more after the initiation of penicillin treatment in a tissue accessible to systemic penicillin, is clear evidence either of inadequate dosage or of penicillin-resistance of the staphylococcus concerned. When the organism is insensitive, the temperature continues high, but this is not in itself a criterion of resistance, for even in cases where the organism is penicillin-sensitive, the temperature does not finally fall, as a rule, until after a week.

When the penicillin-resistance of the responsible organism is clinically or bacteriologically beyond doubt, there is a tendency, as there used to be in prepenicillin days, for the surgeon to rush to radical operation if the patient's general condition becomes progressively dangerous. There was statistical evidence even before World War II that that tendency should be resisted, and operation should be withheld until a subperiosteal abscess is obvious. Radical operation is more likely to lead to general dissemination of the infection than to lessen the systemic disturbance. It seems better patiently to continue all available measures for the combat of septicaemia: sulphatherapy, forced fluids and intravenous fluids if necessary, complete immobilization of the affected part, and watchfulness for the development of metastatic foci. When a subperiosteal abscess forms, it may be opened and drained and the limb, after operation, may be enclosed in plaster. Patients who survive until the periosteal abscess is drained usually recover from the infection. A proportion of patients will die before the subperiosteal abscess forms, but the total mortality will probably be less with this conservative regimen than with the routine performance of early radical drainage of the infected bone marrow.

REFERENCES

[1] Florey, H. W., and Florey, M. E. (1943) *Lancet*, **1**, 387.
[2] Aird, I. (1945) *Proc. R. Soc. Med.*, **38**, 569.
[3] McAdam, I. W. J. (1945) *Brit. J. Surg.*, **33**, 167.
[4] Hudson, V. (1946) *Lancet*, **1**, 236.
[5] Trueta, J. (1946) *Lancet*, **1**, 236.
[6] Bodian, M. (1945) *Proc. R. Soc. Med.*, **38**, 572.
[7] Altemeier, W. A., and Helmsworth, J. A. (1945) *Surg. Gynec. Obstet.*, **81**, 138.
[8] Butler, R. W. (1946) *Lancet*, **1**, 237.

HAND INFECTIONS

By E. C. B. Butler, F.R.C.S.
Surgeon, London Hospital

During the period in which I have been in charge of the septic block at the London Hospital careful records have been kept of all patients with infections of the hand admitted to hospital, and especial note taken of the functional results. From 1945 penicillin has been available in sufficient amounts for the treatment of the majority of in-patients, so that we have been able to assess its value.

Bacteriology

In 140 consecutive cases in which the causative organisms were identified, 118 were due to *Staph. aureus,* 21 to the haemolytic streptococcus and one to anaerobic streptococci and fusiform bacilli. All these organisms are normally penicillin-sensitive.

Methods of administration

Penicillin can be used either locally as a cream or solution (1,000 units per millilitre) or systemically by continuous or repeated intramuscular injections.

Penicillin cream

Early reports[1] were very favourable on the use of penicillin cream as a postoperative application for hand infections. The cream is introduced into the wound by means of a sterile spatula or syringe, and the treatment is repeated every day or every other day until the infection has cleared. We have found this method very useful in superficial lesions of the fingers, but in other sites it is difficult to ensure that the cream gets into the depths of the wound. Repeated dressings are required, which increases the danger of secondary infection.

Penicillin solution

Before supplies of penicillin were adequate, cases of palmar infection were treated by repeated injection of penicillin solution, down a small rubber tube which was kept in place by a suture, every 3 or 4 hours. This method was not very efficient, since the wounds were often too shallow to allow the tube to be introduced satisfactorily and considerable leakage occurred.

In one male patient with multiple web-space infections, pressure of the rubber tube undoubtedly caused a secondary tendon sheath infection. Primary suppurative tenosynovitis has been successfully treated by the injection of penicillin solution down a ureteric catheter, but this method is being superseded by systemic treatment.

Systemic penicillin

This method, in addition to local therapy, is now used in most cases admitted to hospital. The usual dose is 100,000 units every 24 hours for from 5 to 10 days, depending on the severity of the infection.

We are now extending this form of therapy to out-patients, who receive 100,000 units daily in a single injection, but we have not, as yet, any cases to report.

The effects are general and local. The general condition improves and the rare fatalities seen in the past from blood stream infection are prevented. We have seen one staphylococcal and one streptococcal blood infection, both of which were fatal. Locally, penicillin does not replace surgery, which is needed when pus or increased tension is present.

Paronychia

These cases rarely require admission to hospital—early infections frequently resolve if penicillin cream is applied locally—but should pus form, the usual flap operation must be performed with removal of the proximal half of the nail if the pus has tracked deep to it.

Before the introduction of local penicillin these infections often took many days and sometimes weeks to heal. We have found that repeated application of penicillin cream is of considerable value in accelerating the rate of recovery after operation.

A patient with 3 weeks' painful swelling round the nail bed of right thumb was admitted.

A flap operation was performed but the nail was not removed. A culture was taken which showed the presence of *Staph. aureus*. A gauze drain impregnated with penicillin cream was placed under the flap. Two days later the drain was removed, and the flap allowed to heal. Penicillin cream was applied. The wound was redressed with cream after a further 2 days. It healed with restoration of function in 9 days.

Cellulitis of the fingers

Pulp infections.—These infections are usually caused by small perforating wounds. The inflammation may rapidly be followed by osteomyelitis of a part of the terminal phalanx unless the tension inside the pulp is relieved by an incision. Osteomyelitis is frequently followed by the separation of part of the infected bone as a sequestrum. The results of some cases treated as in-patients before the introduction of penicillin are shown.

Number of cases	*Staph. aureus*	H. strept.	Osteomyelitis	Results good	Deformity	Average hospital stay (days)
30	10	2	16	8	18	12

Most of the cases were admitted late, which accounts for the high incidence of osteomyelitis.

If tension is present the treatment is surgical. The pulp should be drained freely by one or two lateral incisions; any slough found at operation should be excised. Penicillin cream may be used as a postoperative dressing, but we have not found that its use causes any appreciable improvement in the rate of healing. Patients sufficiently ill to be admitted to hospital have received systemic penicillin for from 5 to 7 days. Healing has been rapid when there has been no osteomyelitis and provided that no slough has been left in the pulp. Systemic penicillin has not replaced surgery in this group because it is still necessary to relieve the tension in the pulp even in the absence of pus. It is possible that very early cases might resolve with adequate systemic treatment, but we have not had any experience of this. In order to improve the results of this group, early diagnosis is imperative so that adequate treatment may be given before the onset of osteomyelitis or of pulp necrosis. There is no doubt that systemic and local penicillin are valuable in preventing spread of the infection if used in conjunction with adequate drainage.

The following case reports are quoted.

One patient gave a history of 3 days of pain in the middle finger. A lateral incision was made and pus was found. A culture was taken and *Staph. aureus* was identified. Penicillin cream was applied. The cream was reapplied 2 days later, and dressed again with cream after a further 2 days. The finger healed with full function restored in 7 days.

A second patient complained of pain in the thumb of 7 days' duration. It was incised in out-patients' department and the patient was admitted. The wound was enlarged, the slough removed, and systemic penicillin was given for 5 days. The patient was discharged after 11 days, with the thumb healed and good restoration of function. The essential part of the treatment was the removal of the slough; after this penicillin therapy probably hastened recovery.

A third patient was admitted with a history of 11 days of swelling in the thumb, and an incision was made in out-patients' department. An x-ray plate taken later revealed the presence of osteomyelitis. The patient was admitted and a sequestrectomy was performed. Systemic penicillin was given for 5 days. The patient was discharged in 12 days, healed but with limited movement of the thumb. It would have been useless to give this patient penicillin without excising the dead bone.

Subcutaneous infections of proximal and middle phalanges

In this group tension is absent, so that it is safe to wait until there is a localized abscess before advising operation. Many of these patients have a diffuse cellulitis which often resolves with appropriate treatment; early incision only spreads the infection.

The Table shows the results of cases which required incision before penicillin was introduced.

Number of cases	*Staph. aureus*	H. strept.	Results good	Deformity	Average hospital stay (days)
19	12	3	14	3	13

The functional result was good, and healing was usually rapid. Systemic penicillin is valuable in early cases and complete resolution often occurs. Local treatment should consist of immobilization, by means of a light plaster splint on the infected finger. The rest of the hand should be elevated and kept at rest. Postoperatively, systemic penicillin should be used in all but the mildest cases as it may limit the spread of the infection into the neighbouring tendon, joint, or bone and prevent the inflammation tracking into the web spaces of the hand. These complications not infrequently occur in late or neglected cases. Penicillin cream may be applied locally as a postoperative dressing. Three cases are reported.

(1) A patient was admitted with a subcutaneous infection of the proximal phalanx of the ring finger, which was drained. A culture was taken and *Staph. aureus* was present. Penicillin cream was applied. It was redressed with cream after 2 days. The slough was removed and the part was redressed 3 times with penicillin cream at 2-day intervals. The wound healed, and restoration of function was complete in 11 days. The infection appeared to clear rapidly, 2 days less than the average time required in the case of untreated patients.

(2) A patient was admitted with a history of 2 days' pain in the right thumb which was diagnosed as diffuse cellulitis of the proximal phalanx. Systemic penicillin was given for 7 days, and at the end of treatment the infection had subsided.

(3) The patient had pricked her finger with a fish bone and was admitted with signs of cellulitis with abscess formation. The pus was drained, a culture was examined, and *Staph. aureus* was present. Treatment was given by systemic penicillin for 8 days. After 3 days a further abscess was drained on the dorsum of the finger. After a further 18 days the wounds healed, and active movement was possible. This was a severe infection. The healing required 21 days, a longer time than the average, but systemic treatment was valuable because further spread of the infection might easily have occurred with chemotherapy alone.

Erysipeloid infection.—This infection is a subacute cellulitis of the fingers which occurs in butchers and men working in allied trades. The causative organism is *Erysipelothrix rhusiopathiae,* which causes swine erysipelas. It is penicillin-sensitive.

Infection usually occurs through a small abrasion in the skin.

Suppuration is uncommon. The infected finger swells up with considerable induration and the affected segments have a purplish appearance. In the past resolution often took many weeks. Sulphonamide therapy was unsuccessful.

Recently[2], of 5 cases reported, 3 were treated by intramuscular penicillin, which appeared to effect a complete cure in 48 hours.

It is possible these cases are not all due to the organism of swine fever. Similar cases have been seen which have occurred in hospital attendants. In these men the causative organism was thought to be a streptococcus. Their clinical course was similar to that of the first group, but we have had no opportunity of treating them with penicillin.

Space infections

These infections are all examples of cellulitis of the hand, and it is convenient to name these spaces individually because the signs of each are characteristic and the surgical treatment is well established.

Primary cellulitis of the hand rarely gives rise to secondary sheath or bone infection unless it is neglected or wrongly incised, so that there is little danger in conservative treatment in the early stages of the infection provided that the diagnosis has been made correctly. When pus is present drainage is always needed. Healing should be rapid and the restoration of function complete. Systemic penicillin may cause resolution of the cellulitis if it is given before an abscess has formed. Postoperatively it may cause rapid sterilization of the wounds so that secondary suture is sometimes practicable. Systemic treatment also helps to prevent the spread of infection to other parts of the hand. Penicillin cream is a useful postoperative dressing but it has not appreciably altered the course of these infections.

Web space infections.—These infections are hour-glass abscesses between the extensions of the palmar fascia which are going to the fingers. Drainage is generally required. The incision should be free but care must be taken to avoid cutting the digital vessels or nerves.

The results of treatment of this infection were good before the use of penicillin, as shown in the Table.

Number of cases	*Staph. aureus*	H. strept.	Results good	Deformity	Days in hospital
28	23	3	24	4	9

(1) The patient was admitted with a multiple web infection which had been incised between index and middle fingers in the out-patients' department. The incision was reopened and a counter incision made between the little finger and ring finger. A culture was taken and *Staph. aureus* was present. A small rubber tube was sewn into the wound. 2,000 units of peni-

cillin was then injected 4-hourly for 5 days. A culture of the pus then showed the presence of *B. proteus*, and penicillin therapy was discontinued. Later this man developed a tendon sheath infection of the ring finger, which was attributed to the pressure on the sheath by the rubber tube as it lay across the palm. This case illustrates 2 disadvantages of local therapy: (a) secondary infection with penicillin-resistant organisms and (b) pressure necrosis from a rubber tube. Secondary haemorrhage might easily have occurred also.

(2) A web infection of 9 days' duration was incised in the out-patients' department. The patient was admitted with a discharging web space. A culture showed the presence of *Staph. aureus*. Considerable cellulitis was also seen. Systemic penicillin was given for 5 days, after which the patient was discharged with the infection healed. Systemic penicillin was valuable as there was considerable cellulitis of the hand in addition to a local abscess.

Dorsal infections.—Infection frequently spreads from the fingers on to the dorsum of the hand to form a large subcutaneous abscess. Occasionally an abscess forms deep to the extensor tendons (subaponeurotic). This is usually a secondary condition to osteomyelitis of one of the metacarpal bones.

Both types of infection need drainage. In the past, results have been good but the wound has taken a considerable time to heal and return of function has been rather slow.

A man was admitted with infective gangrene of the little finger with cellulitis of the dorsum of his hand. Systemic penicillin was given for 14 days. Two days after admission the base of the finger, web space and dorsum of the hand were incised. A culture was taken and *Staph. aureus* was present. A week later amputation of the finger at the metacarpophalangeal joint was performed with immediate suture and secondary suture of the wound on the dorsum of the hand. The wounds healed, and the patient was discharged.

Systemic treatment was useful in this case because amputation of the dead finger could be performed early and an immediate suture was made instead of leaving the flaps open; it was also possible to perform a secondary suture on the dorsum of the hand; return of function was accelerated by the early healing of the wounds.

Anterior subaponeurotic infections.—These are hour-glass abscesses which arise between the central part of the palmar fascia and the flexor tendons.

There is always a superficial loculus of pus between the fascia and the skin and generally there is a wound in the palm through which the infection has gained entry.

The treatment is surgical and the palmar fascia must be incised to establish free drainage. In the past the majority of cases did well.

Number of cases	*Staph. aureus*	Results good	Days in hospital
11	11	11	9

One patient was treated with local penicillin and the wound healed in 9 days; another who was treated with systemic penicillin took 14 days to recover. In both patients recovery was perfect, but was not quicker than the average rate of recovery in untreated subjects.

Thenar space infections.—These infections usually result from spread of infection from the thumb or index finger. Diagnosis is usually easy owing to the typical ballooning of the thenar space.

Surgical treatment is necessary once pus has formed. The results have previously been excellent.

Number of cases	*Staph. aureus*	H. strept.	Results good	Deformity	Days in hospital
11	8	2	10	1	14

The following cases are reported.

(1) The patient gave a history of pain in the thumb of 8 days' duration. The thenar space was drained and a culture showed *Staph. aureus*. Penicillin cream was applied locally on alternate days until the wound healed in a week.

(2) A diabetic patient complained of pain in the thumb lasting 5 days. The thenar space was incised and a culture was taken showing the presence of *Staph. aureus*. Systemic penicillin was given for 5 days and the diabetes was controlled with insulin. The infection healed with full restoration of function in 18 days.

The first case healed very quickly. The second took longer but systemic treatment was probably helpful since spread of the infection might easily have occurred owing to the presence of diabetes.

Mid-palmar space infections.—Infection of the mid-palmar space is unusual. We have only three cases on record before the introduction of penicillin.

Number of cases	*Staph. aureus*	H. strept.	Results good	Deformity	Days in hospital
3	2	1	2	1	21

The end results depend on the presence or absence of tendon infection.

We have not treated any of these cases with penicillin but undoubtedly systemic treatment should be employed because infection of this space is often associated with severe toxaemia; moreover the infection may spread proximally into the forearm and penicillin might be expected to prevent this complication.

Primary tendon sheath infection

Primary suppurative tenosynovitis is an uncommon condition. Since 1937 only 16 cases have been admitted to the London Hospital; none has been treated since the introduction of penicillin. Secondary infection of the tendons is much more common and it may result from cellulitis, osteomyelitis or bad surgery.

It is probable that the incidence of primary infection is higher than our figures indicate because other clinics have been able to report the results of a considerable number of cases treated since penicillin became available.

The diagnosis of this condition can be made with certainty only in the first few days of the infection. Once pus has ruptured out of the tendon sheath, secondary bone infection readily occurs. Abscesses in the subcutaneous tissues also confuse the clinical picture.

Before describing the results obtained by treatment with penicillin, mention must be made of those lesions treated before the drug became available. The cases can be divided into either those due to the haemolytic streptococcus or those due to the *Staph. aureus.* The distinction is important because the functional results were found to differ considerably.

PRIMARY HAEMOLYTIC STREPTOCOCCAL TENOSYNOVITIS

Site	Operation (drainage)	Bone	Joint	Result
(1) Thumb	Radial bursa	—	—	Stiff thumb
	Ulnar bursa			Stiff little finger
(2) Finger	Sheath	—	—	Bacteriaemia (patient died)
(3) Finger	Sheath	—	—	Stiff
(4) Finger	Sheath	—	—	Movable
(5) Finger	—	—	—	Movable
(6) Finger	Sheath	—	—	Patient died (pulmonary embolism)
(7) Finger	Ulnar bursa	—	—	Stiff
(8) Finger	Sheath	—	—	Movable

Note—Cases (1), (4), (5), (7), (8) were treated with sulphonamides.

PRIMARY STAPHYLOCOCCAL TENOSYNOVITIS

Site	Operation (drainage)	Bone	Joint	Result
(1) Finger	Sheath	Yes	Yes	Amputation
(2) Finger	Sheath	—	—	Stiff
(3) Finger	Sheath	—	—	Stiff
(4) Finger	Sheath	—	Yes	Stiff
(5) Finger	Sheath	Yes	Yes	Stiff
(6) Finger	Sheath	—	—	Stiff
(7) Finger	Sheath	Yes	Yes	Stiff
(8) Finger	Sheath	—	—	Stiff

Streptococcal infection was characterized by a very acute onset but with appropriate treatment the infection rapidly subsided, leaving sometimes a tendon capable of function. Secondary bone and joint infection was rare so that tendon graft operations were sometimes possible after the infection had cleared.

Both of the fatal cases occurred before the value of the sulphonamides had become recognized.

After the introduction of the sulphonamides treatment consisted of a small incision at the base of the sheath in order to relieve tension and to obtain pus for culture. The finger was immobilized in plaster and a full course of sulphonamides given by mouth. In 3 cases in which there was recovery, finger movement was restored.

Infection by *Staph. aureus* always caused a stiff finger. Secondary bone and joint infection was common and amputation often necessary. Reconstructive surgery was impracticable because secondary bone infection caused ankylosis. Sulphonamide therapy did not produce any better result.

When penicillin therapy was first introduced local therapy was chiefly employed. Among the first reports of successful treatment

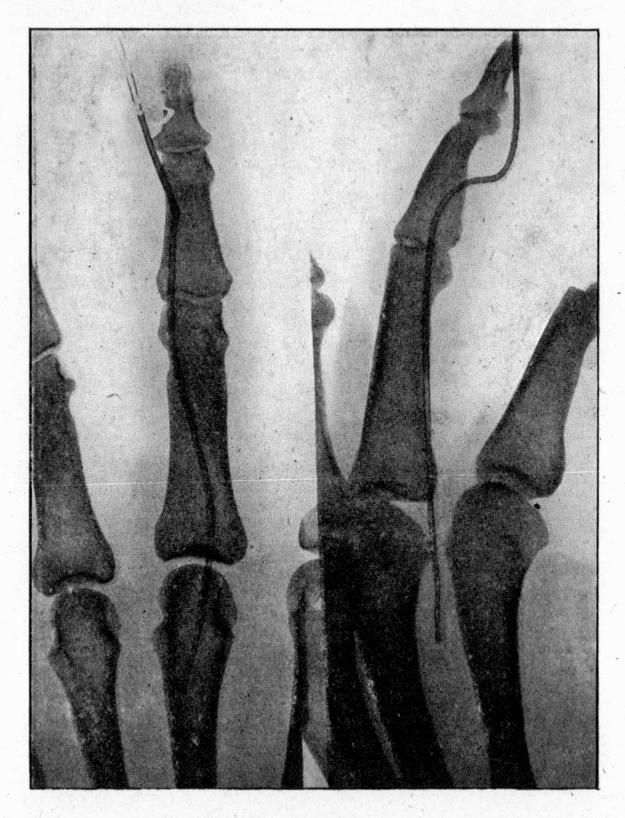

FIG. 44.—The catheter is shown in antero-posterior and lateral views traversing the wound in the front of the finger and passing the whole length of the tendon sheath (*Proc. R. Soc. Med.*)

were those of Mr. Dickson Wright[3] at St. Mary's Hospital, London, to whom I am indebted for the following description of the patients he has treated.

Treatment of tendon sheath infection and local penicillin.—Case reports.

(1) Case of puncture wound of tendon sheath—staphylococcal tenosynovitis.

A factory worker pricked his finger with a sliver of wood. The finger became swollen, red, and tender and movements were very painful. On examination the tendon sheath was obviously infected and there was a small septic wound over the terminal phalangeal joint. The wound was slightly enlarged and a ureteric catheter passed up the sheath. (See Fig. 44.) Synovial fluid and the pus from which *Staph. aureus* was identified were washed out and 1 millilitre of penicillin solution instilled every day for 8 days. Temperature and all symptoms vanished and a well-functioning finger was the result.

(2) A prick with a sewing needle in the index finger was followed by swelling and tenderness along the tendon sheath and by loss of function. The tendon sheath was opened through the site of the puncture and pus containing mixed pyogenic organisms was washed out with a ureteric catheter. Daily instillations of 1 millilitre of penicillin solution for 7 days resulted in a cure.

Two further cases of a similar type have been successfully treated.

When penicillin became more plentiful systemic treatment was tried in place of local therapy. The following case reports sent by Professor R. S. Pilcher of University College Hospital, London, adequately illustrate the method adopted and the results achieved.

Three cases of suppurative tenosynovitis.—

Case (1)

1st day

The patient was admitted to hospital with a history of a painful right index of 2 days' duration. There was no injury and no pain the day before. On the day before admission incision was made in the middle segment by a private doctor without relief of pain. The patient had signs of a tendon sheath infection and a small superficial incision in middle segment of the finger, which was not discharging. Systemic penicillin was started immediately. 30,000 units was given 3 hourly for 5 days. An operation was performed and the proximal end of sheath opened through a transverse palmar incision. Thin pus under tension was ejected and a culture taken. The digital incision was examined and found to lead to a small opening in the sheath. Vaselined calico strips were placed in the wounds and a plaster splint applied. The hand was then elevated.

3rd day

Only slight discomfort was felt since operation. The calico strips were removed.

5th day

The finger could be moved actively without any pain. A clear serous discharge was ejected from the palm. A further culture was taken.

13th day

The wounds healed and the splint was removed.

15th day

The patient was discharged from hospital.

The patient has attended clinic regularly since discharge. The finger remains swollen but it has a good range of movement without pain. There is crepitus in the tendon sheath. (See Fig. 45.)

A swab taken from the tendon sheath at operation showed the presence of haemolytic streptococci which were penicillin-sensitive.

A further swab was taken from wound on the 6th day and growth was not shown.

In view of the sudden onset of the infection and rapid progress made this was probably a primary sheath infection but it may have been secondary to the small incision. There was no evidence of a primary skin lesion and a slough was not present at the site of first incision.

Case (2) 1st day

The patient, a fitter, was admitted to hospital with a history of pain in left ring finger which was of a few days' duration. There was no injury and no previous treatment had been given. Signs of a tendon sheath infection were present. There was no visible skin lesion.

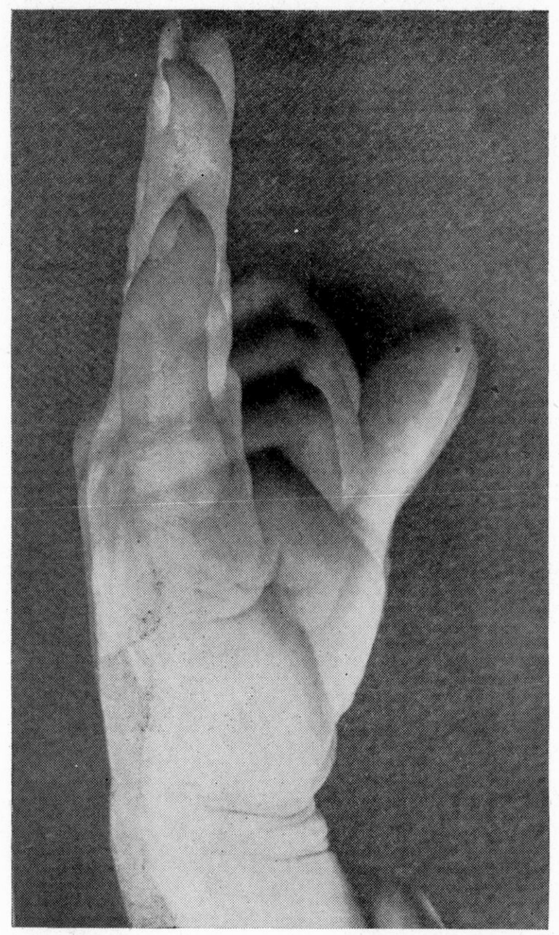

FIG. 45.—Case of suppurative tenosynovitis showing range of movement of the fingers after treatment

The proximal end of the sheath was opened through a transverse palmar incision and the sheath was found to be distended containing a thin yellow pus. Part of the fibrous sheath was slit and the edges of the wound were held open with sutures. A plaster splint was applied and the hand elevated. A culture was taken from the tendon sheath and systemic penicillin was started, 30,000 units 3 hourly for 48 hours, after operation.

3rd day

The sutures holding the wound open were removed and the finger could be moved freely without pain.

4th day

A further culture was taken from the wound.

9th day

The wound was clean but apparently not healing. The finger movements were free and painless. The wound was sutured.

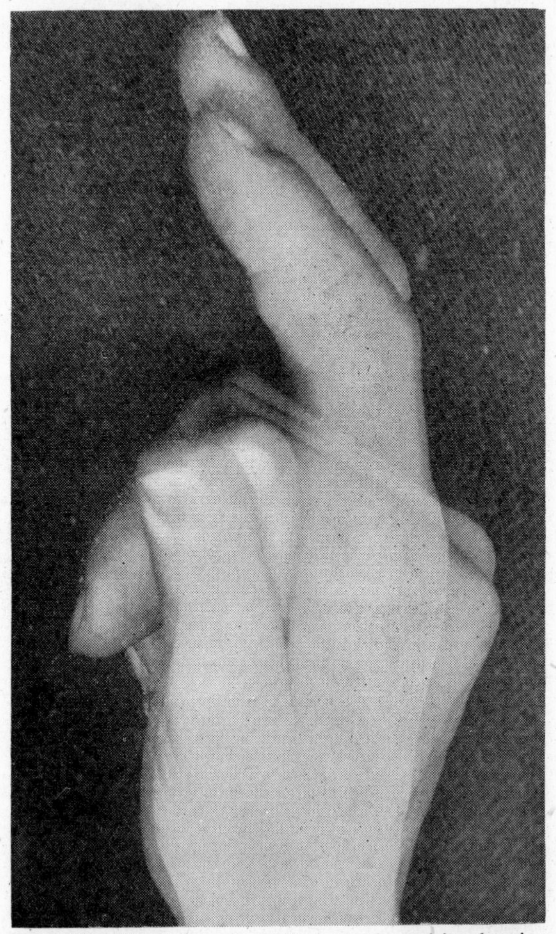

FIG. 46.—Case of suppurative tenosynovitis showing almost full movements of the fingers after treatment

23rd day

The patient was discharged with the wound healed and nearly full movement without pain was obtained. (See Fig. 46.)

Later the patient reported full function of the finger.

Swabs from the tendon sheath taken at operation and after the fourth day showed no growth.

Case (3)

1st day

The patient, a celery washer, was admitted to hospital with a history of pain in the right fifth finger of 5 days' duration. There was no trauma. On the third day a pustule was noticed in the distal crease of the finger, which he had nicked with a razor blade and squeezed, causing the liberation of blood and pus. He had several sleepless nights and felt ill. There were signs of tendon sheath infection of the finger without spread to the ulnar bursa. A superficial dry incision was made in the distal crease.

The proximal end of the sheath was opened through a transverse palmar incision. A thick pus was liberated. A culture was taken. An incision in the crease was examined and a small amount of slough was removed. No opening was found in the sheath. A vaselined calico strip was inserted into the palmar wound, a plaster splint applied, and the hand elevated. Systemic penicillin, 30,000 units 3-hourly for 5 days, was started at operation.

5th day

There was no pain and the patient could move all fingers without pain. The calico strip was removed and a culture taken.

7th day

Both wounds were clean and there was a limited range of movement without pain. The splint was removed.

14th day

The wound healed with little swelling and there was good range of movement without pain. The patient was discharged.

26th day

Full range of movement without pain except for a few degrees was obtained with loss of extension at the proximal interphalangeal joint. A swab taken from the sheath at operation showed *Staph. aureus* agglutination + and penicillin-sensitive.

A swab taken from the wound on the fourth day after operation still showed *Staph. aureus*.

In this case the tendon sheath infection was probably secondary to a distal crease abscess but no opening was found in the sheath at this point and the pus was under tension.

In penicillin, it is evident that we now have a drug which will, when combined with surgery, cure acute pyogenic tenosynovitis and leave the patient with a perfect finger.

Early diagnosis is still essential. Once the tendon has died penicillin therapy will be of no value in restoring the function of the finger, although by its use further spread of the infection may be checked.

Bone and joint infections

In the past the functional results have been bad.

BONE AND JOINT INFECTIONS

Site	Operation	Bone	Joint	Result
(1) Finger	—	Yes	Yes	Stiff
(2) Finger	Sheath drained	Yes	—	Stiff
(3) Finger	Lateral incision	Yes	Yes	Stiff
(4) Finger	Lateral incision	Yes	Yes	Amputation
(5) Thumb	Sheath drained	Yes	—	Stiff
(6) Finger	Lateral incision	Yes	Yes	Stiff
(7) Finger	Lateral incision	Yes	—	Stiff
(8) Thumb	Lateral incision	Yes	—	Stiff
(9) Finger	Lateral incision	Yes	Yes	Stiff
(10) Thumb	Sheath drained	Yes	Yes	Stiff
(11) Finger	Sheath drained	Yes	Yes	Stiff
(12) Finger	Lateral incision	Yes	Yes	Amputation

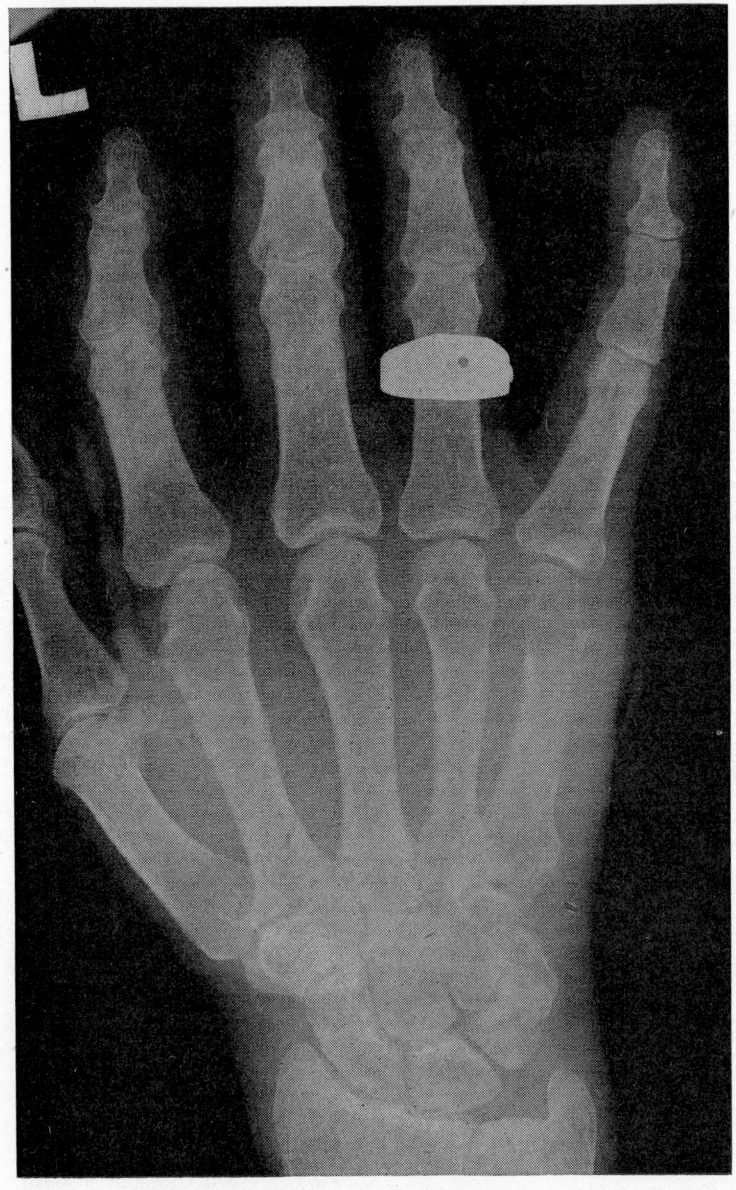

Fig. 47.—Osteomyelitis of the head of the fifth metacarpal with necrosis of a portion of the bone

It is hoped that the routine use of penicillin in hand infections may reduce the incidence of this group by preventing the spread of infection from cellulitis or tendon infection.

Once the bone or joint has become infected surgical treatment is usually required to remove dead bone or drain local abscesses. Systemic penicillin is of value in preventing the spread of infection

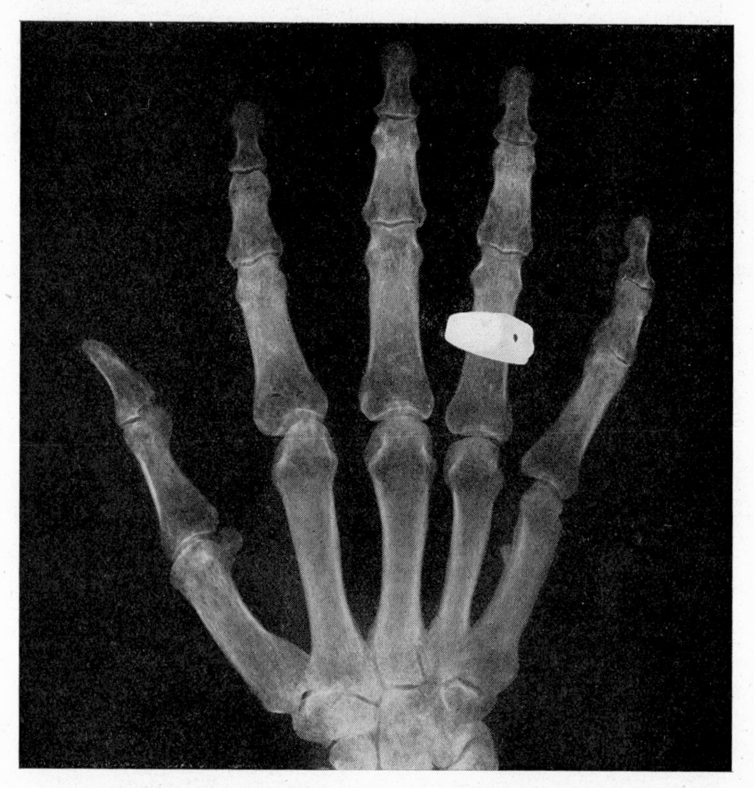

FIG. 48.—Reformation of the head of the fifth metacarpal bone

to other parts of the hand. Despite the unfavourable skiagrams in some of these cases, a good deal of the infected bone may recalcify after systemic treatment. Similar observations have been recorded following the systemic treatment of acute osteomyelitis of the long bones.

Healing is usually rapid once dead bone has been removed but return of function depends on the amount of tissue destroyed.

The following 2 cases are quoted.

(1) Eight weeks' painful swelling of index finger was treated by rest and heat. After 8 days pain and swelling were still present, but there was some

passive movement. Examination of skiagrams proved negative. Further treatment was given by rest, heat and sulphonamides. Five days later pus was drained by lateral incisions over the middle and after a further 8 days distal phalanges. The culture showed *Staph. aureus*. A skiagram showed osteomyelitis of the whole of the middle phalanx with arthritis of the terminal joint. Penicillin 100,000 units daily was given for 10 days. By the end of the course all wounds healed except one over the terminal joint. One month later all healed and some flexion was possible at the proximal joint. The terminal phalanx was removed as a sequestrum. The distal joint was destroyed but the rest of the middle phalanx was sound and there was still flexion at the proximal joint. This case was a severe one and it is possible that the finger would have been lost but for penicillin therapy.

(2) Two weeks' painful swelling on back of hand following a boil. Induration was observed over the head of the fifth metacarpal bone. A skiagram showed osteomyelitis of the head of the fifth metacarpal bone with necrosis of a portion of the bone. (See Fig. 47.) Systemic penicillin was given for 7 days. A sequestrectomy was performed and most of head of fifth metacarpal bone was removed. The wound healed rapidly. On dismissal from hospital the metacarpophalangeal joint gave good movement and the skiagram (see Fig. 48) showed reformation of the head of the bone. Once the dead bone had been removed healing was rapid. It is probable that the patient would have had a stiff joint if penicillin had not been employed.

Anaerobic infection

Infection generally follows human or animal bites; the causative organisms are mixed, anaerobic streptococci and fusiform bacilli being common.

Formerly the prognosis was bad, and several deaths have been reported. Multiple operations and even amputation of an arm have been employed to arrest the spread of infection in other cases.

Two of our cases were treated without penicillin, one that of a lunatic who died following amputation of the arm; the other patient, a porter, recovered after many extensive operations on his hand.

Two other cases were treated with a combination of systemic and local penicillin, and both recovered rapidly without surgical intervention.

Six days before the patient was admitted she had been bitten on the index finger by a man. She was an ill woman. The index finger was swollen, and foul pus was discharged from the terminal phalanx. A culture showed anaerobic streptococci, fusiform bacilli and *Staph. aureus*, which were all penicillin-sensitive. Systemic penicillin was given daily for a week, and penicillin cream applied locally. At the end of a week the swelling had subsided and the discharge had ceased. Four weeks after admission she was dismissed completely healed. In the meantime a fragment of the terminal phalanx had separated and was extruded spontaneously at the site of the original bite. The effects of penicillin on this case were as dramatic as those noted in tendon sheath infections.

Foreign bodies in the hand

In many of these cases cellulitis occurs around the foreign body, making early removal impracticable. The following case history illustrates the value of pre-operative and postoperative systemic penicillin in these cases.

The patient, having cut his hand on a barrel 6 days previously, was admitted with cellulitis of the hypothenar space. A skiagram was taken and 2 metal fragments visualized. Tetanus antitoxin was given. Intramuscular penicillin was administered for 7 days, and at the end of 3 days the signs of cellulitis had subsided. The foreign bodies were removed and a primary suture performed. The patient was dismissed after 14 days with full function.

Infective arthritis of wrist and carpus

Suppurative arthritis of the wrist and carpus is uncommon. These infections usually follow penetrating wounds but occasionally accompany soft tissue infections.

Drainage is difficult and necrosis of one or more of the carpal bones may occur; the end result is usually ankylosis. Only one case has been treated by us with penicillin, and the result was encouraging.

Six days previous to admission the patient had run a needle, which was later removed, into her hand. Throbbing pain in the hand soon developed. There was swelling and oedema of the dorsum of the hand with limited movement of wrist joint. A small abscess pointed at site of needle entry. A culture was taken and showed *Staph. aureus*. Two weeks later the sinus was explored and bare bone was felt in the carpus. A skiagram showed osteoporosis but no definite bone destruction. Following operation intramuscular penicillin was given for 5 days. The patient then refused any more systemic treatment so 4,000 units of penicillin solution was injected twice daily for a week down the sinus. There appeared to be at the time little response; her pain and pyrexia persisted. The patient's wrist and forearm were immobilized in plaster which soon relieved her symptoms. At the end of 3 months the plaster was removed. The sinus had healed, the skiagram showed no permanent bone damage and full function rapidly returned. Complete rest in plaster was probably the most important factor in the treatment, but rest alone usually results in ankylosis so that the course of penicillin may have been valuable by helping to prevent further spread into the carpus.

Infection of the forearm

Infection of the forearm may occur following the spread upwards of a cellulitis or tenosynovitis of the hand. An abscess rapidly forms between the deep and superficial muscles of the forearm. Treatment is drainage by an incision along the subcutaneous border of the ulna deep to the vessels and nerve. Counter drainage may be required. In the past patients usually did well after operation but systemic penicillin should be used in all cases of forearm infection as they are invariably associated with severe hand infection. We have treated one case of this type with local penicillin only, and the results were inconclusive.

The patient was admitted with a thenar space infection which was drained. A culture showed haemolytic streptococci. There were signs of a forearm infection which was drained. The wound was filled with penicillin cream daily for 8 days and no dramatic change was noticed; after a further 7 days the wounds were irrigated with penicillin solution 2,000 units twice daily by means of a rubber catheter and there was a decided improvement. Some days later there was a flare up of infection following attempted active movements. The patient was treated by rest in plaster and sulphonamides, and the condition rapidly subsided. All wounds healed, but there was a stiff terminal joint to her thumb and limited movement of her wrist.

It is probable that this patient would have responded very quickly to systemic penicillin but none was available at the time.

REFERENCES

[1] Florey, M. E., and Williams, R. E. O. (1944) *Lancet*, **1**, 73.
[2] Barber, Mary, Nellen, M., and Zoob, M. (1946) *Lancet*, **1**, 125.
[3] Wright, A. D. (1944) *Proc. R. Soc. Med.*, **37**, 504.

ABDOMINAL INFECTIONS

By R. M. Handfield-Jones, M.S., F.R.C.S.
Surgeon, St. Mary's Hospital, London

GENERAL CONSIDERATIONS

Although the alimentary canal is the normal habitat of an immense number of micro-organisms, the nature and potential pathogenicity of which may vary widely, a great number—including many of the important ones—are insensitive to penicillin. Moreover, the commoner pathogenic invaders are likewise to be numbered in the same category. Reference to Table on page 19 makes this clear, for a glance at the second column reveals the presence of *Esch. coli communis* and its associated forms, *Str. faecalis*, *B. proteus*, the organisms of typhoid and paratyphoid fevers and of bacillary dysentery, together with those of the salmonella group. Inasmuch as the dominant infections of the abdominal viscera are usually due to organisms derived from the intestinal tract, it is apparent that this great field of human pathology affords comparatively little scope for the use of penicillin. It is all the more important, therefore, that its limited uses should be clearly defined and understood, lest we fall into the grievous error of assuming that penicillin has no place at all in abdominal disease. Furthermore, it is justifiable to indicate those fields in which further research may yield an abundant harvest.

This subject covers so wide a field as to require definition. It includes all the contents of the abdominal cavity together with the male genito-urinary organs and those of the female urinary system. It does not touch on venereal infections, which are described later in the book, or on diseases of the female adnexa, which are dealt with elsewhere.

Peritoneum

Peritonitis.—Inflammation of the peritoneum is almost invariably due to bacterial invasion and some degree of acute localized peritonitis is the inevitable concomitant of all infective intra-abdominal disease, which may be conveniently grouped as follows.

(1) Acute infections, for example, appendicitis, diverticulitis, cholecystitis, salpingitis.

(2) Acute perforation of ulcers, for example, peptic, typhoid and stercoral.

(3) Injuries to hollow viscera, for example, penetrating wounds and rupture without external wound.

(4) Injuries to solid viscera, for example, liver, spleen, and ectopic gestation, in which the resulting intraperitoneal haematoma becomes secondarily infected.

(5) Ascending infections from the female genital tract, for example, gonococcal, pneumococcal and streptococcal lesions (particularly puerperal sepsis).

(6) Torsion, strangulation and gangrene of solid and hollow viscera.

(7) Blood stream infections, for example, pneumococcal invasion during pneumonia.

(8) Irritation by sterile fluids, for example, bile, urine or pancreatic juice.

This aetiological review will serve as a reminder that the treatment of peritonitis is that of the causative disease. The peritoneum possesses the most marvellous powers of defence and recuperation provided it is relieved of continued irritation and reinfection. Penicillin may be a valued ancillary treatment but it cannot replace routine surgical methods.

Diffusion into the peritoneal cavity.—In view of statements that systemic penicillin does not diffuse through serous membranes, it is essential that this objection should be answered before attempting to assess the value of penicillin therapy in peritonitis. The reports of Hughes[1], Foster and Colquhoun[2] and Heatley[3], together with those of Miller and Foster[4], prove beyond doubt that diffusion does take place into the peritoneal cavity. The level may not be quite so high as in the blood stream but it is therapeutically adequate.

Traumatic peritonitis.—This lesion following penetrating wounds is dealt with elsewhere.

Acute localized peritonitis.—Early diagnosis and prompt treatment of the cause will lead to so rapid a resolution of the inflammatory process that chemotherapy will hardly be required. It is unlikely that penicillin can be usefully employed in these cases, since the majority are due to those intestinal bacteria which are penicillin-insensitive. If frank pus be present at operation, it should be cultured and tested for penicillin-sensitivity, so that in the unfortunate event of complications occurring, the drug can be employed in suitable cases.

Acute diffuse or general peritonitis.—This condition is an expression of an unusually virulent strain of organism attacking a patient whose resistance is low. At operation a condition is found with which every surgeon is familiar. Instead of thick yellow pus, with an unmistakable smell of coliform organisms, a severe inflammatory lesion is accompanied by a thin, dirty-looking fluid with little odour. Usually these exudates are heavily laden with streptococci, which are not always of the insensitive *faecalis* type. So grave are the implications of this variety of peritonitis that penicillin should be used in addition to sulphonamide powder to dust the whole operation area. A test swab will have been taken and, should this prove sensitivity, full penicillin therapy should be instituted.

Pneumococcal peritonitis.—This may result from a blood-stream infection during an attack of pneumonia, but more commonly is an ascending infection *via* the vagina, uterus and uterine tubes of children below the age of 12 years. Before the introduction of chemotherapy prognosis was so bad that the mortality was over 50 per cent. Although its incidence has always been low, this is a dread disease of childhood and penicillin will save many lives. If the diagnosis has been correctly made, the abdomen should not be opened but penicillin should be given intramuscularly in large doses. If, however, doubt regarding a diagnosis has led to a laparotomy, penicillin powder should be applied locally and the wound closed without drainage. Systemic penicillin will be commenced immediately the child is returned to bed.

Streptococcal peritonitis.—This condition has been referred to above under the heading of diffuse peritonitis. An improvement in prognosis can confidently be expected if the organism is sensitive to penicillin.

Gonococcal peritonitis.—This condition is discussed elsewhere.

Local intraperitoneal abscess.—Theoretically a local plastic peritonitis may seal off a collection of pus in any part of the abdominal cavity; in practice, however, localized abscesses are seen in well defined situations either above the colic shelf in the subphrenic or subhepatic situation, or below the colic shelf in the right iliac fossa, the left iliac fossa, or the pelvis. Each undoubtedly presents problems of diagnostic interest, but none raises any special difficulties with regard to penicillin therapy. Treatment follows general principles and penicillin will be used only in those cases in which sensitive organisms are identified; these are likely to be few.

Paralytic ileus.—Although this condition is well recognized as a manifestation of certain toxic states, for example, uraemia, it is more usually associated with diffuse peritonitis, and it is with this latter type that we are concerned. Although suction drainage of the proximal intestine combined with continuous intravenous saline transfusion has greatly improved prognosis, this dire complication remains a source of grave anxiety to the surgeon. Administration of penicillin is likely to be based on purely empirical grounds, but in spite of our insistence upon sensitivity controls, we believe its use to be justified in this way in this most dangerous condition. Real assessment of its value is difficult to obtain, because several aetiological factors are likely to be at work, bacteriological control may not be easy owing to the mixture of organisms present, several methods of treatment are being applied concurrently and, finally, improvement in early diagnosis and treatment has greatly reduced the incidence of this condition. Further reports will be awaited with interest.

Retroperitoneal cellulitis.—Reports from all theatres of war have amply confirmed the long-established fact that the retroperitoneal cellular tissues are singularly ill equipped to defend themselves against infection. This subject belongs chiefly to the domain of war surgery and is especially associated with wounds of the fixed parts of the colon. Occasional cases occur, however, unassociated with disease or injury of the intestinal tract and these possibly may be due to sensitive organisms. Such patients will, of course, be subjected to full penicillin therapy.

Pelvic cellulitis.—The very term conjures up a mental picture of an obstetrician faced with the grave complications of a septic puerperium or abortion. Chemotherapy has proved to be an ally of inestimable value to him in his anxieties and this aspect is ably dealt with in the Chapter on Obstetrics and Gynaecology. Not every case of pelvic cellulitis, however, is necessarily associated with obstetric disasters or is indeed confined to females. Infection of the pelvic cellular tissues may result from spread from any component of the osseomuscular walls or from the retroperitoneal structures contained therein. Injuries and diseases of the urinary bladder and ureters leading to spread of infection or extravasation of urine, diseases of the prostate and vesicles penetrating Denonvilliers's aponeurosis, osteomyelitis of any part of the bony pelvis and sacrum, infective processes of the lower sigmoid colon, of the rectum and ischiorectal fossae are all examples of this type of pelvic cellulitis. Each demands its special treatment, but in every case penicillin may be a useful adjuvant if the organisms prove to be sensitive.

Stomach and duodenum

No intrinsic disease of either stomach or duodenum is likely to benefit from penicillin.

Small and large intestine

Enteritis.—A study of the table of insensitive organisms shows that little good can be expected to come from penicillin therapy in this type of disease.

Colitis.—Ulcerative colitis is a most intractable disease, but some encouraging results have come from local sulphonamide treatment, although many patients prove resistant to it. A careful bacteriological examination of material taken direct by sigmoidoscopy from ulcers is certain to reveal a mixed growth of organisms;

amongst these may be one or more penicillin-sensitive strains, in which circumstance an improvement may be expected from its use. Unfortunately, in practice it has been found that penicillin is useless in this disease except in those very rare cases which are of staphylococcal origin.

Diverticulitis.—The predominance of insensitive organisms in this and similar intestinal inflammations precludes any hope that peniciliin will play a large part in their treatment. Some cases of diverticulitis, however, with local abscess formation are due to streptococci and, should these be sensitive, penicillin therapy will radically curtail convalescence.

Anthrax.—Intestinal involvement in anthrax is the rarest of its manifestations. In the past treatment was of no avail and death rapidly ensued. Anthrax patients might well be saved by penicillin but unfortunately the true diagnosis is likely to be unsuspected until too late. Herrell[5] reports successful results in animal experiments, but at present published reports in human disease are confined to cutaneous lesions, in which brilliant results have been obtained.

Appendix and ileocaecal angle

Acute appendicitis.—This is due either to invasion from its lumen by one or other of the usual intestinal organisms or, less commonly, to blood-borne streptococci. Clearly this is not a condition in which penicillin can replace routine surgical practice, but it may be a useful ally in certain circumstances. Whatever personal views surgeons may hold concerning the controversy of expectant treatment *versus* immediate operation, none will deny that an untreated acute appendicitis of 72–96 hours' duration with a palpable tumour in the right iliac fossa is a source of real anxiety. Four such cases are reported by Heatley[3], who at the time was working on the intensive intravenous method of therapy, consisting of 600,000 units given within $2\frac{1}{4}$ hours on each of 3 successive days. All these patients became afebrile within 3 hours of the commencement of treatment and in each case the abscess rapidly decreased in size. Four cases are insufficient for balanced judgment, but they are certainly an inspiration for further investigation.

Actinomycosis.—This condition is dealt with elsewhere, but as the ileocaecal angle is one of the sites most commonly attacked, a few notes must be included here. On test culture *Actinomyces* is noticeably penicillin-sensitive and earlier disappointments in treatment were due presumably to insufficient knowledge of correct dosage and more especially to the length of time over which administration must continue. Abdominal and thoracic actinomycosis must inevitably present difficult problems of management, but recent experience suggests that greatly improved results may be expected.

Cope[6] has recently treated a patient who both abroad and on his return to Great Britain was diagnosed as having a carcinoma of the caecum which was regarded as inoperable. A small area of abdominal wall above and to the right of the symphysis pubis began to soften and eventually broke down, discharging pus containing the tell-tale granules. Prolonged treatment with penicillin continued over many weeks has led apparently to a complete disappearance of the disease from the abdomen.

Rectum and anal canal

Injuries and infections of the buttocks and perineum.—When these involve the lower part of the rectum and anal canal, they present certain features of surgical interest which will be dealt with on general principles of wound treatment. In civil practice, however, there is one aspect of this type of injury which demands special notice, more especially as its incidence is not appreciated as widely as it should be. I refer to those unusual cases of "autogenous" gas gangrene in which the infection is introduced not from without but by faecal contamination from the patient's rectum. Two cases amply illustrate this condition.

A woman sitting in the front seat of an open motor car was involved in an accident, with the result that she was thrown into the air, and descended, still in a sitting position, upon the windscreen. A projecting metal fitment tore a jagged hole in one buttock which involved the rectum. Her body fell across the bonnet and remained there, so that there was no question of soiling from the ground. Within 48 hours a virulent gas gangrene infection was established in the perirectal tissue.

In another woman, who had sustained a tear of the rectal mucosa from a fragment of rabbit bone, a submucous abscess developed which contained *Cl. welchii*. Within a few hours infection had spread into the isolateral buttock, carried there presumably *via* the lymphatic vessels.

These 2 cases occurred before the advent of chemotherapy and show that all wounds of this type should be regarded as of potentially grave significance. These tragedies will be averted by the routine use of penicillin both as a prophylactic measure and as a means of active treatment.

Ulceration of the rectum.—The lesion may be due to many types of infecting organism, few of which are likely to be penicillin-sensitive. What has been said of ulcerative colitis applies with equal force here.

Ischiorectal abscesses.—These are classified into 3 groups, according to the channels by which organisms reach the ischiorectal fossa: (1) from the rectum, (2) from the skin of the peri-anal region and neighbouring buttock and (3) *via* the blood stream. Whereas in group (1) most of the causative organisms will be insensitive, those in groups (2) and (3) are likely to be sensitive. Although an ischiorectal abscess involves the skin and subcutaneous tissue and is therefore pathologically analagous to other superficial inflammations, for example, breast abscess, prognosis is overshadowed by the subsequent danger of fistula in ano formation, for which reason incision and drainage at the earliest opportunity must remain correct surgical treatment. Penicillin, nevertheless, will be of great assistance in a rapid clearing of the infection and shortening of convalescence.

Fissure and fistula in ano.—The mechanical conditions underlying these two lesions are such that penicillin cannot be usefully employed until after operation. Treatment in each case is followed by a tedious period when open wounds are granulating and vigilant watch is kept to prevent too early healing of the skin across the surface, in case the lesion recurs. The type of dressing to apply to these raw areas has always been a matter in dispute, but recent experience has convinced me that penicillin cream cannot be surpassed.

Liver and gallbladder

Penicillin has been shown to be excreted in the bile in experiments both on animals and on human subjects (Abraham and others[7]; Rammelkamp and Helm[8]; Struble and Bellows[9]). The reports prove that the concentration is higher in bile than in serum or in any other tissue except the kidney. Provided, therefore, that the causative organisms are sensitive, infections of the liver should be readily controlled by penicillin. Once again we are confronted with the fact that insensitive intestinal organisms are likely to predominate in these lesions.

Acute suppurative cholangitis.—This is usually associated with a gallstone impacted in the common bile duct, and treatment is surgical by removal of the stone and drainage of the duct. When the duct is first opened bile will gush out; this should be taken for culture and, should sensitive organisms be present, penicillin therapy will hasten recovery. Unfortunately we are more likely to find insensitive bacteria.

Acute pylephlebitis.—Portal pyaemia resulting from a suppurative thrombophlebitis of some radical of the portal vein, for example, appendicular or rectal, is a very serious disease; indeed it is doubtful whether in an established case the patient has survived. Although the organisms concerned are of the usual intestinal types and therefore insensitive, it would be justifiable to try the effect of intensive penicillin therapy in an attempt to avoid an otherwise certain death.

Multiple liver abscesses.—When these result from systemic

pyaemia *via* the hepatic artery they are in an entirely different category. The patient will have been ill for sufficient time for the bacteriology of the causative disease to have been worked out. In the case of penicillin-sensitive organisms, generalized pyaemia will rarely be seen in the future except in neglected patients; in other cases due to insensitive organisms the prognosis is fatal and penicillin will not be of any value.

Weil's disease.—This disease is produced by a leptospira and is spread by infected rats who pass the organism in their urine. Bulmer[10] reports on an epidemic in Normandy in 1944 in which 39 patients were seen. Of these, 16 received penicillin, one dying of uraemia. From this series certain facts emerged. (1) Early treatment with penicillin has a favourable influence in shortening the disease and controlling the number of febrile relapses. (2) Early diagnosis is seldom possible and is unlikely to be, except during an epidemic when practitioners are alive to the possibility. (3) Penicillin has not any effect upon liver and kidney damage, once this has been inflicted. (4) Every effort must be made to diagnose cases in the pre-icteric stage. (5) Large doses of penicillin are needed, 1,250,000 units being given in 4 days.

Acute cholecystitis.—Streptococcal invasion is a frequent cause of this condition. There are two schools of thought concerning the surgical treatment of this disease, operative and expectant. The latter is in fact a policy of standing by with folded arms hoping the patient will do all the necessary defensive and reparative work. None will deny that this technique is accompanied by much anxiety. If operation is to be withheld, it would be a solace to know that penicillin could help us. There is too little material upon which to form a sound judgment. Heatley[3], however, has one encouraging case to report.

An officer was admitted gravely ill with acute cholecystitis (temperature 103·4° F., pulse 140), and in great pain. On examination an extremely large gallbladder could be felt. He was given intensive therapy and within 4 hours his temperature and pulse returned to normal levels, at which they remained; pain disappeared and appetite returned. This case unfortunately was not followed up owing to the patient's evacuation to the United Kingdom.

While this was being written I have had a similar experience.

A man of 34 years with upper abdominal pain, vomiting and pyrexia was admitted as an emergency case; on examination a large tender mass was felt in the upper right quadrant of the abdomen, having all the characteristic appearances of an acute cholecystitis. Intensive penicillin therapy brought the temperature down from 102·6° F. to normal within 24 hours and all pain and tenderness had disappeared. On the fourth day the general condition was good but there was little change in the swelling and it seemed probable that operation would be needed. On the seventh day, however, the swelling had greatly decreased and the decision to operate was postponed. On the eleventh day nothing abnormal in the abdomen could be found; the patient was discharged and requested to report at fortnightly intervals.

These two cases are a very meagre contribution but at least suffice to stimulate further investigation.

Pancreas and spleen

Acute pancreatitis.—Such varying severity attends this disease that it is likely to set problems of diagnosis which are often incorrectly answered. As a result the abdomen will be opened and the real pathology recognized by the presence of fat necrosis. It has been claimed that, should a correct diagnosis be made, operation should not be performed and the patient should be treated on expectant lines. There is little doubt that this disease is definitely an inflammatory one and Hiren De[11] has recently recorded a case which suggests that penicillin might reasonably be used in this condition. His patient was so gravely collapsed when the abdomen was opened that nothing could be attempted, and she was returned to bed to die. Within 24 hours, however, she had rallied and a full course of sulphadiazine was started. The final recovery was rapid and complete. Little can be claimed from this one case, but it is an incentive to test the efficacy of penicillin in this disease.

In no other disease of either pancreas or spleen can penicillin be usefully employed.

GENERAL THERAPEUTIC CONSIDERATIONS

The foregoing account of abdominal diseases illustrates the truth that in abdominal cases we cannot expect such consistent and dramatic results from the use of penicillin as we can in some others. In spite, however, of the unfavourable bacteriology of the intestinal canal, there is sufficient evidence to warrant carefully controlled clinical experiments in the use of penicillin in certain types of intraperitoneal disease even when it is impossible to obtain pus for test culture. The intensive intravenous method of therapy tried by surgeons of the 21st Army Group has much to recommend it, and I believe that in these doubtful cases of abdominal disease large doses will be required within short periods of time if favourable results are to ensue.

GENITO-URINARY SYSTEM

So close is the inter-relationship between the various components of the genito-urinary system in the male and, to a lesser degree, in the female, that infections of one unit of the system are likely to spread to other units. A more comprehensive understanding of the problem involved, therefore, will be given if we approach it in a general way.

Urinary infections in general.—These may be divided into those introduced by the blood stream or those carried in from below *via* the urethra. Apart from tuberculosis, blood-borne organisms fall into two main groups, namely, *Esch. coli* and pyogenic cocci; although others introduced from below will include gonococci and many other pyogenic organisms, the coliform group will not usually figure in this category. The rôle of penicillin in the treatment of urinary infections is made clear by this clean-cut division, for it will be valueless in cases of invasion by *Esch. coli*, *B. proteus* and other intestinal organisms but of the greatest help in coccal infections.

Kidney

Pyelitis.—The very word, unless specifically qualified, implies an infection due to *Esch. coli*, the commonest of all urinary invaders. Penicillin has no place in the treatment of this disease, which yields readily to sulphadiazine.

Pyelitis, however, is not always of coliform origin. Should the urine contain penicillin-sensitive organisms, the drug will yield good results. Among this group will be cases of staphylococcal bacteriaemia or septicaemia with widespread involvement of all components of the genito-urinary system in the male and the urinary system in the female.

Perinephric abscess and carbuncle of the kidney.—In adults staphylococci in the blood stream exhibit a well known predilection for the kidney and one of two lesions may follow. Either a small subcapsular abscess is formed which ruptures into the perinephric fat or a low-grade chronic indurative process spreads in the kidney parenchyma. The main interest in these two conditions lies in the difficulty of diagnosis. Whereas the former demands incision and drainage, no surgical interference is indicated for the latter, unless the destruction of tissue is sufficient to demand a nephrectomy. In both diseases penicillin is used immediately the diagnosis has been made. In perinephric abscess the results are dramatic and rapid resolution and healing may be confidently expected. In carbuncle, however, response is certain but slow and penicillin therapy should be continued over a long period—possibly 3–4 weeks—if recurrences are to be avoided. Normal temperature and pulse, together with a feeling of well-being, are not sufficient indications to cease therapy, but the pyelographic picture also must have returned to normal.

Bladder

Cystitis.—Introduction of infection into the bladder from below *via* the urethra results in a higher percentage of penicillin-sensitive organisms being found in cystitis than in renal lesions. Nevertheless a large number of cases of infection by *Esch. coli* and *B.*

proteus will be seen and in these penicillin cannot be of any value. In many others it will bring about a rapid improvement.

Prostate and vesicles

Although the gonococcus is so common an invader, the prostate is not infrequently infected with a variety of other organisms; amongst these will be certain strains of streptococci, some of which are sensitive. This type of lesion is sometimes associated with low-grade arthritis, dermatitis and other metastatic conditions, which present great difficulties in treatment. Should the organism be penicillin-sensitive a problem will not arise, but an insensitive organism proves extremely resistant.

Penicillin will be usefully employed in postoperative control of urinary infection following prostatectomy. Many patients both before and after operation have staphylococcus-laden urine. In two of my patients septicaemia developed. Penicillin is of inestimable value in cases of this nature.

Testis

Acute epididymo-orchitis may arise as a complication of any genito-urinary infection and a variety of organisms may be found, upon the sensitivity of which the usefulness of penicillin depends. Subacute and chronic non-specific epididymitis, now forming a well recognized group, present peculiar difficulties in diagnosis and treatment. If the urine be sterile, identification of the organisms in the lesion may be difficult or even impossible and treatment may have to be based upon empirical grounds alone. In the presence of penicillin-sensitive organisms it will, of course, be used in the ordinary way; in other cases in which the organisms cannot be identified or in which they prove resistant to sulphadiazine, penicillin therapy is justifiable.

The venereal diseases which figure prominently among the infections of the genital system are now treated with penicillin, but this aspect is dealt with at length elsewhere.

REFERENCES

[1] Hughes, K. E. A. (1945) *Penicillin Therapy and Control in* 21 *Army Group*. Numerous articles.

[2] Foster, J. N., and Colquhoun, J. (1945) "*Penicillin Content of Body Fluids in Penicillinised Patients*". *Penicillin Therapy and Control in* 21 *Army Group*, p. 339.

[3] Heatley, S. (1945) "*Intensive Intravenous Penicillin Therapy*". *Penicillin Therapy and Control in* 21 *Army Group*, p. 157.

[4] Miller, C. P., and Foster, Alice Z. (1944) *Proc. Soc. exp. Biol., N.Y.*, **56**, 166.

[5] Herrell, W. E. (1945) *Penicillin and Other Antibiotic Agents*, p. 247. W. B. Saunders Co., Philadelphia and London.

[6] Cope, V. Z. (1946) Personal communication.

[7] Abraham, E. P., Chain, E., Fletcher, C. M., Florey, H. W., Gardner, A. D., Heatley, N. G., and Jennings, M. A. (1941) *Lancet*, **2**, 177.
[8] Rammelkamp, C. H., and Helm, J. D., Jun. (1943) *Proc. Soc. exp. Biol., N.Y.*, **54**, 31.
[9] Struble, G. C., and Bellows, J. G. (1944) *J. Amer. med. Ass.*, **125**, 685.
[10] Bulmer, E. (1945) "Weil's Disease". *Penicillin Therapy and Control in* 21 *Army Group*, p. 245.
[11] Hiren De (1946) *Brit. med. J.*, **1**, 367.

OBSTETRICS AND GYNAECOLOGY

By Leslie Williams, M.D., M.S., F.R.C.S., F.R.C.O.G.
Obstetric Surgeon to Out-patients, St. Mary's Hospital;
Consulting Obstetric Surgeon, Queen Charlotte's Maternity Hospital;
Gynaecological Surgeon, The Samaritan Hospital, London

OBSTETRICS

Prenatal use of penicillin

Penicillin can be used safely in the case of a pregnant woman suffering from any intercurrent disease—for example, carbuncle—for which such therapy would normally be indicated. True, there has been made the suggestion that penicillin injections can, in non-pregnant women, sometimes bring on menstruation at a time when it is not due, or, in the case of a pregnant woman, that it can bring on premature labour. We ourselves have had one case of an expectant mother who, having received an intensive course of penicillin for congenital syphilis, which was discovered during pregnancy, came into premature labour shortly after the completion of the course. The bulk of evidence, however, goes to show that such an occurrence is merely coincidental. Admittedly the earlier observers were rather impressed by this danger. Thus Lentz and others[1] noted 2 cases of threatened abortion after penicillin treatment for syphilis in pregnant women. Leavitt[2] mentioned the observation of Lentz and commented on the effect of penicillin in inducing premature menstruation in non-pregnant women or in prolonging menstruation already started. He went on to survey cases in which his patients had been treated with penicillin during pregnancy and, although he found a considerable number who showed uterine overactivity while under treatment, he suggested that this effect might be due to an impurity since, in one series of 8 cases in which such overactivity was shown, 7 patients had been treated with the same batch of penicillin. On the other hand, Leavitt suggested that there is more evidence that penicillin therapy in heavy dosage may in itself initiate premature menstruation in non-pregnant women. Even this last suggestion is denied, however, by Speiser and Thomas[3], who did not find any significant alteration in menstrual rhythm in non-pregnant women; nor did they find, in the case of pregnant women, any undue tendency to ante-partum haemorrhage or to premature labour which could be attributed to penicillin treatment, however intensive it might have been.

In gonorrhoea.—It would appear, therefore, that altered menstrual rhythm or interruption of pregnancy in a woman receiving penicillin treatment is either coincidental or the result of impurities in the penicillin. In the latter event, as therapeutic penicillin becomes more and more pure, the risk should now be very much less than it was some time ago. It is permissible to conclude that we can dismiss the suggestion that this treatment may be undesirable during pregnancy. Indeed everything points strongly the other way. Thus a pregnant woman infected with gonorrhoea can be successfully treated with penicillin. This form of treatment is especially called for in the case of an expectant mother infected with a sulphonamide-resistant strain of gonococcus, and even more particularly when the time of delivery is near, otherwise an unsuccessfully treated woman might infect her baby with ophthalmia neonatorum. The treatment does not differ in any way from that given to a non-pregnant woman with gonorrhoea; the details will be found in the chapter which deals particularly with that disease. Very briefly, the idea is to give enough penicillin to cure the gonorrhoea but not enough to mask syphilis, with which the woman may also be infected. It is now customary to give one injection of 100,000 units in a beeswax-oil medium at night and a further 50,000 units in the same medium the following morning. This completes the course.

In syphilis.—Syphilis too is a strong indication for penicillin therapy when a pregnant woman is found to be so infected. The modern tendency seems to be to give massive doses over a comparatively short space of time, that is, 500,000 units daily for 7 days. The medium for the injection is again a beeswax-oil suspension which delays the absorption of penicillin, produces a very high blood level for a short space of time and keeps a reasonably high blood level present throughout the 24 hours. At the same time there is started a course of 10 injections of neoarsphenamine (Neoarsphenamina B.P. and U.S.P. XII) at 4-day intervals, together with 10 injections of bismuth (Injectio Bismuthi B.P., which contains 20 per cent *w/v* of precipitated bismuth). For the details of treatment for this disease the reader is referred to the appropriate chapter. The treatment for pregnant and non-pregnant women is identical.

The results of treatment appear to be very promising; thus Lentz and others[4] reported that although in cases of early syphilis untreated pregnant women almost uniformly gave birth to dead or diseased children, among 14 syphilitic mothers who were treated with penicillin not a single stillbirth or neonatal death occurred. Seven of the infants were known to be serologically negative and clinically healthy for periods up to 101 days *post partum.*

This illustrates the point that the foetus of an infected mother can be protected from certain diseases by the giving of adequate penicillin therapy to the mother. Penicillin has been shown by Herrell and others[5] and by Greene and Hobby[6] to pass through the placenta and to enter the foetal circulation. In some instances the foetal cord blood contained an amount of penicillin which was approximately half the amount present in the mother's blood. In general, the ratio of the amount of penicillin in the treated mother's blood to the amount in the blood of her foetus can be presumed to be approximately 2 : 1. It should therefore be possible by antenatal treatment of a syphilitic mother to protect her foetus from congenital syphylis. In practice the result seems to be achieved. Furthermore, a healthy and protected baby should be born even in the case of a mother suffering from, for instance, a severe generalized septicaemia, always provided that she receives intensive and adequate penicillin dosage.

Doubtless many other illustrations of foetal protection from some maternal disease contracted during pregnancy and adequately treated by penicillin will come to light in due course. At this point it might be convenient to mention that, although ideally all babies should be protected from congenital syphilis by penicillin treatment given to the mother, should a case be missed and a baby be born and later found to be infected with congenital syphilis, such a baby can suitably be treated with, and will respond satisfactorily to, penicillin. This subject is more fully discussed elsewhere.

Intranatal use of penicillin

Caesarean section and its risks.—One of the most significant points of value in penicillin therapy in obstetrics is the fact that we are now able to accept a certain degree of risk of maternal sepsis when such acceptance would give advantage to the baby. In such cases the prophylactic use of full doses of penicillin will usually prevent the development of any septic complications in the mother. Even in the unfortunate event of sepsis ensuing in consequence of some risky obstetric procedure, we have in penicillin so powerful a weapon that our fear of infection is considerably lightened.

The following type of case is an example. All obstetricians encounter from time to time a case in which labour has become obstructed with the foetal head deeply impacted in the pelvic cavity. This may be the result of outlet contraction or may follow labour in which there has been some malpresentation, for example, a face presentation in which the chin has rotated posteriorly. Perhaps even more common would be deep transverse arrest of an occipito-posterior position of the vertex complicated, it might be, by a minor degree of outlet contraction, so that attempts at the more usual methods of delivery have proved to be unsuccessful. In many of these cases there will have been considerable interference—attempts perhaps at manual rotation or forceps delivery or both. In such cases the obstetrician is faced with the choice of the performance of Caesarean section or of craniotomy. The latter course is, naturally, abhorrent if the child is living, and may be even the more dangerous of the two when modern weapons against sepsis are taken into consideration. The choice, in quite a considerable number of cases every year, will therefore be Caesarean section. The usual obstetric procedure would be to perform this operation by the lower segment route. Any obstetrician who has had to deliver a deeply impacted head through a lower segment incision is aware of the difficulties encountered in getting the head up out of the pelvis. The difficulties result in foetal death in a very great number of such cases. One has only to talk to anaesthetists who have witnessed these struggles, to get an impartial observer's view on the obstetric difficulties and the frequency of occurrence of stillbirths. These troubles and foetal dangers could be eliminated by the performance of the classical operation. The extraction of the baby is greatly facilitated by traction from above, and the birth of a living baby is almost certain provided that the foetal heart is beating well at the beginning of the operation. The classical operation in such a case, however, carries a tremendous risk of sepsis and until recently has been abandoned in cases in which the patient is in labour. Every obstetrician will agree that the lower segment operation is far and away the best operation for the patient in labour when the head is high and there is obstruction at the brim and a thin lower segment. Some obstetricians even go so far as to deny any place to the classical operation, and to say that the lower segment should be the chosen route in all cases, whether or not the mother is in labour. The more level-headed would probably consider that this was merely exalting technique at the expense of judgment and that there was still a place for the classical operation in modern obstetrics. The idea of doing the classical operation for the case late in labour and after operative attempts at vaginal delivery would rightly, however, have filled any surgeon with horror prior to the advent of penicillin. Now, for the type of case discussed at the beginning of this paragraph, it is suggested that the classical operation should again be adopted. It will save many foetal lives and will be justified in that the maternal risk is largely eliminated by a full 7-day course of systemic penicillin, which is started, if possible, before the operation is undertaken. Up to now, our personal experience is limited to one case, but in that one case the foetal extraction was found to be relatively easy, the baby cried almost immediately after birth and progressed satisfactorily. The mother had a satisfactory and afebrile puerperium. Obviously, judgment cannot be based on one isolated case, but success in that one case encourages further trial.

As an indication of the dosage that should be used in a prophylactic course of penicillin directed against septic infection likely to ensue after a risky classical Caesarean section, as in the above example or in any other obstetric interference which is judged to be particularly likely to be followed by infection, it is suggested that 20,000-40,000 units be given 3-hourly or 4-hourly for 7 days.

The prophylactic value of penicillin in obstetrics.—Puerperal sepsis has been the great bugbear of obstetricians for many centuries. Fear of it, in recent years, has diminished largely because of the successful therapeutic results achieved first by the sulphonamides and more recently by penicillin. There is, however, another factor, and that is the diminished virulence of the streptococcus in recent times. We see this not only in the lessened severity of cases of puerperal sepsis, but also in the lessened virulence of scarlet fever and erysipelas. There is not any reason, however, to believe that the impaired virulence of the streptococcus will persist for ever. One of these days it will regain full potency, and we may then expect an increase in the incidence and severity of puerperal infection.

Prevention of puerperal sepsis is now largely a matter of aseptic and antiseptic midwifery, of guarding against droplet infection from the respiratory tracts of attendants, of minimizing the danger of disseminating organisms from unsterilized blankets and of the prevention of epidemic spread. Despite all this, there are certain cases in which the danger of puerperal infection seems to be a real one. For example, there is the case in which there has been much bruising and laceration of soft tissues, the case of repeated operative attempts at delivery, the case of manual removal of the placenta, the obstetric patient whose resistance has been lowered by illness or haemorrhage, and the patient who has had the misfortune to be attended by a doctor or nurse in whom an infected respiratory tract or some other focus of infection has been discovered. These and many others may be regarded as patients for whom some special effort to ward off the threatened danger of sepsis would be justified. These are the cases in which a prophylactic course of penicillin therapy is advisable. It is suggested that such patients be given 20,000 or 40,000 units every 4 hours for 4 or even for 7 days. Alternatively, the slow absorption method of giving 200,000 units in beeswax-oil once a day for 4 days may be employed. The present time is not one when prophylactic penicillin on any wider scale would be suggested. The time may come, however, when the streptococcus is more virulent, when penicillin is more plentiful, and when some method of administration will have been devised whereby a high blood level of penicillin can be obtained by some relatively simple and infrequent method of administration. When this time arrives it may perhaps be practicable to give prophylactic penicillin treatment to all mothers as part of the routine obstetric management of the case.

Post-partum use of penicillin

In prophylaxis against ophthalmia neonatorum.—In chronological order, the first use for penicillin after delivery of the baby is as an instillation into its eyes as a prophylactic against ophthalmia neonatorum. Sorsby[7] has shown that all the common organisms which cause ophthalmia neonatorum seem to respond to penicillin therapy. In this treatment he advises the frequent instillation of strong preparations of penicillin and he advocates the use of a solution in the strength of 2,500 units per millilitre. This is not the place to discuss in detail the treatment of established ophthalmia neonatorum; it is dealt with elsewhere. The successful treatment of the established disease and the fact that the common causative organisms are penicillin-sensitive, clearly point to the possible use of penicillin as a prophylactic in the place of the silver salts at present in vogue—a prophylaxis which is, in fact, now on trial. A few drops of a solution of penicillin in the strength of 2,500 units per millilitre are instilled into the eyes of infants as soon after birth as is possible. The drops are well tolerated, but a practical difficulty is the keeping of a solution in a state of unimpaired activity when it has to be used day after day and often several times in one day. This means storage under refrigerator conditions and the constant preparation of fresh solutions. Because of these difficulties an attempt was made to use lamellae containing penicillin instead of a solution. The lamellae proved to be unsatisfactory since they were frequently extruded from the child's eyes very shortly after their—none too easy—introduction into the conjunctival space. The drop method therefore continues to be used, but some time must elapse before one can say whether or not the prophylaxis is complete.

In prophylaxis against puerperal sepsis.—The next important use for penicillin subsequent to delivery is in cases of puerperal sepsis. There are many reports of the effectiveness of penicillin in the treatment of severe puerperal infections by *Staph. aureus* or *Str. pyogenes* even in some cases in which heroic doses of the sulphonamides have failed[8,9,10]. The value of penicillin in these infections is so well known that it needs little further mention here. Herrell, in his book (p. 197)[11], states that he is inclined to believe that penicillin is one of the most effective agents yet available for the treatment of anaerobic streptococcal infections in the puerperium. Here is yet another type of puerperal sepsis in which good results can be expected from penicillin therapy.

There still remain the gas gangrene organisms as important causes of puerperal infection, and these too would presumably respond satisfactorily to penicillin treatment. For this infection, however, penicillin would have to be reinforced by the administration of antitoxin in heavy dosage. In puerperal gas gangrene, excision of necrotic and infected tissues, desirable as it would be, is not as simple a process, unfortunately, as it is in many cases of gunshot wound. Judging from the recommendation of Florey and Cairns[12] the penicillin should be given systemically in large dosage aggregating perhaps 1,000,000 units. In addition, any infected local vulval or vaginal laceration should receive local penicillin treatment with the powdered calcium salt or with a solution in the strength of at least 1,000 units per millilitre.

In the treatment of cases of puerperal sepsis caused by the commoner organisms, therapy on similar lines would seem to be indicated, although there is now some evidence that even heavier penicillin dosage may be desirable. Thus Hudson and his colleagues[13] stress the value of 60,000 units administered every 3 hours in severe cases of generalized sepsis of any type, including puerperal. This means that a patient receiving this dosage for 4 days—which can be only minimal—receives about 2,000,000 units.

In treatment of cracked nipples.—Another type of puerperal case which responds well to administration of penicillin is the common one of a mother with cracked nipples. Various dressings for the lesion have been recommended, but perhaps more valuable than any of the older remedies is penicillin cream. This is made up in the strength of at least 200 units per gramme of a base which is a mixture of Lanette wax SX and castor oil. Treatment of a cracked nipple consists in cessation of breast feeding for 48 hours, emptying of the breast by massage or breast pump whenever it gets uncomfortably distended, frequent cleansing of the crack and application of penicillin cream.

In treatment of breast abscess.—Breast abscess is yet another clear-cut indication for penicillin therapy. This unfortunate complication of the puerperium and the subsequent months is probably more common and more troublesome than it is realized to be by many of us who see the majority of our obstetrical cases in hospital. It is not always realized that breast abscess may appear weeks or months after lactation has been established. In any event, when it does occur it causes the patient great suffering and the doctor great anxiety. When we first began to treat this condition with penicillin we had great hopes that needling of the abscess, aspiration of the pus and the replacement of it by an equal volume of penicillin solution in the strength of 500–1,000 units to the millilitre, would prove to be sufficient. In some cases it is sufficient; but in this, as in the case of other abscess cavities, it is often found that although the contained pus is rendered sterile, there form sloughs which line the cavity and have to separate and to be discharged through a drainage incision. Or again, it may be found that one aspiration and replacement by penicillin may be followed by a re-accumulation of pus, so that a second aspiration and replacement has to be done. If pus should again accumulate, it will from time to time seep out through the old needle punctures, and again incision and drainage will be indicated. The wise treatment for a breast abscess is therefore rather more intensive than mere needling and replacement of pus by penicillin solution. This can, and should, be done as a first step; but, in addition, a course of systemic penicillin in the dosage of 20,000-40,000 units according to the severity of the case, given 4-hourly for 7 days, should be initiated. If the abscess cavity should again be found to be filled with pus at a second—certainly at a third—aspiration, an incision should be made and drainage should be established. This surgical attack will also probably be required in any case when the cavity is obviously large and there is likely to be difficulty in collapsing it. Incision and drainage expedites the cure in these cases and, as well, shows its value by facilitating the separation and discharge of any sloughs which may have formed.

GYNAECOLOGY

There are not as many interesting indications for the use of penicillin in gynaecology as there are in obstetrics. The substance can, however, be put to many valuable uses, and it will be obvious that any infection by the penicillin-sensitive organisms occurring as a complication during the course of a gynaecological case will be appropriately treated by this therapy. The purely gynaecological cases which respond best to this treatment are postoperative sepsis, pelvic cellulitis and salpingo-oophoritis.

Postoperative sepsis

This may be evidenced by abdominal wall suppuration or by suppuration spreading from a vaginal repair operation. The success of penicillin may be very striking, even in cases in which the sulphonamide drugs have failed. This is illustrated in a case of blood stream infection after a vaginal plastic operation, which is reported on by Hellman and Guilfoil[14]. For such cases, for abdominal wall suppuration or for other evidence of postoperative sepsis, a full 7-day course of penicillin injections every 3 hours day and night, in doses of 20,000–60,000 units on each occasion, are indicated.

Pelvic cellulitis

Pelvic cellulitis manifests itself as an inflammatory mass in the base of the broad ligament which bulges down the vaginal fornix on the affected side, displaces the uterus to the opposite side and tends to spread. The directions of spread are as follows. Usually the inflammatory mass enlarges laterally over the psoas and iliacus muscles and becomes palpable in the groin above the inguinal ligament; more rarely, the cellulitis spreads into the buttock through the lesser sciatic notch or down into the thigh along the femoral vessels or through the obturator foramen. Sometimes these masses resolve, sometimes suppuration occurs with subsequent pointing either into the vagina or the rectum, or in the line of spread. This condition may occur after childbirth, but is also found as a gynaecological complication, particularly of vaginal plastic operations or of hysterectomy, or when the cervix has been lacerated by attempts at dilatation. The sulphonamides have proved to be of considerable value in the treatment of acute and subacute pelvic cellulitis[11], but they have not been of special value in the treatment of some anaerobic streptococcal infections which occur after surgical procedures in the pelvis as well as after abortions and confinements. For these cases the full 7-day routine course of systemic penicillin is indicated. Forty thousand units given intramuscularly every 3 hours would be a suitable dose for a moderately severe case. If suppuration should occur, aspiration of the pus and replacement by penicillin solution, 5,000 units per millilitre, may be tried. Even after sterilization of the abscess cavity in this way, incision and drainage may be required for a few days in order to allow separation of sloughs.

Salpingitis, salpingo-oophoritis, pelvic peritonitis

By whichever name this condition is known, it is a condition of inflammation in the uterine appendages; usually it occurs *post abortum, post partum,* or as a complication of gonorrhoea. It follows, therefore, that the majority of cases of this disease should respond to penicillin therapy—and this response indeed occurs.

Some cases of salpingitis, however, are tuberculous in origin and may be diagnosable clinically by their subacute course and by associated uterine or other tuberculous lesions. Such cases would not respond to penicillin therapy; nor would cases of *Esch. coli* infection of the uterine tubes after some bowel lesion such as appendicitis or diverticulitis. The majority of tubo-ovarian infections, however, are caused by penicillin-sensitive organisms.

It is now accepted that surgical interference is hardly ever required for a case of acute salpingitis. These cases respond very well indeed to simple palliative treatment such as rest in bed, application of warmth to the lower abdomen, and administration of morphia or other analgesics. Recovery, especially in the early case before there is pus formation, is greatly assisted by the giving of sulphonamides, since the causative organism is usually the gonococcus or one of the pyogenic group, and these organisms, unless they have acquired resistance, are sulphonamide-sensitive. It is in the sulphonamide-resistant case that penicillin will be found to be particularly useful. Equally valuable is it for the patient who has already received so much of the sulphonamide group of drugs in the treatment of, say, postabortal uterine sepsis, as to have reached the limit of safe dosage. Yet a third indication would be the severe case which shows threatening indication of spread rather than of localization to the pelvic cavity. In all these cases systemic penicillin will be found very valuable. The substance could be given by continuous intramuscular drip, using 100,000 units in about 500 millilitres of physiological saline every day for 7 days; or 3-hourly or 4-hourly intramuscular injection of 20,000 units could be used. As much as 60,000 units given 3-hourly might be indicated for some exceptionally severe cases.

It has been said that penicillin has difficulty in passing the serous membrane barrier of the peritoneal and other serous cavities. Such statements can be disregarded. It is now clear that after intramuscular injection, penicillin rapidly diffuses into the peritoneal cavity. Miller and Foster[15] state that it is found in higher concentration there than in the blood. The appearance of penicillin in peritoneal fluid has been confirmed by Hughes[16], and he indicates that in cases in which penicillin cannot be found in peritoneal fluid after intramuscular injection, the absence may be because of the destruction of penicillin brought about by penicillinase produced by the infecting organism, which may be of the coliform group. This is not likely to happen in cases of salpingitis, and the beneficial effect of penicillin in these cases may perhaps be due in part to the appearance of penicillin in the peritoneal fluid. In any event, this form of therapy will be found to be very satisfactory in the majority of cases of salpingo-oophoritis. It will not be of benefit in the tuberculous case, however.

Infections of the vulva

Finally, there are two other suggested possible uses for penicillin. The first of these is in the case of a chronic pyogenic vulval infection which is sometimes implanted on senile degenerative changes in the vulva and the vagina. A large enough number of these cases has been treated to make it plain that the local application of penicillin cream advantageously reinforces the oral administration of the synthetic oesterogens which preferably should be given for a period not exceeding 10 days a month. The second suggestion is that the incorporation of penicillin in bougies which could be inserted into the cervical canal would be a suitable treatment for chronic cervicitis when the infection is caused by a penicillin-sensitive organism. This suggestion is under trial, and it is anticipated that good results will be secured.

REFERENCES

[1] Lentz, J. W., Ingraham, N. R., Jun., Beerman, H., and Stokes, J. H. (1944) *J. Amer. med. Ass.*, **126**, 408.
[2] Leavitt, H. M. (1945) *J. vener. Dis. Inform.*, **26**, 150.
[3] Speiser, M. D., and Thomas, E. W. (1946) *J. vener. Dis. Inform.*, **27**, 20.
[4] Lentz, J. W., Ingraham, N. R., Jun., Beerman, H., and Stokes, J. H. (1944) *J. Amer. med. Ass.*, **126**, 408.
[5] Herrell, W. E., Nichols, D. R., and Heilman, Dorothy H. (1944) *J. Amer. med. Ass.*, **125**, 1003.
[6] Greene, H. J., and Hobby, Gladys L. (1944) *Proc. Soc. exp. Biol., N.Y.*, **57**, 282.
[7] Sorsby, A. (1945) *Brit. J. Ophthal.*, **29**, 511.
[8] Keefer, C. S., Blake, F. G., Marshall, E. K., Jun., Lockwood, J. S., and Wood, W. B., Jun. (1943) *J. Amer. med. Ass.*, **122**, 1217.
[9] Mitchell, R. McN., and Kaminester, S. (1944) *Amer. J. Surg. N.S.*, **63**, 136.
[10] White, R. A. (1944) *Sth. med. J.*, **37**, 524.
[11] Herrell, W. E. (1945) *Penicillin and other Antibiotic Agents.* W. B. Saunders Co., Philadelphia and London.
[12] Florey, H. W., and Cairns, H. (1943) A preliminary report to the War Office and Medical Research Council on Investigations concerning the use of penicillin in war wounds. *Brit. med. J.*, **2**, 755.
[13] Hudson, R. V., Meanock, R. I., McIntosh, J., and Selbie, F. R. (1946) *Lancet*, **1**, 409.
[14] Hellman, A. M., and Guilfoil, E. F. (1944) *Amer. J. Obstet. Gynec.*, **47**, 125.
[15] Miller, C. P., and Foster, Alice Z. (1944) *Proc. Soc. exp. Biol., N.Y.*, **56**, 166.
[16] Hughes, K. E. A., *Penicillin Therapy and Control in* 21 *Army Group*, p. 333.

SEPSIS NEONATORUM

By Donald Paterson, M.D., F.R.C.P.

Physician, Hospital for Sick Children, Great Ormond Street; Physician for Children's Diseases, Westminster Hospital, London

and

Martin Bodian, M.D. Vienna, L.R.C.P. & S. Ed.

Pathologist, Hospital for Sick Children, Great Ormond Street, London

GENERAL CONSIDERATIONS

The newborn infant, particularly the premature infant, appears to be extremely susceptible to infections and these may manifest themselves in an obscure fashion. The generally recognized signs of infections in older infants and children may be entirely absent. There may not be any temperature, in fact, a high degree of fever in such infants is uncommon. The sepsis may show itself merely by limpness, apathy, a poor colour, failure of the infant to take feed or to thrive, diarrhoea or vomiting. From the foregoing it is clear that, in the past, infections in neonates, particularly of the blood stream, have often gone unrecognized.

Incidence of infections

Of 269 neonates admitted to the Hospital for Sick Children, Great Ormond Street, London, during the years 1943 and 1945, 40·7 per cent were found to be suffering from infections. These figures are also borne out by an analysis of 706 necropsies on neonates at the Children's Hospital, Birmingham[1], during which infections were found in 42 per cent of the cases. A slightly lower incidence was noted by Macgregor in Edinburgh[2], who found infections in 30 per cent of 465 neonatal deaths. Cruickshank[3] analysed 800 neonatal deaths, and found that 29·75 per cent of these were due to infections.

Bacteriology

The advent of chemotherapy has greatly stimulated research into the bacteriology of neonatal infections. Bodian[4], working at the Hospital for Sick Children, Great Ormond Street, found in a series of 78 patients under the age of one year, who were selected for penicillin treatment, that in 75 per cent of the cases the infecting organism was *Staph. aureus,* coagulase-positive. Of his 78 cases, 37 were investigated during the neonatal period, and of these 81 per cent were infected by *Staph. aureus*. Positive blood cultures were obtained in 25 of the 78 cases, and in 19 of these 25 cases (76 per cent) the organism was *Staph. aureus*.

Sixty-nine neonates were admitted to the Hospital for Sick Children, Great Ormond Street, during 1945, suffering from infections; 60 of these (an unselected series) were investigated bacteriologically and showed the following distribution of causative organism: (1) *Staph. aureus,* coagulase-positive, found to be entirely responsible or in conjunction with other organisms in 66·6 per cent of cases; (2) coliform organisms, alone or in conjunction with other organisms in 20 per cent of cases; (3) streptococci in 15 per cent of cases. A variety of other organisms made up the remainder. Of this series, 6 cases gave positive blood cultures, in 4 of which *Staph. aureus,* coagulase-positive, was isolated. Bodian suggests that the high rate of incidence of staphylococcal infection is not generally recognized by paediatricians.

The introduction of the sulphonamide group of drugs was a great advance, but, from the above figures, it is obvious that in this particular period of the infant's life, penicillin must be the therapeutic agent of choice.

Portal of entry of infection

There are 4 portals of entry: (1) the upper respiratory tract; (2) the umbilicus; (3) the skin; (4) the alimentary tract. From any of these sites a generalized blood stream infection may result which is due to the neonate's poor ability to localize its infection.

The investigation of an infected infant will therefore consist in obtaining bacteriological evidence from all these potential sites, that is, from material taken by swab from the eye, the nose, the throat, from the nasopharynx, from the umbilicus and from the rectum; in many cases a blood culture will be made and, in addition, swabs taken from any other obvious site of infection.

Clinical manifestations of sepsis in the newborn

Of the 69 neonates admitted to the Hospital for Sick Children during 1945, 56 were treated with penicillin. The clinical manifestations were as follows.

Umbilical infection	12
Diarrhoea and vomiting	10
Nasopharyngitis (including 1 diphtheritic)	10
Pneumonia (including bronchiolitis)	9
Septicaemia	9
Skin sepsis	8
Eye infections	6
Otitis media	4
Pyelitis	4
Thrush	2
Meningitis	1
Pericarditis	1
Tetanus	1

(In some cases more than one manifestation was present)

SPECIFIC DISEASES

Ophthalmia neonatorum (conjunctivitis)

This may be of a severe or virulent type, depending upon the organism involved and the state of nutrition of the infant. The duration of the infection before treatment has been instituted is also of importance. Sorsby[5] advocates the instillation of penicillin drops in the strength of 2,500 units per millilitre at very frequent intervals, even as often as every minute. His contention is that as fast as the drops are instilled they tend to be washed away, and unless they are continually replaced the treatment is of no avail. We have not had experience of this method of treatment, and it has been our custom to use penicillin drops in the strength of 500 units per millilitre every 3-4 hours, but in addition to give full doses of penicillin systemically at 4-hourly intervals (for dosage see p. 294). Sometimes the conjunctivitis occurs as part of a nasopharyngeal infection; in such circumstances the treatment is similar.

Example of a treated case

Female, aged 13 days. Birth weight 6 lbs. 14 ozs. Weight on admission 7 lbs. Abscess on chest wall, with severe conjunctivitis of 3 days' standing. General condition good. Eye swab and pus from abscess grew *Staph. aureus*, coagulase-positive; blood culture negative. Treatment was by 15,000 units of penicillin daily, given systemically, for 3 days, together with penicillin drops, 500 units per millilitre, 4-hourly for 3 days; abscess incised. Complete and rapid recovery.

Nasopharyngitis

This is an extremely common and important clinical manifestation, the diagnosis of which is too often missed. There may be slight nasal catarrh; the fauces are reddened; frequently there may be an otitis media of varying severity which may even show involvement of the mastoid cells. Accompanying the nasopharyngitis, symptomatic diarrhoea or vomiting, or both, are common. Too often attention is paid to the diarrhoea and vomiting, and the cause—the nasopharyngitis—is missed. The causative organism is usually the haemolytic streptococcus or *Staph. aureus,* but we have met one case in which the nasal swab yielded a growth of virulent Klebs-Löffler bacillus. The treatment consists in the giving of penicillin systemically together with one of the sulphonamides (for dosage see p. 304).

Example of a treated case

Male, aged 9 days. Birth weight 5 lbs. 4 ozs. One month premature. Weight on admission 5 lbs. Taking poorly; purulent nasopharyngitis; stools green and offensive. Nasal swab yielded a mixed, heavy growth of haemolytic streptococci and virulent K.L.B. of the intermedialis type, which was about 10 times less sensitive to penicillin than the Oxford standard strain of *Staph. aureus*. Anti-diphtheritic serum 10,000 units was given, also penicillin systemically 9,000 units per day for 10 days. Rapid clinical recovery followed by 3 negative K.L.B. swabs. No contact established.

See also *infra*, **Umbilical sepsis.**

Otitis media

The tympanic cavity and if necessary the mastoid processes should be dealt with surgically in conformity with the general principle that pus when present should be evacuated; any such surgical treatment should be covered by the systemic administration of penicillin.

Example of a treated case

Male, aged 5 weeks. Birth weight 3 lbs. 5 ozs. Weight on admission 2 lbs. 12 ozs. Three weeks premature. Subnormal temperature. Did not suck well; very tiny, wasted infant. Found to have a discharging right ear. Swab from ear gave a good growth of *Staph. aureus*, coagulase-positive. Blood culture yielded the same organism. Right mastoidectomy performed on the fifth day; yielded pus which on culture showed a good growth of *Staph. aureus*, coagulase-positive. Penicillin was given systemically from the day of admission for 9 days, 4,500 units each day. The blood culture was negative on the seventh day. Subsequent treatment comprised 3 blood transfusions for the persistent anaemia. R.B.C.s raised from 1,800,000 to 4,200,000. Discharged one month after admission weighing 5 lbs. 1 oz. Seven weeks later reported to be very well and had gained a further 4 lbs. 11 ozs.

Lung infections (including pneumonia)

In the neonate this condition is often quite unsuspected until revealed by x-ray. The treatment consists in the administration of one of the sulphonamides together with penicillin systemically. In staphylococcal pneumonia which has become well established prior to the commencement of treatment the prognosis is distinctly poor.

Example of a treated case

Male, aged 3 weeks. Birth weight 6 lbs. 13 ozs. Weight on admission 7 lbs. 6 ozs. Went off feeds 2 days prior to admission to hospital. Cough for one day. On examination pneumonic facies; right lung solid. Treated with Sulphamezathine and penicillin for 2 days and subsequently with penicillin only. 9,000 units of penicillin were given systemically, each day, for a total period of 18 days. On admission the postnasal swab grew *Staph. aureus*, coagulase-positive. The temperature settled in a few days, but the general condition remained poor. Final x-ray of the chest was suggestive of gangrene of the lung. At necropsy the whole of the right lung was adherent to the chest wall; the central part of the lower lobe formed a large multilocular abscess cavity from which *Ps. aeruginosa* was cultured. The lower lobe of the left lung was completely solid.

Umbilical sepsis

Infections may occur at the umbilicus both before and after the cord separates; it is often found that, when it is infected, the cord does not separate for a week or two, or even longer, and on the whole late separation must be looked upon as unsatisfactory. Accompanying the infection of the umbilicus there may be a general blood infection, with a variety of manifestations. The infection present at the umbilicus may pass to the liver *via* the umbilical vessels, and as a result liver necrosis accompanied by jaundice and sometimes gastro-enteritis may be present. In treatment, local penicillin is not recommended; it is better to dry the umbilicus with applications of rectified spirit and dusting powder, and to give penicillin systemically.

Example of a treated case

Male, aged 2 weeks. Birth weight 8½ lbs. Weight on admission 7½ lbs. Circumcised on the fourth day. Sucking poorly; very lethargic; septic spots on skin; umbilicus red and discharging pus; right tympanum red and bulging; tonsils also red. Umbilical swab, throat swab and swab of pus from right ear (myringotomy) all grew haemolytic streptococci, Lancefield Group A. Blood culture negative. Penicillin was given systemically—8,000 units daily for 4 days; bacteriology then negative, and the infant was discharged 5 days after admission to hospital gaining weight and his clinical condition most satisfactory.

Skin sepsis (pemphigus neonatorum; generalized furunculosis; cellulitis)

When the infection is not severe the application of penicillin cream, 500 units per gramme of base (see p. 53), is recommended. When the infection is severe and widespread the giving of penicillin systemically in addition to local application is desirable. Occasionally an infant may be found to be hypersensitive to the local application of penicillin; in such cases local application should be immediately discontinued and the penicillin given systemically.

Example of a treated case

Female, aged 3 weeks. Birth weight 6 lbs. Weight on admission 7 lbs. Vomiting for 5 days. Diagnosis of pyloric stenosis made and Ramstedt's operation performed under local anaesthesia. Three days later the abdominal wound was noticed to be infected with pus formation. *Staph. aureus*, coagulase-positive, was found to be the infecting organism. Penicillin was given systemically, 9,000 units daily. Three days after the beginning of penicillin therapy, 4 septic stitches were removed from the wound, and it was noted that the cellulitis was localizing. Penicillin was continued for a total period of 10 days. The infant was discharged having made a complete recovery.

Septicaemia and pyaemia

This may result from an infection which has gained entrance through the nasopharynx, the umbilicus, the skin, the alimentary tract or other portals. The manifestations of a septicaemia may be masked and clinically may be quite slight, the infant being merely listless, apyrexial, or failing to take its feeds or thrive. On the other hand, there may be gross manifestations of the blood infection, for example, diarrhoea and vomiting, bullous lesions of the skin, and multiple abscesses of the skin, subcutaneous tissues and internal organs. The treatment consists in the systemic administration of penicillin.

Example of a treated case

Male, aged 15 days. Birth weight 5 lbs. 14 ozs. Weight on admission 5 lbs. Three weeks premature. Took well for the first 2–3 days only. Since then had been gradually becoming more drowsy. Jaundiced from the third day. Kapilon (Methylnapthoquinone; Menadionum U.S.P. XII) had been given intramuscularly on the sixth and seventh days into the thighs. Abscesses had developed at the site of the injections on the eleventh day, accompanied by diarrhoea and vomiting and a temperature of up to 102° F. The abscesses were incised and haemolytic streptococci were grown from the pus and also from the blood culture. X-ray of the chest showed consolidation of the right lung. The infant was given penicillin systemically: 12,000 units daily for 8 days. On the sixth day of treatment an *Esch. coli* pyelitis developed, with an associated *Esch. coli* bacteriaemia and a temperature of 100° F. The urine and the blood culture were normal after 7 days' treatment with Sulphamezathine; the right lung had also cleared. The infant was discharged, but returned 10 days later with diarrhoea and vomiting. A focus of infection was not found. An intestinal obstruction developed, with large, bile-stained vomits and dehydration. Very gradual improvement took place on intravenous fluid therapy, combined with a further 15 days' systemic penicillin and also Sulphamezathine. This case provides an example of a severe neonatal infection in which during the course of penicillin treatment, Gram negative bacillary complications occurred; we therefore stress the importance of combined penicillin and sulphonamide therapy. At the age of 6 months the infant was reported to be progressing satisfactorily and weighed 16 lbs.

Septic parotitis

Occasionally the parotid gland becomes infected during the neonatal period. The organism is usually *Staph. aureus* or haemolytic streptococcus, and occasionally a positive blood culture may be obtained. The infection shows itself as a firm brawny swelling over the parotid gland; pus may be pressed from the parotid duct. Penicillin should be given systemically.

Example of a treated case

Male, aged 11 days. Birth weight 6 lbs. Weight on admission 6 lbs. 4 ozs. A large hard brawny swelling of the right parotid gland of 3 days' standing was present. Septic spots were present on the back of the head; there was slight jaundice. The umbilicus had not separated. Pus exuded from the parotid duct into the mouth; a growth of *Staph. aureus*, coagulase-positive, was obtained from culture of the pus. The infant was given 9,000 units of penicillin systemically daily for a period of 7 days. He made an uninterrupted recovery and was discharged from hospital after 11 days.

Septic arthritis and osteomyelitis

Although the theory is difficult to substantiate, it would appear that these conditions are due to a blood-borne infection. Only occasionally can a positive blood culture be obtained. Septic arthritis may show itself as a swelling of one or more joints; the knee, shoulder and hip joints are most commonly affected. Aspiration of the joint, followed by the introduction of 2,000 units of penicillin, is indicated, together with the giving of penicillin systemically. Repeated aspirations may be necessary. Arthritis may be accompanied by an osteomyelitis in an adjoining bone or the osteomyelitis may be present in some other part of the body. The treatment should be systemic penicillin, with the aspiration of any subsequent abscess formation, and the instillation of penicillin (2,000 units) into the abscess cavity. Usually it is desirable to continue treatment for a fortnight or longer, until all signs of the infection have completely subsided. The x-ray picture may be misleading and may lag behind the clinical and bacteriological recovery. Should a sequestrum form, this should be removed; penicillin therapy should be continued during this process, and usually the wound may be closed immediately.

Examples of treated cases

Septic arthritis.—Male, aged 18 days. Birth weight 7 lbs. 10 ozs. Weight on admission 7½ lbs. Admitted with pseudoparalysis of the right arm and swollen shoulder joint. Purulent discharge from both eyes. X-ray showed considerable widening of the joint space. Ten millilitres of thick pus were aspirated from the shoulder joint. *Staph. aureus*, coagulase-positive, grown from the pus, the eye swab and from the blood culture. The pus was replaced with 1,500–2,000 units of penicillin daily, and latterly every second day, for a total period of 3 weeks. Cultures from the shoulder joint were negative after 8 days' penicillin treatment. Penicillin was also given intramuscularly: 9,000 units daily for 9 days. Total systemic penicillin, 80,000 units; total local penicillin, 30,000 units. On discharge, 25 days after admission, there were not any signs of inflammation in the neighbourhood of the joint and movement of the arm was slowly returning. Four months later, there was no x-ray evidence of bone disease and the infant had full movement of the arm.

Osteomyelitis.—Female, aged 25 days. Birth weight 7 lbs. 12 ozs. Weight on admission 7 lbs. 6 ozs. For 3 days there had been swelling of the right leg; a septic spot had been noted on the head 15 days previously. X-ray diagnosis: osteomyelitis of fibula with considerable cavitation of bone and raising of periosteum for half of the length of the fibula. The abscess which presented itself was aspirated daily; the pus yielded a growth of *Staph. aureus*; the blood culture was negative on 2 occasions. Penicillin was injected into the abscess cavity each day, 1,500 units being injected daily for a period of 6 days; at the same time penicillin was given systemically. Total systemic penicillin, 50,000 units; total local penicillin, 9,000 units. The temperature of 102° F. subsided on the third day. The infant was discharged at the end of a fortnight with only slight clinical thickening of the lower end of the leg; 4 weeks later there was no clinical evidence of abnormality. At the end of 5 months the x-ray showed thickening of the fibula only but not any evidence of sequestration.

Tetanus

In addition to tetanus antitoxin, which in the neonate has not proved to be very efficacious, the administration of penicillin appears to be of real value since the tetanus bacillus is penicillin-sensitive. Adequate sedation with Avertin (Bromethol B.P. Add. III; Liquor Tribromoaethanolis U.S.P. XII) or phenobarbitone (Phenobarbitonum B.P.; Phenobarbitalum U.S.P. XII) is also most important.

Examples of treated cases

(1) Male, aged 2 weeks. Birth weight 7 lbs. (forceps delivery). One day's history of feeding difficulty with spasm. Clenched mouth and fists; rigidity of abdomen. Cord had separated a week previously and the umbilicus had not been moist since that time. Culture from the umbilical swab did not grow pathogens. Diagnosis of tetanus neonatorum was made. Treated with sedatives: Avertin, paraldehyde and phenobarbitone. 20,000 units of tetanus antitoxin were given intravenously, and penicillin, 1,250 units each 4 hours for a period of 5 days. At necropsy toxaemic changes of the parenchymatous organs were noted; the umbilicus, excised under sterile conditions, was cultured and a mixed growth of haemolytic streptococci and *Cl. tetani* was obtained.

(2) Male, aged 12 days. Birth weight 8¼ lbs. Unwell for 6 days, refused to suck; did not open mouth properly; on admission spasms of breath holding and rigidity of body; spasms whenever handled. Umbilicus dirty. *Cl. tetani* not isolated from umbilical swab. Diagnosis of tetanus neonatorum was made. Intravenous feeding with the addition of phenobarbitone* was begun on the second day after admission and continued for 6 days. Attempt at tube feeding was not made during these 6 days. 60,000 units of tetanus antitoxin given intravenously in 2 doses with a 2-hour interval between the doses. Penicillin was given, 1,500 units each 4 hours, in the first instance by intravenous drip and later intramuscularly, for a total period of 14 days. A total of 79,000 units of penicillin given. Transient oedema developed, but the spasms gradually became less and ultimately the infant made a complete recovery.

*1 gr. i.v. daily for 2 days
$\frac{1}{6}$ gr. orally 4-hourly for 5 days
$\frac{1}{4}$ gr. orally 4-hourly for 5 days
$\frac{1}{4}$ gr. orally 3 times daily for 3 days

Congenital syphilis

This condition is often undiagnosed until after the first month of life (the neonatal period). The general principles of treatment are the administration of penicillin systemically in minimal doses at first, the daily dosage being gradually increased to that advocated in other infections (for dosage see p. 288). This method spreads the average length of treatment over a period of 3 weeks; the total dose will be proportional by body weight to that of the average adult (160 lbs.), bearing in mind that the adult receives 2,400,000 units per course; for example, an infant weighing one-tenth of an adult's body weight would receive a total of 240,000 units during the 3 weeks. When other bacterial infections are present, such as the haemolytic streptococcus in the nasopharynx, it has been found to be advantageous to give one of the sulphonamide drugs in addition during the period of low penicillin dosage.

Example of a treated case

No case of congenital syphilis has been treated at the Hospital for Sick Children, Great Ormond Street during the neonatal period. We therefore quote a specimen case in a young infant treated with penicillin.

Male, aged 3½ months. Birth weight 4 lbs. A premature (7 months) infant; underweight, miserable, with florid congenital syphilis; marked, typical, coppery rash; snuffles. Weight on admission 8 lbs. Hepatosplenomegaly; anaemia (R.B.C. 3,000,000; Hb. 55 per cent); x-ray of long bones: periosteal elevation along the shafts of both tibiae, with notching of the middle border of the proximal end of the shafts. Blood W.R. strongly positive (serum in dilution of 1 in 480 completely fixed complement). Kahn ++. C.S.F.: normal protein and cell count, W.R. negative. Penicillin was given for a period of 3 weeks as follows: 4,500 units daily for 4 days; 6,000 units daily for 2 days; 7,500 units daily for 2 days; 9,000 units daily for 2 days; 10,000 units daily for 11 days. Total penicillin given: 170,000 units. The skin lesions rapidly disappeared; hepatosplenomegaly receded gradually; snuffles disappeared last. The child gained weight satisfactorily. Reaction to penicillin therapy was not noted. The long bones appeared normal on x-ray 2 months after the beginning of treatment; the blood W.R. was negative in

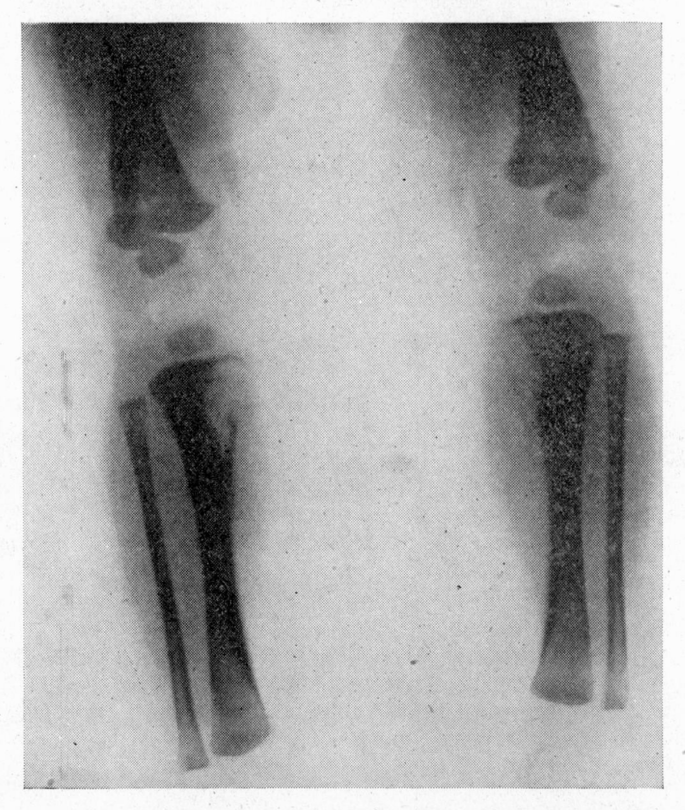

FIG. 49.—Congenital syphilis. X-ray photograph before treatment (*by courtesy of Dr. Bernard Schlesinger*)

10 weeks and the Kahn 7 months after treatment was started. More than one year's follow-up does not show any change in the situation.

We should like to draw attention to the fact that early in our series we did observe severe reactions to penicillin therapy, but this was at the time when treatment was begun with full doses of penicillin; for this reason the suggestion is made that in the treatment of cases of congenital syphilis very small doses should be given to start with, these should be gradually increased to the full dose, and the course of treatment should be spread over a period of 3 weeks.

The very marked improvement in the skiagrams of another case of congenital syphilis which was treated with penicillin is shown in Figs. 49 and 50.

The patient was a male, aged 3 months. The Wassermann reaction was negative 4 months after treatment was begun.

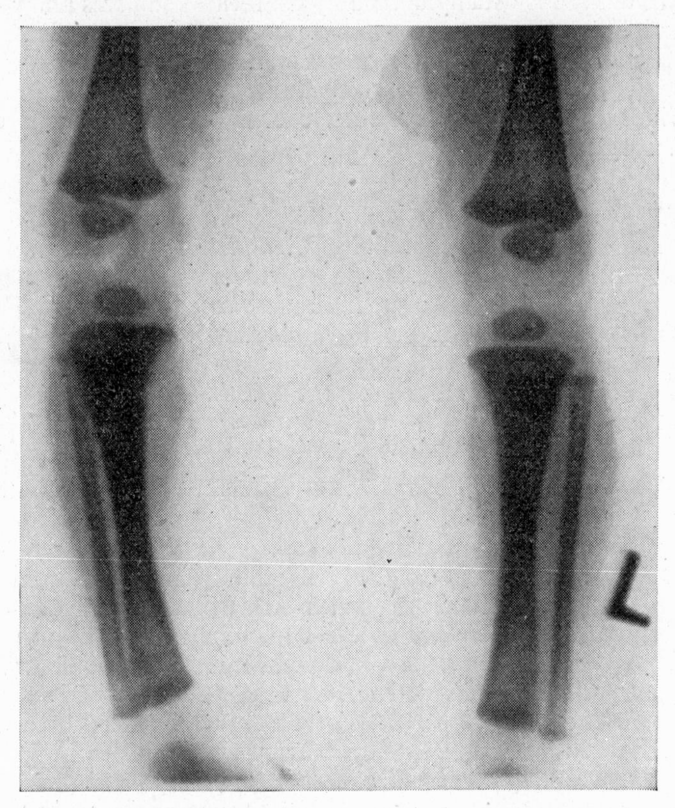

FIG. 50.—Congenital syphilis. X-ray photograph after treatment (5 weeks later) (*by courtesy of Dr. Bernard Schlesinger*)

Meningitis

Streptococcal, pneumococcal, staphylococcal or meningococcal meningitis, as well as some types of *H. influenzae* (Pfeiffer's bacillus) are penicillin-sensitive and therefore may be treated with systemic penicillin; it will be necessary also to give penicillin intrathecally because of the blood-cerebrospinal fluid barrier. A suitable intrathecal dose would be 2,000 units in 1 millilitre twice daily at the beginning; later the dose should be given less often, depending upon the progress made. The intrathecal treatment may require to be prolonged beyond the systemic treatment. It is advisable to administer a suitable sulphonamide at the same time. We personally have not treated any such cases during the neonatal period.

Pyelitis

This disease is usually caused by coliform organisms and one of the sulphonamides will therefore be found to be most efficacious. On the other hand, if the organism is penicillin-sensitive (for example, the streptococcus), penicillin may be given with benefit, provided an associated obstructive element, if present, is dealt with surgically.

Stomatitis

When stomatitis is caused by *M. albicans* (thrush), penicillin treatment is not indicated as this organism is not penicillin-sensitive. In some cases, however, the causative organism may be the haemolytic streptococcus or *Staph. aureus* ; in such circumstances the condition is rapidly cleared with systemic penicillin combined with penicillin painted locally on the lesions.

GENERAL PRINCIPLES OF TREATMENT WITH PENICILLIN

Dosage

The problem of the dosage of penicillin in infants and neonates was investigated at the Hospital for Sick Children, Great Ormond Street, under the auspices of the Penicillin Trials Committee of the Medical Research Council (1944-1945)[6]. Adequate dosage was calculated on the basis of 1,000 units of penicillin per pound of expected body weight per 24 hours. Because of the slower excretion rate of the infant's kidney, it has been found to be possible to space the single penicillin dose at 4-hourly intervals, rather than the 3-hourly intervals as used in the case of adults. In infants, intermittent intramuscular injections are found to be far superior to continuous intramuscular treatment, since the risk of secondary contamination by excreta is thus at a minimum. Intravenous treatment tended to lead to early thrombosis of veins and is not generally recommended. Penicillin appears to be extremely well tolerated by neonates.

An adequate blood penicillin level can be maintained in premature infants for 6 hours, and it is therefore recommended that 6-hourly injections are most suitable for such infants.

Calcium and sodium salts of penicillin are equally suitable in the treatment of neonates.

Many infants tend to pass large quantities of urine while they are having penicillin ; their state of hydration has therefore to be watched very carefully and any dehydration has to be made good.

ANALYSIS OF THE RESULTS IN 69 NEONATES TREATED WITH PENICILLIN AT THE HOSPITAL FOR SICK CHILDREN, GREAT ORMOND STREET, LONDON, DURING 1944–1945

CONDITION	TOTAL NO. OF CASES	CURED	DIED	
Septicaemia	23	17	6	1 *Esch. coli* pyelitis, pneumonia and D & V 1 acute nephritis 1 numerous abscesses 1 prolonged sulphonamide treatment; penicillin for last 4 days of life only 1 premature; came late to hospital 1 with cirrhosis of liver
Nasopharyngitis	10	7	3	1 premature 1 with severe D & V
Umbilical sepsis	9	8	1	(1 with liver necrosis)
Otitis media	8	7 (1 with mastoiditis)	1	(1 with mastoiditis)
Pyodermia	8	8	0	
Lung infections	6	4	2	hospital admission late in the disease
Ophthalmia neonatorum (conjunctivitis)	4	4	0	
Cellulitis	4	3	1	(necropsy showed lung abscesses)
Septic parotitis	3	3	0	
Tetanus neonatorum	2	1	1	
Septic arthritis	2	1	1	1 prolonged sulphonamide treatment; penicillin for last 4 days of life only
Osteomyelitis	1	1	0	
Diphtheria (nasal)	1	1	0	

It should be noted that more than one condition was present in some cases. Of the 69 patients, 14 died, that is, the mortality was 20·3 per cent.

Methods of administration

Systemic administration.—The solution should be made up in physiological saline or distilled water, to contain one calculated dose in 1 millilitre of the solution.

Local application.—This can be, for example, intrathecal in meningitis, intrapleural in empyema, intra-articular in septic arthritis, or into an abscess cavity after the evacuation of pus; 2,000 units per single injection is usually found to be adequate, the solution being made up to contain the 2,000 units in 1 millilitre of physiological saline or distilled water.

Cream.—For application as cream, 500 units are contained in 1 gramme of Lanette wax SX base; this is a non-oily and completely non-irritant base.

Eye drops.—For local application as eye drops, 500 units of penicillin in 1 millilitre of physiological saline should be instilled into the eye each 3-4 hours.

Vapour.—We have very little experience of the method of giving penicillin as vapour for inhalation to infants with infections of the respiratory tract. It is true to say, however, that the penicillin blood level may be maintained at an efficient height by this convenient mode of administration.

REFERENCES

[1] Parsons, L. G. (1944) *Lancet*, **1**, 267.
[2] Macgregor, Agnes R. (1943) *Edinb. med. J.*, **50**, 332.
[3] Cruickshank, J. N. (1930) *Spec. Rep. Ser. Med. Res. Counc. Lond.*, No. 145.
[4] Bodian, M. (1946) *Arch. Dis. Childh.* (in press).
[5] Sorsby, A. (1945) *Brit. J. Ophthal.*, **29**, 511.
[6] Bodian, M. (1945) *Proc. R. Soc. Med.*, **38**, 572.

BRAIN AND MENINGEAL INFECTIONS

By A. Dickson Wright, M.S., F.R.C.S.
Surgeon in Charge of Out-patients, St. Mary's Hospital, London

Sepsis inside the cranial cavity has always exacted a heavier toll than sepsis elsewhere for the following two reasons. (1) The dangerous intracranial pressures and cerebral dislocations produced by inflammatory collections inside the unyielding and partitioned cranial cavity, and (2) the poor defence of the acellular cerebrospinal fluid against bacterial infection.

Penicillin has come as a greater boon in this region than anywhere else, and as the Gram negative bacilli are infrequently encountered practically the whole field of intracranial infection is brought under effective control.

As a large proportion of intracranial abscesses and meningitis is caused by spread from infections of the middle ear and accessory nasal sinuses, the improvement in the treatment of these primary conditions with penicillin will produce a great reduction in the intracranial complications. Furthermore the primary condition should not be forgotten in the struggle with the dangerous secondary intracranial complication and it is essential to keep up a steady systemic administration of penicillin in these cases to control the primary condition, not forgetting the appropriate aural and nasal surgical treatments if required. Furuncles and carbuncles of the head and face when treated in good time with penicillin, will not produce the intracranial thromboses, abscesses and meningitis as of yore. In this connexion the general practitioner has a great opportunity of giving treatment in the early stages of all these septic conditions of the head and face before intracranial mischief is established. Scalp wounds and compound fractures of the vault are also treated with local and general penicillin and primary abacterial healing obtained, so reducing the incidence of another cause of intracranial sepsis. Fracture of the base of the skull with escape of cerebrospinal fluid from the ear should be treated with penicillin ear drops or penicillin and sulphadiazine powder. When the cerebrospinal fluid escapes from the nose a penicillin nose spray will serve to prevent meningitis also.

Osteomyelitis of the skull

This condition generally originates from sepsis in the frontal sinuses. Due to the staphylococcus it was previously a condition with an almost 100 per cent death rate, and it was quite common for the whole of the vault to be reduced to a crepitant shell of sequestra and granulation tissue before death ensued from

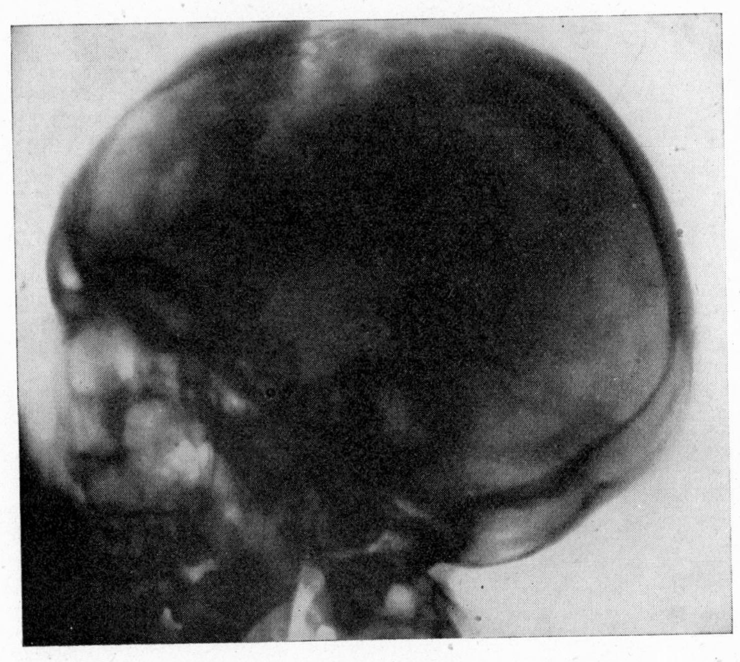

Fig. 51.—Osteomyelitis of skull. Before treatment

intracranial infection (see Fig. 54). Systemic penicillin in the usual doses effectively controls the spread of the sepsis and surgical treatment consists in opening any fluctuation in the scalp and inserting a small tube for penicillin instillations of a strength of 1,000 units to the millilitre. Intracranial complications are treated separately if they appear. A most remarkable restoration of the bony architecture of the vault is possible with penicillin; the bone as shown by skiagram, disorganized and "fluffed" out of recognition, is gradually returned to normal (see Figs. 51 and 52).

Extradural abscess

This is a complication of mastoid and frontal sinus suppuration and also of compound fractures of the skull, especially those involving the frontal and ethmoid sinuses. These large dissecting collections of pus between dura and bone were notoriously difficult to drain as the pus was in a thin layer and stripped up the dura over a large area frequently extending to inaccessible regions over the base of the skull (see Fig. 53). A burr hole is now made over the most accessible part of the abscess and Carrel tubes are passed into the cavity in various directions. Injection of small amounts of penicillin, 1,000 units per millilitre strength, into these tubes once a day, combined with systemic administration, transforms the whole situation in a short time and ready healing is obtained.

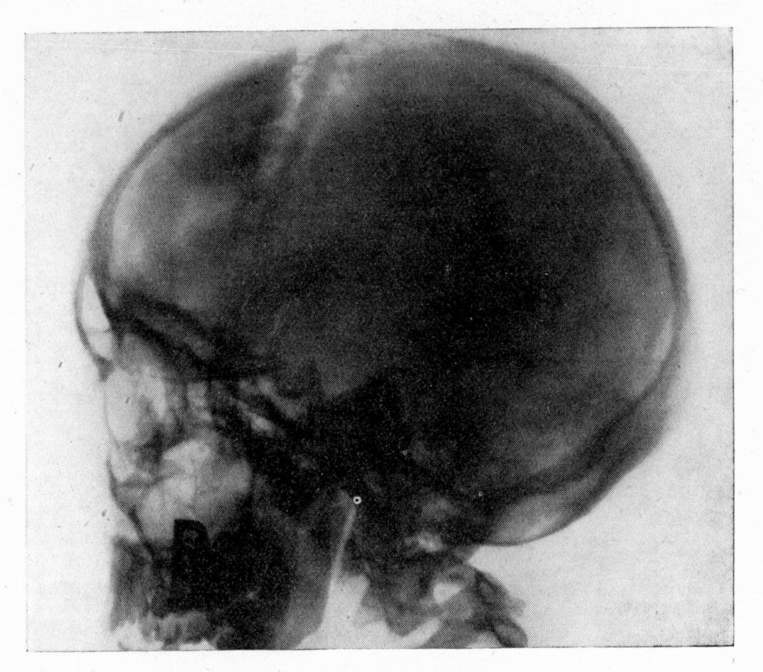

Fig. 52.—Osteomyelitis of skull. After treatment

Brain abscess

In the most expert hands up to the advent of penicillin brain abscess carried a mortality rate of 30–40 per cent. In keeping with this high death rate there was great division of opinion on treatment. Since the advent of penicillin the Dandy method is now established as the best. The abscess is localized clinically or if necessary by ventriculography. A small burr hole is made immediately over it. The abscess is now punctured with a brain needle and the pus sucked out. Penicillin, 1,000 unit strength, is injected into the cavity, half of the volume of the aspirated pus being used, and one millilitre of Thorotrast can be added to the penicillin without any reduction in the antiseptic powers; this will help in the future study of the abscess by skiagrams. The pus is, of course, examined by direct examination and by culture, especially anaerobically, because it is more common to find penicillin-resisters in abscesses than in any other cerebral infection. Mixed infections are also found in abscesses and possibly one organism of two or three is resistant; in these cases sulphonamides can be instilled with penicillin as recommended by de Wet.

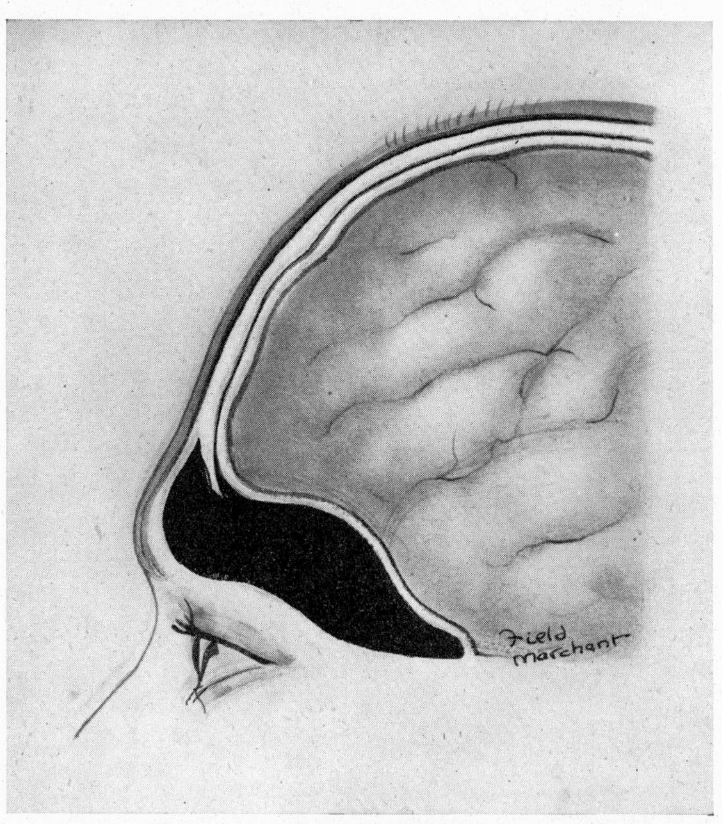

FIG. 53.—Extradural abscess tracking over the base of the skull

The necessity for further aspirations and injections will depend on the patient's degree of consciousness. Any tendency to lapse into coma will demand a repetition of the procedure. If the patient does not improve as expected then the following possibilities must be considered: (1) the pus is too viscid or contains necrotic lumps and aspirates badly; (2) is there another abscess present close to the one already found? A search should be made with the needle to a greater depth so as to pass through the far wall of the already tapped abscess. If this reveals no deeper abscess then the needle should be withdrawn and passed in alternative directions in a search for adjoining loculi (see Fig. 56); (3) is there a remote abscess present in a silent area of the brain? This is most likely to occur when the abscess is secondary to pulmonary suppuration or pyaemia. The ventriculograms should be studied again from this

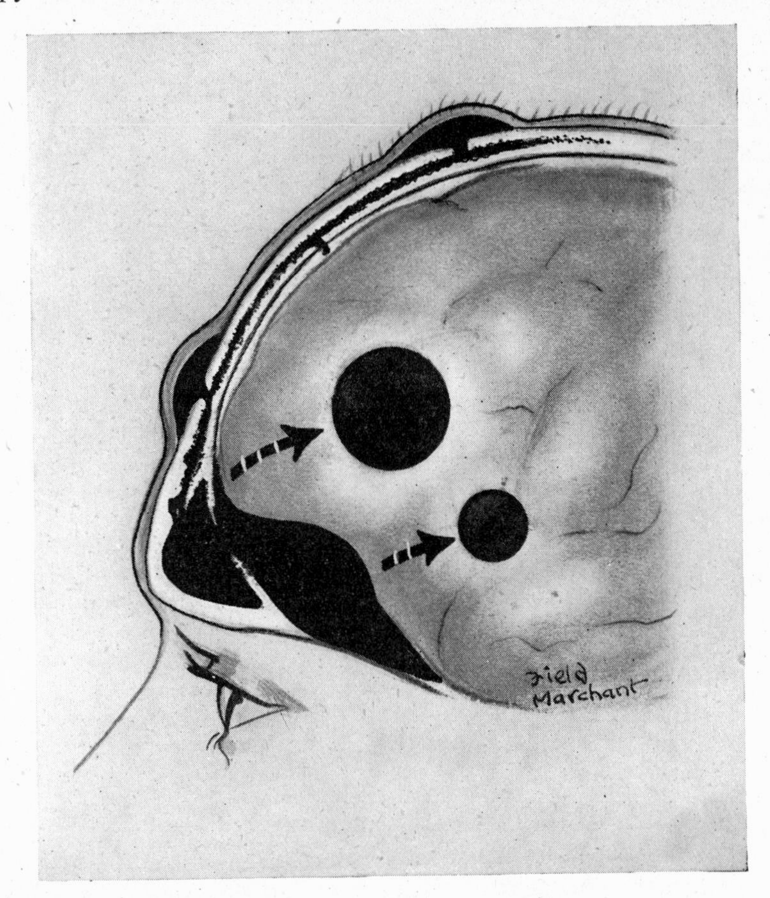

FIG. 54.—Spreading osteomyelitis of the skull illustrating the spread of the infection

point of view, or if the first abscess has been located clinically, ventriculography should now be carried out so as to leave nothing to chance (see Fig. 57); (4) in otogenic cases are there cerebellar and temporosphenoidal abscesses present simultaneously? It often happens that the cerebellar abscess gives less indication of its presence than the other. Needling in the site of a temporosphenoidal abscess is always justified in a case of this kind which does not improve quickly (see Fig. 55); (5) the abscess has formed in conjunction with a breaking-down secondary growth. This is especially liable to occur when the primary growth is a bronchial carcinoma. Careful examination of the pus may reveal malignant cells and even keratin; (6) the organism, or one of the organisms, may be resistant to penicillin or a fresh organism such as *Ps. aeruginosa* has found its way in during the punctures.

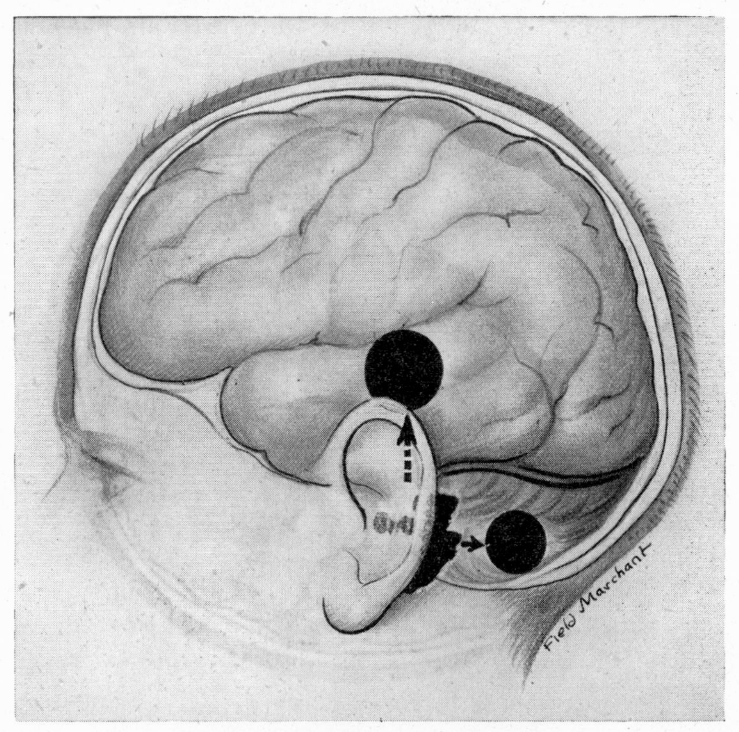

FIG. 55.—In aural cases abscesses may be present both above and below the tentorium

Careful repeat bacteriological examinations should therefore be carried out each time pus is obtained from the abscess.

If all these possibilities have been excluded and the patient does not improve with regard to consciousness, then it is probable that the surrounding oedema and encephalitis are not resolving fast enough after bacterial activity in the central abscess cavity has ceased and a general depletive treatment with rectal magnesium sulphate solution and possibly intravenous hypertonic solutions has been given. There should now be no hesitation in opening the skull widely with the usual bone flap approach and then dissecting the abscess out *en coque*, as recommended by Vincent, without spilling its contents. If the abscess ruptures and contaminates the field this is no longer a catastrophe, and the pus should be carefully sucked out. Careful search must be made for satellite abscesses and these must be removed also. At the end of the operation all the abscess material will have been evacuated. Although the subarachnoid space is opened up, and frequently the lateral ventricles, this is of no great moment because penicillin fluid distributed throughout the wound will care for any remaining

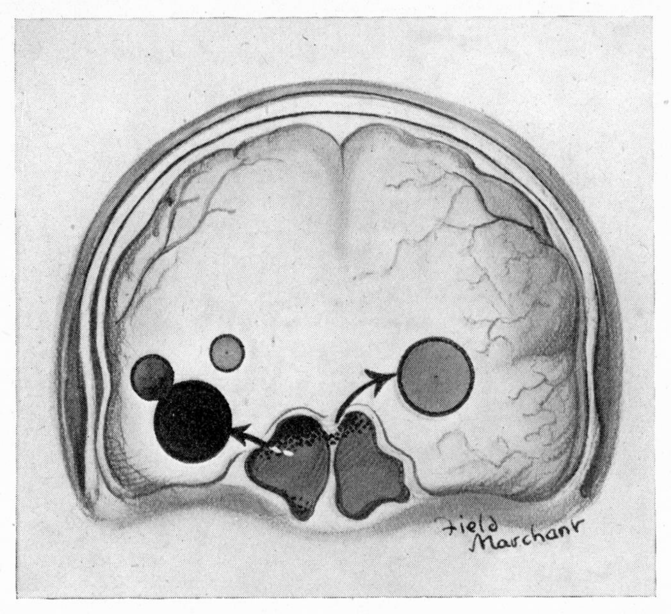

FIG. 56.—Illustrating how an infection in the frontal sinus may cause single or multiple abscesses in the brain with uninvolved brain substance in between

organisms very satisfactorily. During the closure penicillin fluid or penicillin and sulphadiazine powder, if left between the layers of the wound, will deal with any infection in these parts. For the 2 or 3 days following operation a blunt brain needle is insinuated under the flap and a small quantity of 1,000 unit per millilitre strength penicillin fluid introduced strategically into the operation field. Systemic penicillin for 7 days after the operation is an added precaution and prevents osteomyelitis of the bone flap. Any sign of meningitis will be an indication for intrathecal penicillin treatment.

Future series of brain abscess cases will show a reduction of mortality probably to 5 per cent, because 9 out of 10 patients will get well by aspiration alone and in the tenth patient bold exposure with no fear of postoperative sepsis will make all the difference.

Septic intracranial thrombosis

Septic intracranial thrombosis secondary to otic infections, facial carbuncles and dental sepsis were conditions of the greatest danger in prepenicillin days. Cavernous sinus thrombosis carried a mortality rate of almost 100 per cent. A substantial number of

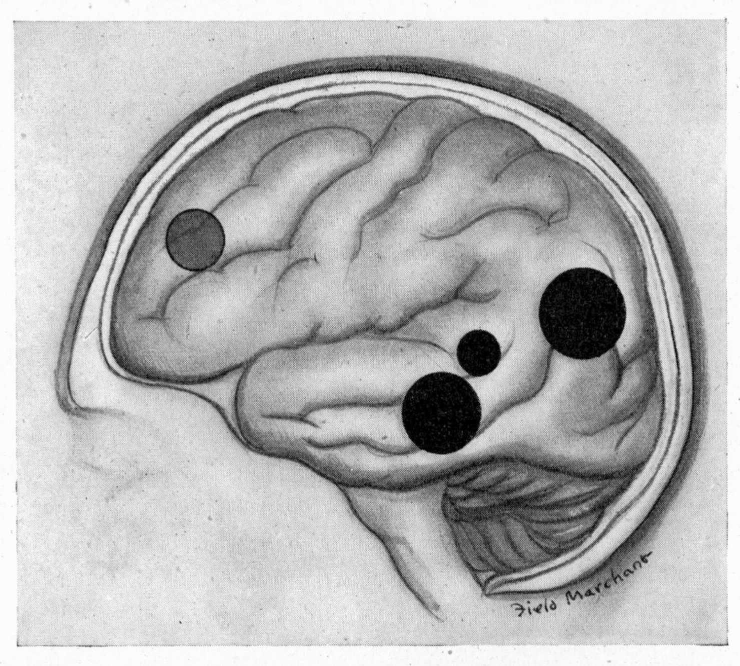

FIG. 57.—Multiple abscesses of the brain secondary to thoracic suppuration. Some may give localization signs and others in silent areas can only be discovered by ventriculography

these patients recover with systemic penicillin therapy and it is reasonable to suppose that with a better realization of the dangers of facial infections and an earlier recourse to penicillin therapy cavernous sinus thrombosis may become of only historical interest. The picture of the extremely toxic patient with intense exophthalmos, immobile chemotic globes and complete loss of vision is well known. The whole aspect seems hopeless in the last degree, yet with routine penicillin treatment I have seen these apparently hopelessly ill patients recover. The swellings all subside, the movements and vision return to the eyes and the patient recovers from the ordeal without any mark. The recovery of the patient from the local condition and its concomitant septicaemia allows complications to appear nowadays which were not seen before because death resulted early. For instance, the orbital swelling may recur, but in a slightly different form, and is now due to a staphylococcal orbital abscess which must be drained. The lungs will show pyaemic staphylococcal abscesses and the larger ones may require drainage because secondary infection from penicillin-resisters may occur and an empyema may form which will also need drainage because of secondary infection. Thromboses in the lateral sinus from mastoid disease did not carry the identical risks as the same condition in the cavernous sinus because the ligation of the jugular vein in the neck often puts an end to the pyaemic spread. It is probable that this operation will not be necessary now because the septic thrombosis will be controlled by penicillin alone.

MENINGITIS

The dread of this disease has been greatly diminished by the advent of the sulphonamides, which pass the blood-brain barrier and obtain a good concentration in the brain tissues and fluids. Although a very satisfactory reduction in mortality and sequelae was obtained by those drugs the death rate was still very considerable, especially in the cases due to the Gram positive cocci and even the meningococcus.

Treatment would have been very simple if systemic penicillin were as effective as sulphonamides in traversing the blood-brain barrier, but this highly selective screen does not permit the passage of penicillin. There is, however, some evidence to show that the blood-brain barrier loses some of its effectiveness in inflammatory diseases of the brain and meninges and permits some penicillin to reach the brain fluids. It is therefore worth while administering systemic penicillin in all cases of Gram positive coccal meningitis not only to secure the benefit of this slight seepage but also to deal with the primary focus so often present in the ears, accessory sinuses, lungs or cardiac valves. Needless to say any incarcerated collection of pus in the tympanic antrum or nasal sinuses should be drained without delay. Although penicillin does accomplish curative miracles that is not any reason why it should produce a lack of watchfulness on the part of the surgeons, who should be ready to help whenever there is a collection of pus to be drained.

Treatment by penicillin is indicated for the following cases: (1) all pneumococcal cases; (2) streptococcal cases with the exception of some due to *Str. viridans* penicillin-resistant strains; (3) all meningococcal cases; (4) all staphylococcal cases; (5) some cases due to Pfeiffer's bacillus (*H. influenzae*) in which the infecting strain is inhibited by high penicillin concentrations which are easily obtained in the closed subarachnoid space.

As the blood-brain barrier stands between the circulating blood

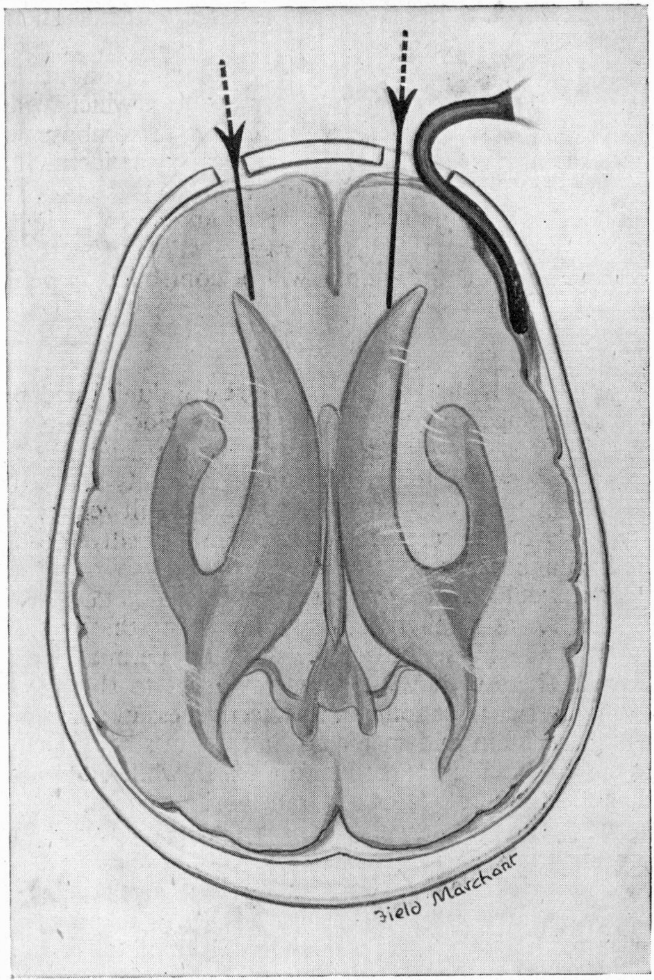

FIG. 58.—Introduction of penicillin in pneumococcal meningitis by means of catheter passed over surface of brain after aspirating the ventricle

and the brain tissues and fluids it is necessary to by-pass this barrier by injecting the penicillin solution directly into the cerebro-spinal fluid by lumbar, cisternal and ventricular puncture. It is noteworthy that this was first done by Fleming in 1941 (on a case due to *Str. viridans*) with complete restoration to health of a moribund patient. It was a bold step to introduce an antiseptic into such a holy of holies as the subarachnoid space, but the bland fluid did not produce any harm. Previously the use of

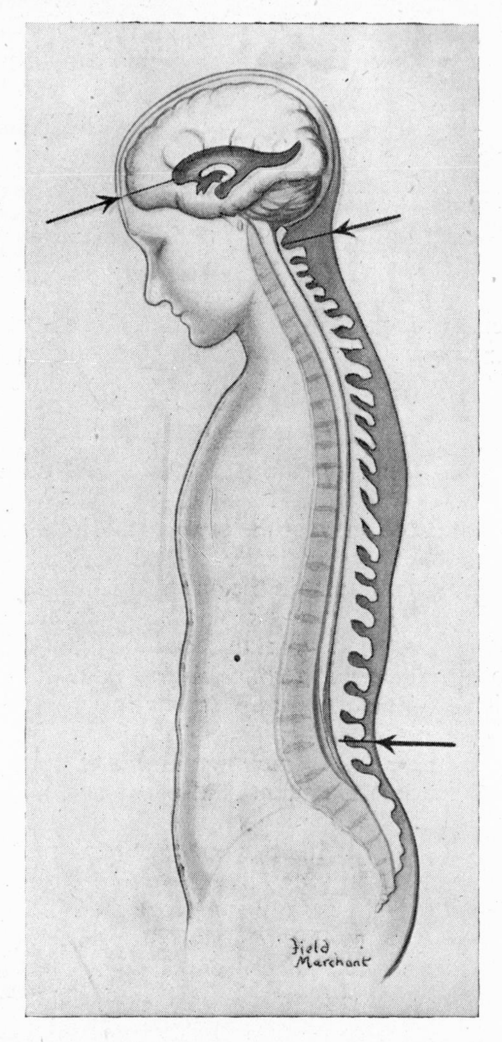

FIG. 59.—Sites for introduction of penicillin in cases of meningitis

antiseptics in the thecal space had led to some sad tragedies. Fleming's patient recovered with lumbar puncture alone, but this could not be hoped for in all cases; for instance, little diffusion of the fluid given by lumbar puncture can be expected in the infected ventricles. Cairns first introduced the fluid into the ventricles and met with great success. Even with the ventricular and lumbar introduction of the fluid patients still died to the extent of 10 per cent; at necropsy flat collections of fibrinous pus were found over the cortex and in the basal cisternae, and once these are formed the penicillin passes round them but does not enter into them. In some other cases associated abscess was the cause of death. To prevent these loculations the manoeuvre shown in Fig. 58 is of value. Both anterior horns are tapped through burr holes and the ventricles emptied; this allows the brain to contract and a space between the cortex and dura is created. A fine flexible catheter is then passed back as far as possible over the surface of the brain and as it is slowly withdrawn penicillin—500 units per millilitre—is distributed over the surface of the cortex. If the patient is cooperative, forced breathing while this is being done will help to draw the solution into all the crevices of the cortex. Finally 5 millilitres of 500 unit strength is injected into each ventricle. On subsequent days it is not possible to reopen the wounds, and the lateral ventricles are tapped between the stitches and 10 millilitres of the solution introduced daily on alternate sides.

Cisternal puncture may be helpful at the initial treatment to prevent basal collections of pus cells and fibrin.

The most important point in the management is early treatment. It is worth while to have ready in all cases of suspected meningitis 10 millilitres of 1,000 unit strength solution, and if the lumbar tap is turbid to introduce this at once. If the fluid does not contain any organisms or penicillin-resisters harm will not have been done, but if the case is a meningococcal or pneumococcal one a quick start is made in the race against fibrin formation in the subarachnoid space; the patient is also put on to sulphonamides and systemic penicillin immediately. If the case is secondary to mastoid disease the daily lumbar puncture with the same dose of penicillin for 7 days will generally suffice.

In a meningococcal case the same routine is followed, but if improvement is not immediate the ventricle should be entered from a burr hole in the forehead and 10 millilitres of 1,000 unit strength introduced; the effect is magical.

If the infecting organism is found to be the pneumococcus then it becomes essential to exert every effort on behalf of the patient with this fulminating disease without any delay; the solution is introduced on the first day into the lumbar theca, and cisterna magna and the ventricles and subarachnoid space of the hemispheres—10,000 units in each location. Only by these heroic measures will the mortality of this dreaded disease be reduced, and there must be no delay in instituting treatment as sometimes the duration of the whole illness may be only 24 hours. It is unwise to introduce more than 10,000 units in 10 millilitres in any of the situations mentioned. This amount is more than adequate, and if stronger solutions are used the impurities introduced produce some side effects such as root pains and retention of urine. Moreover, the blood-brain barrier is now helping the treatment because it prevents the penicillin escaping into the blood stream, and prolonged contact is obtained; as the volume of the cerebrospinal fluid is so small compared with that of the blood and body fluids, very high concentrations are obtained from these small amounts and the penicillin has every opportunity to do its work.

The administration of penicillin into the subarachnoid space must be done with the greatest attention to asepsis, and rubber gloves should always be worn; the organism generally introduced by carelessness is the ubiquitous *Ps. aeruginosa* found in all tap water and frequently in "antiseptic" lotions in common use.

The treatment of the meningitis is generally carried on for 7 days and longer if the patient does not recover completely. The necessity for speed in starting cannot be too strongly emphasized to prevent (1) formation of purulent collections over the cortex and in the basal cisternae; (2) atrophy of the convolutions and mental changes from the prolonged effect of sepsis; (3) obstruction of Magendie's foramen by adhesions and hydrocephalus; (4) obliterative arachnoiditis in the dorsal region of the cord with paraplegia; (5) arachnoiditis in the neighbourhood of the optic chiasma or auditory nerves with resultant blindness or deafness.

The possibility of cerebral abscess should always be borne in mind if the patient is slow to recover. Ventriculography is easily carried out at the daily ventricular tapping if the abscess cannot be localized clinically.

Intracranial operations

These are rather prone to infection because of the long operative period with the wound open to the air and because of the deep scalp follicles harbouring staphylococci.

Penicillin solution introduced into the wound before closure or dusting with penicillin and sulphadiazine powder most effectively prevents invasion by stray staphylococci.

Fulminating postoperative streptococcal infections due to theatre infections are also prevented.

In the future systemic penicillin will doubtless become a 48-hour routine treatment after intracranial operations and will close all the doors to bacterial invasion.

VENEREAL DISEASES

BY G. L. M. McELLIGOTT, M.R.C.S., L.R.C.P.
DIRECTOR, DEPARTMENT OF VENEREAL DISEASES, ST. MARY'S HOSPITAL, LONDON

GONORRHOEA

DURING the last 3 years very extensive trials have shown penicillin to be the most effective known agent in the treatment of gonorrhoea. The *in vitro* experiments of Fleming and of the Oxford workers were clinically confirmed by Mahoney and others[1] in 1943, who cured all but one of 75 cases with 16 injections 3-hourly of 10,000 units (total dosage 160,000 units). Since then many thousands of cases have been successfully treated, and it is now apparent that over 90 per cent of acute infections in men can be rapidly cured with a total dosage of about 150,000 units spread over as short a period as 12 hours and that most of the few patients who fail to react or who relapse, respond to re-treatment with somewhat higher doses[2]. As, however, very few cases of late relapse have been reported, it is probably safer not to carry out tests of cure until 3 months after treatment. There is not at present any certain evidence that the disease is becoming to any extent resistant to penicillin, as it undoubtedly did to the sulphonamides, but a personal communication from one United States Army venereologist[3] suggests that it has been necessary to raise the total dosage to 200,000 units or more in some areas of Europe, in order to obtain optimum results. It is possible, however, that microscopical diagnosis may have become slack and that a proportion of the apparent failures were, in fact, not cases of gonorrhoea, but of non-specific urethritis, a fairly common condition among young soldiers, which rarely responds to penicillin.

The average civil patient usually finds it difficult if not impossible to come into hospital for the treatment of a venereal disease, and in most cases of uncomplicated gonorrhoea it is not necessary for him to do so. Excellent results can be obtained using 3 injections 4-hourly of 50,000 units, and almost as good a result with one injection of 100,000 units followed by another 8 or 9 hours later. When penicillin is suspended in an oil-wax medium such as 2 to 5 per cent beeswax in peanut oil or ethyl oleate, absorption from the tissues is considerably delayed and consequently an effective blood level is maintained for a longer period after each injection[4,5]. The initial blood level for the first half-hour is not so high as after the injection of a watery solution, and it may possibly be because of this, that the results of a single injection of 100,000-150,000 units suspended in an oil-wax medium have not equalled those following multiple injections of an aqueous solution. Some workers[6] have achieved over 90 per cent success rate after single subcutaneous injections of 300,000 units mixed with 0·22 gramme of magnesium sulphate suspended in 1 millilitre of peanut oil. They claim that the magnesium sulphate competes with the penicillin for the available tissue fluids after injection and thus retards its solution and the rate of its absorption. The obvious answer is to try larger doses of penicillin, but it must be remembered that about 3 per cent of all cases of acute gonorrhoea are likely to be incubating a syphilitic infection and that there is a distinct possibility, if not a likelihood, that signs of this second and more important disease would be masked, modified or delayed, were doses of over 200,000 units of this powerful antispirochaetal agent used as a routine for the treatment of recent gonorrhoea. Experience so far suggests that there is little danger of this happening, if a total dosage of 150,000 units is not exceeded, though I have seen one case which presented a secondary syphilitic rash, with apparently total suppression of the primary chancre, 5 months after treatment of gonorrhoea with 100,000 units. The diagnosis was confirmed by positive blood tests, the patient denied a subsequent risk of infection and seemed to be a reliable witness. Such cases must be exceedingly rare, and the vast majority of patients with concurrent syphilitic infections develop a primary sore well within 60 days of infection, in spite of having had 150,000 units of penicillin for their gonorrhoea.

Approximately similar results to those in men have been obtained in women, although up to the present, large-scale carefully controlled trials, such as those carried out in the Forces, have not been possible. There is, however, a growing impression among most venereologists that failures and relapses are commoner in women than in men and that the former need somewhat higher doses and longer periods of administration. It is difficult to see why this should be so, as the infected parts in the female have an excellent blood supply and the gonococci should be readily accessible to the penicillin.

Local complications—males

Acute prostatis, even with abscess formation, usually responds rapidly. Chronic prostatitis responds well, provided that the gonococcus or another penicillin-sensitive organism is responsible for the condition. Thus, prostatitis due to coliform organisms is unaffected by penicillin. In chronic prostatitis it is important that drainage of the infected gland is aided by massage and warm vesical irrigations.

Acute epididymitis[7] does not respond dramatically, although signs of concurrent urethritis rapidly disappear and the pus-laden urine quickly clears. Relapse of the condition is unusual, unless there is a secondary infection, and resolution on the whole seems to be somewhat accelerated.

Local complications—females

Acute bartholinitis with abscess formation does not react well to penicillin, unless the abscess is first drained. Although some authorities recommend aspiration and injection of penicillin into the abscess cavity, I have had far better results after incision and drainage, no penicillin being given until this has been done. Then 30,000 units 3-hourly to a total of from 150,000 to 300,000 units will almost invariably effect a cure.

Acute salpingitis of gonococcal origin reacts well to penicillin; pain, tenderness and constitutional disturbance subside rapidly after the commencement of treatment. Although the palpable tube rapidly decreases in size, complete resolution does not occur for some weeks and occasionally the condition passes into the chronic stage. Chronic salpingitis reacts capriciously to penicillin, results being sometimes dramatic, while on other occasions little or no effect is noticeable. This may well depend on whether a secondary infection with a resistant organism is present and, as this cannot be ascertained in advance, trial treatment is always justifiable. The blood sedimentation rate is a good index of response or of resistance to treatment. In both acute and chronic salpingitis dosage should be on the high side and at least 400,000 units should be given over a period of 3 days. Gonococcal vulvovaginitis in small girls reacts well, 75,000-100,000 units being given over a period of about 24 hours. No local treatment, except warm sitz baths, is advisable. Because of the well known tendency of this condition to relapse and the danger of reinfection from contaminated towels and clothing, frequent smears and cultures of the vaginal secretion should be examined for an absolute minimum of 3 months after treatment. Non-gonococcal vulvovaginitis is not uncommon and is often unaffected by penicillin. It is, however, advisable to give it in addition to any other treatment, as gonococci may be difficult to discover in smears and cultures from a case that has become heavily contaminated with secondary organisms.

Metastatic complications

Gonococcal iritis rapidly subsides under routine penicillin treatment, but local atropine must always be used to prevent adhesions. Acute and chronic arthritis associated with gonorrhoea do not usually respond dramatically, although the accompanying urethral infection almost invariably does so. In some cases, however, the response is immediate; pain, tenderness and swelling subside rapidly after treatment. This would suggest that many cases of "gonorrhoeal rheumatism" may not be gonococcal in origin, but are caused by secondary infection with penicillin-resistant organisms, or the condition may in some cases be an allergic response to the original infection which takes its own time to subside. Reports of the results of the instillation of 10,000 units in physiological saline into the infected joint cavity are conflicting and unless gonococci have been cultured from the joint fluid and parenteral penicillin has failed, this is not recommended. The risk of introducing penicillin-resistant organisms, such as *Ps. aeruginosa,* is not inconsiderable. Even if, however, gonococci are cultured from the joint fluid, it is probably better practice in persistent hydrarthrosis or pyarthrosis to continue to give large doses of penicillin intramuscularly, 100,000 units 4-hourly, and to aspirate the joint daily. This will assist the secretion of penicillin into the synovial cavity as the joint refills with fluid.

Gonococcal endocarditis

This very unusual and almost invariably fatal complication is rarely diagnosed in its early stages, when penicillin might be expected to do good. By the time large infected vegetations have developed, the outlook is bad but treatment similar to that recommended for acute bacterial endocarditis should be instituted.

Proof of cure

It is impossible to overemphasize the importance of careful tests of cure after an adequate period of observation. This in males should never be less than 12 weeks, during which time the patient and his urine should be periodically examined for signs of relapse. At the end of the period the prostatovesicular secretion is examined microscopically and if possible culturally, a full-sized metal sound passed into the bladder and the urethra palpated thereon for signs of littritis or infiltration. If any abnormality is suspected, urethroscopy is carried out. Provided signs of relapse do not appear within a week after these tests, cure may be presumed. In women, urethral and cervical cultures and smears are examined weekly for the first 3 weeks after treatment and thereafter monthly for at least 4 and preferably 6 months. A persisting urethritis or cervicitis should be regarded with grave suspicion, even when gonococci are not isolated, and the patient should not be pronounced cured until she has been free from all signs and symptoms for a minimum of 3 months. A bimanual examination must be carried out before final dismissal, in order that infection of the uterine tubes can be reasonably excluded. The possibility of a concurrent syphilitic infection having been masked by the penicillin must not be forgotten and it is always advisable to have a serum test for syphilis made at 3 and 6 months after treatment.

Non-gonococcal urethritis

Penicillin does not usually affect the course of this disease except when it is caused by a pure pyococcal infection. These cases are rare, although in the urethral smear staphylococci from the fossa navicularis are often seen with many other varieties of bacteria. It should be remembered that a slight non-gonococcal discharge is sometimes the presenting sign of an intra-urethral chancre; consequently, it is best not to try penicillin in this condition, except in cases where syphilis has been excluded or which have resisted all other forms of treatment.

SYPHILIS

In 1943 Mahoney, Arnold and Harris[8] began to treat syphilis with penicillin. It soon became apparent that the immediate results of treatment equalled if they did not excel those following treatment with arsenicals and bismuth, even when the latter drugs had been given intensively. Various dosage schemes were tried and clinical and serological relapses occurred where subminimal doses were used[9]. By the spring of 1944, it was established that good results in early syphilis could be expected to follow the intramuscular injection of a total of 1,200,000 units given in divided doses over a period of 8 days (25,000 units 4-hourly)[10]. The early results of this treatment are summarized as follows. (1) Treponemata are no longer found in primary lesions 12-16 hours after the commencement of treatment; (2) primary sores heal in an average of 7 days and the accompanying regional adenitis subsides within this time; (3) secondary manifestations on skin and mucous membranes disappear within 10-21 days; (4) positive serological reactions usually become negative within 4-6 months, although generally the older the infection the longer the serology takes to revert[9]. This rate of serological response is similar to that noted after either standard or intensive treatment with arsenicals and bismuth; (5) the incidence of early relapse is approximately inversely proportional to the total dosage of penicillin when this is less than 1,200,000 units. Relapse was found to be much more frequent after intravenous than after intramuscular injections, even when a constant intravenous drip technique was used; consequently this route was abandoned at an early stage.

In June 1944, penicillin was adopted as the "drug of choice" for the treatment of early syphilis in the United States Army (European Theatre of Operations), and in the autumn of the same year by the Royal Navy, the British Army and the Royal Air Force. As by this time it had become apparent that a small but constant number of relapses were to be expected, the dosage was empirically doubled and the standard course of treatment for early syphilis in the British and American Forces fixed at 2,400,000 units in 7½ days (60 injections 3-hourly of 40,000 units).

It is still too early to foretell the ultimate results of this treatment, though it is thought that a relapse rate of 15 per cent is to be anticipated. It is certain, however, that the decision to use it in early syphilis in the Forces on active service was completely justifiable. Its immediate and early results equalled if they did not excel those obtained by time-honoured methods, treatment was completed in little over a week, and many thousands of man-hours were saved for the war effort. It is not generally known that under active service conditions not more than 50 per cent of patients complete treatment with arsenicals and bismuth owing to toxic effects, default or other causes.

In order to economize in the use of penicillin, treatment with doses much higher than 2,400,000 units has not been tried on a large scale, and there is now a general tendency to treat early syphilis with 2-3 mega-units of penicillin over a period of about a week, in addition to about 10 injections of both an arsenical and a bismuth preparation at weekly intervals. It is known that as small a dose as 5 grammes of neoarsphenamine and 2 grammes of bismuth will cure about 60 per cent of all cases of early syphilis, but in the interests of the minority it has in the past been necessary to overtreat the majority, even at the risk of subjecting them to possible toxic effects. Animal experiments[11] have shown that, as well as the additive effect of combining these two types of treatment, there is probably a true synergistic action between them, so that it is advisable to give the first 3 injections of the arsenical and bismuth compounds during the week of penicillin treatment.

With the present acute shortage of hospital beds, the admission of every case of early syphilis for penicillin treatment is impracticable. Even if this were possible, it is doubtful whether many patients would consent to the consequent family publicity and to the loss of a week's wages. Thus, it is imperative that a satisfactory rapid out-patient treatment be evolved as soon as possible. Most authorities believe it to be desirable, if not essential, that an adequate penicillin blood level be maintained throughout the period of treatment, but it is by no means certain that this is necessary[12]. In the Royal Navy results comparable with those following 60 injections 3-hourly of 40,000 units have been achieved with 8 daily injections of from 300,000 to 500,000 units in a watery solution, although no trace of penicillin is detected in the blood 13 hours after each injection. When, however, a suspension of 500,000 units in an oil-wax medium, such as 5 per cent beeswax in ethyl oleate, is used, an appreciable blood level is easily maintained for more than 24 hours. It would therefore seem that if the maintenance of a constant blood level is important, oil-wax suspensions or other preparations ensuring slow release of penicillin from the tissues should always be used in the out-patient treatment of syphilis.

In the present state of knowledge, the following schedules of combined treatment, using penicillin, arsenicals and bismuth, for syphilis of less than 6 months' duration, can be recommended with some confidence, but it is emphasized that it may become necessary to modify them later in the light of future experience. These recommendations are made without prejudice to any future reports on the treatment of syphilis with penicillin alone, using larger doses for longer periods. When supplies are unlimited, the potentialities of this almost completely non-toxic agent will doubtless be more thoroughly investigated. The assessment of the thousands of cases treated in the Forces with penicillin alone is still in progress and it is impossible to foretell with accuracy how many of them are still likely to relapse.

Recommended treatment of primary and early secondary syphilis

Penicillin.—40,000 units in water 3-hourly for 7½ days (intramuscularly or deep subcutaneously), or 500,000 units in an oil-wax suspension daily for 6 days.

Arsenicals.—Neoarsphenamine 0·45 gramme or Mapharside (Mapharsen) 0·06 gramme or arsphenoxide tartrate (Neo-Halarsine) 0·09 gramme intravenously every 4 days for 40 days.

Bismuth metal.—0·2 gramme intramuscularly every 4 days for 40 days.

Treatment should be commenced with all 3 agents on the same day in order that the benefit of any synergistic action of penicillin and the arsenicals may be obtained.

Follow-up

All cases of early syphilis must be observed for at least 2 and preferably 5 years after treatment. At least 3 serological tests should be made during the first 6 months and a further 6 at 3-monthly intervals for 2 years. A full examination of the cerebrospinal fluid should be made at the sixth and twenty-fourth months and the skin and mucous membranes examined periodically for signs of mucocutaneous relapse. This is particularly important, as clinical relapse may occasionally occur before the blood tests become positive. Seropositive cases may take anything up to 6 months after treatment before they revert to negative. In the meantime, the serologist can aid the clinician by informing him whether the titre is rising or falling. If it is still rising at the end of 4 months, it is safest to presume a failure, and after examination of the cerebrospinal fluid to exclude asymptomatic neurosyphilis, to recommence treatment more strenuously, with at least 2 courses of penicillin, arsenicals and bismuth with 28 days' interval between courses.

Reactions to treatment

About 50 per cent of patients treated with penicillin for early syphilis[18] experience varying degrees of malaise on the first day of treatment. There is usually some pyrexia, and in some cases the primary sore, the secondary rash and adenitis become temporarily more pronounced. This phenomenon, known as the Herxheimer reaction, can in early cases be ignored and invariably subsides within 24 hours. It is said to be due to a large-scale destruction of spirochaetes in the lesions resulting in a sudden release of toxins with a consequent exacerbation of signs and symptoms.

Local reactions at the site of injection are rarely met, and few patients complain of more than a slight soreness which soon passes away. Oily suspensions are generally as well tolerated as are watery solutions, although very occasionally a tender induration appears about 3 days after an injection of the former. It is possible that the patients may be sensitive to some constituent or impurity in the penicillin or in the vehicle.

Generalized urticaria, with or without a slight constitutional upset, very occasionally occurs about a week after the first injection, but it is not an indication for discontinuing treatment.

Very few instances of rather more severe systemic reactions have been reported[14]; these have included severe malaise, pyrexia and various toxicodermal reactions, but in the course of 2 years' experience I have not encountered any of them. It must, however, be remembered that a diffuse generalized erythema sometimes occurs about 9 days after the first injection of an arsenical preparation. This is always an indication for discontinuing the arsenical drug, and treatment should be completed with bismuth and penicillin alone.

Late syphilis

So rapid and favourable has been the response to penicillin of the late cutaneous manifestations of syphilis that, although a decade must pass before its ultimate effect on late syphilis can be accurately evaluated, it seems certain that, even at the present stage, all cases with the possible exception of gross cardiovascular disease should have the benefit of penicillin in addition to whatever other treatment is necessary. It must, however, never be forgotten that, whereas in early syphilis a Herxheimer reaction can be ignored, in late disease it can be a very real danger. This is especially the case where hidden lesions are present in the heart and great vessels, and to an appreciable although lesser extent in the brain or spinal cord. For this reason, treatment of late or latent syphilis should always be commenced very cautiously, even if there is not any obvious disease of the two "vital systems", and 6-10 injections of bismuth with concurrent iodides by the mouth every 4 or 5 days should always precede penicillin or even arsenicals. In addition, a complete clinical examination should be made, a full examination of the cerebrospinal fluid done, and the heart and great vessels investigated radiologically, before treatment is commenced.

Latent syphilis

The diagnosis of latent syphilis is one of exclusion and is difficult to make with accuracy. It will depend largely on the clinical experience of the examining doctor, on negative results of radiological and cerebrospinal fluid examinations and on verification by repetition of positive blood findings. The condition is usually diagnosed by routine blood tests done on the apparently fit, such as expectant mothers and blood transfusion donors, and most syphilologists are agreed that, although the prospect of reversing the seropositive results is usually remote, they should always receive a minimum amount of "insurance" treatment. In prepenicillin days this usually consisted of about 30 injections of both bismuth and an arsenical preparation, bismuth alone being given for the first 6 weeks, in order to minimize the risk of a possible cardiovascular Herxheimer reaction. It is impossible at this stage to say how much of this treatment could be replaced by penicillin, but if one may draw comparisons between it and arsenicals and bismuth from their results in early syphilis, it would appear that from 2–3 mega-units given over a period of about a week is therapeutically equal, if not superior, to 20 injections each of standard arsenical and bismuth compounds. It must, however, be remembered that a minimum of 6 weeks' preliminary bismuth treatment will still be necessary, whether penicillin or arsenicals or both are given later.

Late cutaneous, mucocutaneous, visceral and osseous syphilis.—These conditions respond well to penicillin, and when disease of the nervous and cardiovascular systems has been excluded, and preliminary bismuth treatment given[15], it seems that at least half, if not more, of the treatment previously considered necessary for these cases could be replaced by penicillin on the scale suggested above. In syphilis of the larynx, preparatory bismuth is especially necessary, as an exacerbation of the lesion may lead to the disastrous results of obstruction of the air passage. Penicillin, being completely non-toxic, would appear to be especially suitable in the treatment of syphilis of the liver, but here again great care should be taken to avoid a too rapid therapeutic effect. If healing with fibrosis occurs too quickly, strangulation of the portal circulation with a resulting ascites may occur—a true "therapeutic paradox".

Cardiovascular syphilis

Because of the risk of Herxheimer reactions, there has been up to the present considerable reluctance to treat cardiovascular syphilis with penicillin, and reports of its use in this condition are awaited with interest.

Neurosyphilis

Improvement in both the clinical condition and the cerebrospinal fluid in many types of neurosyphilis has already been reported, and it is especially encouraging to learn that the cerebrospinal fluid often continues to improve for as long as 4 months after a standard 8-day course of from 2 to 4 mega-units. The best results seem to follow 2 or more courses with an interval of 3 weeks between the courses, which augurs well for the success of multiple course techniques in the future. Dramatic improvement has been reported in both the clinical condition and the cerebrospinal fluid in acute meningovascular syphilis, but where there has been no preparatory treatment with bismuth, severe Herxheimer reactions, such as acute transverse myelitis, have occurred. In tabes dorsalis no dramatic clinical changes can be expected, although the progress of primary optic atrophy is said to have been arrested and in most cases the cerebrospinal fluid improves. It is interesting to note that, before this improvement begins, there is often an immediate increase in the cell count and total protein together with a temporary exacerbation of symptoms, for example, lightning pains. Such reactions in a condition so superlatively chronic as tabes dorsalis, underlines the exceptional potency of penicillin as a spirochaeticidal substance. In the treatment of general paralysis of the insane, although some workers claim an improvement in the clinical condition after penicillin alone, the drug is used by most others only in combination with arsenicals, bismuth or artificial fever therapy. Reports of results are conflicting, but all agree that, even when penicillin alone is used, some improvement occurs in the cerebrospinal fluid of more than half the number of patients treated.

In asymptomatic neurosyphilis results are excellent, fluids becoming normal in a very large proportion of the cases treated with penicillin alone. Nevertheless, preparatory bismuth should always be given in previously untreated cases, and at this stage it is probably safer not to curtail such treatment with arsenicals and bismuth as is usually considered necessary for this serious condition.

Intrathecal injections of penicillin have not yet been used to any great extent in the treatment of neurosyphilis and it is still uncertain whether better results would follow administration by this route than by the usual parenteral ones.

Congenital syphilis

In infantile congenital syphilis the clinical response to penicillin is as spectacular as it is in the early stages of the acquired disease, serum tests becoming negative within 2 or 3 months or even earlier. Herxheimer reactions are common on the first day of treatment and in puny or marasmic infants are always dangerous. Some authorities commence the treatment with small doses of penicillin while others prefer to administer mercury or bismuth for the first few days. A total penicillin dosage of up to 100,000 units per kilogram of body weight is then given over a period of about 8 days, injections being given at 4-hourly intervals during this time. It would appear that daily injections of oil-wax suspensions in proportionate doses would be a preferable method of treating very young children. Although the early results of treatment are so good, it would at this stage be unwise to rely on penicillin alone and at least 10 injections each of an arsenical and a bismuth preparation should be given in addition. The importance of a careful and prolonged follow-up in such cases is obvious.

Late congenital syphilis responds equivocally to penicillin and the literature on the subject is conflicting. Dramatic improvement has, however, been reported in 4 of a series of 14 cases of interstitial keratitis.

It is obvious that much work spread over a lengthy period must be done before the place of penicillin in the treatment of syphilis can be accurately designated. Prolonged massive dosage, multiple courses, and possibly combined treatment with aqueous solutions and oil-wax suspensions have yet to be tried and found wanting, before it can be said with certainty that penicillin alone is not to be relied upon. Up to now it has been necessary to economize in the use of the supplies, and present-day opinion of the potentialities of penicillin in syphilis is largely, if not entirely, formed from the results of treatment with 2,400,000 units in 8 days in many thousands of Service cases. In early syphilis, whether congenital or acquired, moderate doses of penicillin combined with a short course of arsenicals and bismuth, would seem to give results equal if not superior to those achieved by time-honoured methods, with the added advantages that the period of treatment is considerably shortened and the risk of toxic effects greatly reduced. In late syphilis, the position is far more obscure, and until the equivalent therapeutic values of penicillin, the arsenicals and bismuth have been more accurately determined, it will not be possible to utilize to the full the accumulated experience of the last 25 years. Meanwhile, as new schemes of dosage are tried, it is to be hoped that the necessity for a long and careful follow-up will be impressed on all patients and that Government-inspired propaganda will bring this need to the notice of the public. In the words of Dr. J. Earle Moore[15] of Johns Hopkins Hospital, " . . . we are still in the process of learning how to use this drug. We don't know yet, and it is going to be some time before we are sure".

Other venereal diseases

Penicillin has been tried in the treatment of chancroid and granuloma venereum, and in these conditions it has proved to be ineffective. It gives good results in acute streptococcal genital ulceration, in which condition, however, its use is not generally advisable, except when sulphonamides and local treatment have failed, as there is here a considerable danger of masking an underlying syphilitic infection[16].

REFERENCES

1 Mahoney, J. F., Ferguson, C., Buchholtz, M., Van Slyke, C. J. (1943) *Amer. J. Syph.*, **27**, 525.

2 Sternberg, T. H., and Turner, T. B. (1944) *J. Amer. med. Ass.*, **126**, 157.

3 Padgett, P. (1945) Personal Communication.

4 Romansky, M. J., Rittman, G. E. (1944) *Bull. U.S. Army Med. Dept.* No. 81, p. 43.

5 Romansky, M. J., Rittman, G. E. (1944) *Science*, **100**, 196.

6 Lloyd-Jones, T. R., Donaldson, E. M., Allen, S. J. (1946) *Lancet*, Vol. 1, pp. 526–29.

7 Marshall, J. (1945) *Brit. Jour. Ven. Dis.*, Vol. XXI, No. 4, pp. 150–56.

8 Mahoney, J. F., Arnold, R. C., and Harris, A. (1943) *Vener. Dis. Inform.*, **24**, 355.

9 Mahoney, J. F., Arnold, R. C., Sterner, B. L., Harris, A., and Zwally, M. R. (1944) *J. Amer. med. Ass.*, **126**, 63.

[10] Moore, J. E., Mahoney, J. F., Schwartz, W., Sternberg, T., and Wood, W. B. (1944) *J. Amer. med. Ass.*, **126**, 67.
[11] Eagle, H., Magnuson, H. J., and Fleischman, R. (1946) *J. vener. Dis. Inform.*, **27**, 3.
[12] Jones, T. R. L., Maitland, F. G. (1945) *Brit. J. vener. Dis.*, **21**, 166.
[13] Pillsbury, D. M. (1945) *Brit. J. vener. Dis.*, **21**, 139.
[14] Kolodny, M. H., Denhoff, E. (1946) *J. Amer. med. Ass.*, **130**, 1058.
[15] Stokes, J. H., Sternberg, T. H., Schwartz, W. H., Mahoney, J. F., Moore, J. E., and Wood, W. B., Jun. (1944) *J. Amer. med. Ass.*, **126**, 73.
[16] Willox, R. R. (1946) Post Grad. med. J., **22**, 97.

OPHTHALMOLOGY

By Arnold Sorsby, M.D., F.R.C.S.
Research Professor in Ophthalmology at the Royal College of Surgeons and the Royal Eye Hospital, London

THEORETICAL CONSIDERATIONS

Physiologically and pathologically the eye is a double organ. The lids, conjunctiva and sclera are nourished in the same way as are most other tissues, excluding the central nervous system; they are freely supplied by blood vessels, and substances circulating in the blood stream readily reach them. In contrast, the cornea and the interior of the eye constitute—as does the brain—a largely insulated system. Although blood freely reaches the eye through the central retinal artery, the long and short posterior ciliary arteries and the anterior ciliary vessels, the nutrition of the globe depends largely not upon blood bathing the tissues but upon highly selected filtrates of the blood. This is strikingly seen in the case of the aqueous humour which is a derivative of plasma and which nourishes the lens and the cornea. Although the choroid is a rich vascular network and the retina contains its own arterial system, the nutrition of the retina is probably as selective as is that of brain tissue, in which the blood-brain barrier shields the central nervous system from many constituents in the blood stream. In consequence a high concentration of a drug in the blood stream does not necessarily mean that the drug reaches the interior of the eye or the cornea. If penicillin is administered systemically it may be expected to reach the lids, orbital contents, conjunctiva and sclera in a concentration not dissimilar to that obtaining in the blood stream, but it cannot be assumed that it will also be present in the interior of the eye.

Experimentally, penicillin has in fact been found to belong to the large group of agents which do not penetrate into the interior of the eye. If clinical doses are injected intravenously into the dog, cat and rabbit, penicillin cannot be recovered from the aqueous humour or the vitreous body. When a massive dose corresponding to 10 or more times the usual clinical dose is injected into the dog, a low concentration of penicillin can be established in the ocular interior, as described by Struble and Bellows[1]. That the physiological barrier to the penetration of penicillin into the interior of the eye is not absolute is also suggested by some evidence on the inflamed eye (Leopold and La Motte[2]). Nevertheless, on both experimental and clinical evidence it would appear that the systemic administration of penicillin in intra-ocular infections is unlikely to give satisfactory results.

The impermeability of the eye to penicillin injected systemically raises the question of the direct introduction of the agent into the aqueous humour or the vitreous body. Such procedures involve several uncertainties. Presumably one application of penicillin is not likely to be effective, since it is probably rapidly excreted from the eye. Moreover, a massive quantity will have to be applied in view of the undesirability of repeated puncture of the eye. The procedure can be justified only if the eye readily tolerates a single injection of a highly concentrated solution of penicillin, or several less concentrated injections at frequent intervals.

A less drastic procedure is to inject penicillin subconjunctivally. Experimentally it has been found that the injection by this route of 2,500 units gives low values in the interior of the eye within 1½ hours (Struble and Bellows[1]; Rycroft[3]). It seems that most of this absorbed penicillin is largely excreted within 3 hours. Clinically such massive doses are not tolerated. An injection of 600 units of unpurified penicillin is relatively painless, but generally cannot be repeated until after 48 hours (Sorsby[4]). Still less drastic, but even more unpromising for any level of intra-ocular concentration, is the instillation of penicillin into the conjunctival sac. Whether applied in the form of drops or of ointment penicillin cannot be recovered from the aqueous humour. Wetting agents do not materially increase penetration.

The use of penicillin in ophthalmology is, therefore, largely confined to infections of the outer eye and the adnexa oculi. As these are readily accessible to local applications, local therapy is the main method of administering penicillin.

CLINICAL APPLICATIONS

On account of the limitations indicated, the use of penicillin in clinical ophthalmology may be conveniently considered under 5 headings: local therapy, subconjunctival injection, intra-ocular injection, systemic therapy, and various tentative procedures.

Local therapy

Since no satisfactory standard experimental lesion of the outer eye is available to help in establishing the best ways of applying penicillin locally, present-day practice has been evolved by clinical trial. Concentration and frequency of application have been found to be determining factors in obtaining adequate results.

Concentration.—Since the penicillin-sensitivity of different organisms varies considerably, the concentration to be used clinically is best standardized to correspond with the least sensitive organisms commonly met with in infections of the outer eye. The staphylococcus, which is highly sensitive to penicillin, is often a causal organism; the pneumococcus, which is less sensitive, is not uncommon, and neither are various bacilli with a low penicillin-sensitivity. An upper limit of concentration is, however, fixed by the relative intolerance of the outer eye to the current samples of unpurified penicillin. Most of these samples in a concentration of 10,000 units per millilitre produce damage to the corneal epithelium, and considerable conjunctival hyperaemia. A concentration of 5,000 units per millilitre is likewise prone to produce hyperaemia. In practice it has been found that concentrations of 2,500 units per millilitre are well tolerated and effective. There is not, therefore, anything to be gained by the use of solutions of a weaker potency.

Frequency of application.—Commonly, penicillin is used in the form of drops. These, however, are rapidly washed out from the eye and there is little antibacterial activity in the conjunctival secretion within 2 minutes after instillation of drops. Frequent applications are, therefore, essential for consistent results. In practice it has been found that severe conjunctival infections can be overcome by the instillation of drops at intervals of an hour. Better results are obtained if the frequency is increased to half-hourly intervals, and results are even better if the drops are instilled at intervals of 5 minutes. When drops are instilled at intervals of one minute the severest forms of conjunctival infection are brought under control within less than half an hour.

Ointments and lamellae.—In order to obviate the need for such frequent instillation some vehicle other than water or physiological saline is necessary. It is possible that an adequate ointment base will serve, but for the present it is not certain whether this has as yet been evolved. A suitable ointment base has to possess many qualities: it should be neutral, as any excess of alkalinity or acidity destroys the penicillin; it should readily lend itself to sterilization since a contaminated ointment base also destroys penicillin; sterilization should not affect its *p*H concentration; it should not irritate the conjunctiva; it should fairly readily take up penicillin, and also liberate it fairly readily; it should not be washed out from the eye, or melt too readily in the conjunctival sac. Lanette wax SX, which at one time gained favour, is not suitable for ophthalmic use for it is not too stable and it is readily washed out from the eye. For the present, Eucerin ointment base, and the Oculentum base of the 1932 Pharmacopoeia appear to be the most satisfactory, but it is possible that Vaseline or soft paraffin (petrolatum U.S.P. XII) will prove to be better.

Lamellae have proved to be unsatisfactory; they either dissolve so readily as to be little different from drops, or they are largely ineffective in that they remain undissolved, or are expelled, or do not readily liberate penicillin.

Mode of application.—For the present conjunctival infections are, therefore, best treated by the instillation of penicillin drops in a concentration of 2,500 units per millilitre at frequent intervals; for infections of the lid and lid margin the current ointment bases have proved to be satisfactory. In ointments, concentrations of 2,500 units per gramme are unnecessary, as the usual infecting organisms are staphylococci, and concentrations of 400-800 units per gramme have proved to be effective.

Clinical conditions amenable to local therapy

Ophthalmia neonatorum.—The gonococcus is responsible for about 20 per cent of all cases of ophthalmia neonatorum, staphylococci for about 35 per cent, viruses morphologically similar to that causing trachoma and inclusion conjunctivitis for about 15-20 per cent, and various coccal organisms and bacilli for most of the remainder. Ophthalmia neonatorum, with its severe purulent reaction and its multiplicity of causal organisms with their varying sensitivity to penicillin, is a good test condition for assessing optimal concentration and frequency of application of penicillin in conjunctival infections. The standards evolved in the treatment of this affection are, therefore, of special interest (Sorsby[5]).

Recovery can be obtained in some cases when drops are used in a concentration of 500 units per millilitre at intervals of one hour. The best results, as already indicated, are obtained when concentrations of 2,500 units per millilitre are used at intervals of one minute. Intermediate concentrations applied at intermediate frequencies all give positive results, but neither consistently nor quickly.

In the treatment of ophthalmia neonatorum the following routine procedure should be used. When the baby is admitted to hospital the eye is irrigated with half-strength physiological saline at room temperature in order to remove the profuse pus. Two drops of freshly—or relatively freshly—prepared penicillin solution in a strength of 2,500 units per millilitre are instilled, and the infant is allowed to close its lids. The irrigation is best carried out with the baby on a table, or in a specially prepared trough such as is available in most ophthalmia neonatorum units. After the first instillation of penicillin the baby is held by a nurse on her lap, while another nurse is responsible for instilling penicillin, 2 drops at intervals of a minute. Generally pus does not re-form in any quantity during the treatment, so that further irrigation is unnecessary. Within 20-30 minutes all tendency to pus formation is completely suppressed. Any purulent material present can be wiped off with a pledget of cottonwool, both during the treatment and at the end of the first half hour. The baby is now transferred to its cot, and the instillation of penicillin is continued at 5-minute intervals for half an hour, half-hourly intervals for 3 hours, and at hourly intervals for a further 6 hours. As a safety measure instillation is continued at 2-hourly intervals for a further 12 hours.

The process of recovery has two distinct phases. The suppression of the pus is rapid, but the oedema of the conjunctiva and lids persists for much longer. A clinical cure is generally obtained within 12-24 hours.

The dreaded corneal complications of ophthalmia neonatorum, which were so common when the affection was allowed to run its course for weeks, are now exceptional. It is unnecessary to use atropine as a routine, but one drop of atropine sulphate 1 per cent should be instilled in any case in which haze of the cornea is seen after the first few instillations of penicillin have allowed a clear view of that structure. When corneal ulceration is present the atropine should be repeated at 3-hourly intervals. No other special measures are needed. In one case in which purulent infiltration of the cornea was present when the child was admitted to hospital, penicillin, although it rapidly cleared the conjunctival infection, did not seem to influence materially the corneal lesion.

Acute purulent conjunctivitis in adults.—The treatment should be the same as for ophthalmia neonatorum.

Mucopurulent conjunctivitis.—Ten instillations of penicillin drops at intervals of one minute bring most of these cases under control. In order to consolidate the effect 4-6 further instillations of drops at intervals of half an hour may be used, or more conveniently, penicillin ointment made in a concentration of 800 units per gramme may be instilled at intervals of 2 hours for 12 hours.

Hypopyon ulcer.—This is a composite group of affections, and the results of penicillin administration are not equally effective in the different varieties. The best results are obtained in infected traumatic ulcers in which the causal organism is generally the pneumococcus. In hypopyon ulcer seen in neuroparalytic keratitis the results are not impressive, and good results have not been obtained in 2 cases of recurrent hypopyon iritis. None the less penicillin may be regarded as an effective remedy in most cases of hypopyon ulcer (Juler and Young[6]) and, apart from the use of atropine drops, it can be employed exclusively. When the patient is first seen, penicillin in a concentration of 5,000 units per millilitre should be dropped on to the infected ulcer, and this procedure is repeated 5 times at intervals of one minute. Thereafter, penicillin ointment, 800 units per gramme, should be instilled at hourly intervals. In most cases the hypopyon will have greatly diminished or will have disappeared altogether within 12 hours. If there is no response to penicillin treatment within 24 hours, other forms of therapy should be used. Occasionally oral sulphonamide therapy succeeds when penicillin fails.

Infected corneal ulcers.—These generally respond well to penicillin when treatment is the same as for hypopyon keratitis.

Trachoma.—Although experience is limited, penicillin has shown considerable promise in the treatment of trachoma (Sorsby[4]). This is not altogether unexpected on account of the satisfactory response of virus ophthalmia neonatorum to penicillin. Any follicles in the fornices should first be expressed, and penicillin in a concentration of 2,500 units per millilitre should be vigorously painted on the expressed surfaces. Thereafter penicillin ointment, 800 units per gramme, should be instilled at 3-hourly intervals. Atropine should also be used when the corneal condition calls for it. Marked improvement should be noticeable within a week.

Dendritic ulcer.—It is possible that penicillin applied as for hypopyon ulcer is effective in at least some forms of dendritic keratitis.

Blepharitis.—Results in blepharitis are particularly good, and are not unexpected on account of the fact that the causal organism is generally *Staph. aureus.* First, all the crusts should be freely removed by soaking them with either sodium bicarbonate solution or hydrogen peroxide (10 volumes) (Liquor Hydrogenii Peroxidi B.P. and U.S.P. XII). The cleansed lid margin should be washed with sterile water and penicillin ointment in a concentration of 400-800 units per gramme applied at 3-hourly intervals. Even longstanding and severe cases will respond within a period of days. A few cases which do not readily respond generally show persistent chronic conjunctivitis with watering. If this is bacterial in origin a short course of intensive treatment with penicillin ointment, 800 units per gramme, applied to the conjunctiva at 2-hourly intervals may be effective. Relapse after penicillin cure is not uncommon in debilitated children. Attention must therefore be paid to the general condition.

Other conditions.—When purulent and mucopurulent infection of the conjunctiva and cornea is present either as a primary lesion or as a secondary effect, penicillin may be used as indicated; it will either cure or alleviate the condition. Penicillin may help in infected socket and in dacryocystitis. There is not, however, a place for penicillin in the treatment of phlyctenular ophthalmia, epidemic keratoconjunctivitis and most virus infections, and in allergic and metabolic reactions such as spring catarrh and acne rosacea keratitis.

Intra-ocular injection

The current samples of unpurified penicillin are not well tolerated in large quantities when they are directly injected into the anterior chamber, and are hardly tolerated at all when they are injected into the vitreous body (Sallmann, Meyer and Di Grandi[7]; Sorsby[4]; Mann[8]). Injections into the anterior chamber tend to produce a reaction of the iris. The maximal quantity which can be injected would appear to be 0·15 millilitre, and it does not seem to be safe to inject more than 500 units per millilitre. There are reports of recovery of infected eyes after irrigation of the anterior chamber with penicillin, and by leaving quantities of penicillin—up to 1,000 units—in the space. Personal experience of this procedure has been disappointing.

As for injection into the vitreous body, experimentally a severe endophthalmitis leading to shrinkage of the eye is produced by the injection of 5,000 units of unpurified penicillin in 0·1 or 0·2 millilitre of physiological saline. The upper limit of safety would appear to be about 200 units of unpurified penicillin, and personal experience in one case in which 2 injections of this dose were made at intervals of 3 days, has been disappointing. Moreover, experimental evidence shows that in spite of the relatively rapid excretion, damage to both the retina and the lens is likely to follow the energetic use of penicillin injected directly into the vitreous body. It is possible that purified samples of penicillin may allow a larger scope for this method.

Subconjunctival injection

For the present this has little application, for unpurified penicillin injected subconjunctivally is not well tolerated. As already indicated, the upper limit is an injection of 600 units which can be repeated after 48 hours. Since such penicillin as is absorbed appears to be rapidly excreted from the eye, this time interval is too long for the maintenance of an adequate intra-ocular concentration. Up to the present time there has been little clinical experience with this procedure, but there is some promise that it may be useful in interstitial keratitis (Sorsby[4]), and possibly in infections within the anterior chamber. It appears that pure penicillin is tolerated much better, so that it may be possible to inject larger quantities at more frequent intervals.

Systemic administration

A number of case reports would suggest that recovery is possible from the systemic use of penicillin in endophthalmitis after septic abortion, and in gonococcal choroiditis. Alternatively, failures in iridocyclitis, choroiditis, endophthalmitis, and threatening panophthalmitis, are also on record. It is difficult to see how satisfactory results are likely to be obtained on account of the low penetration of penicillin into the interior of the eye on systemic injection. The possibility that penicillin passes more readily into the inflamed eye, however, must not be overlooked, nor the fact that considerable quantities do reach the choroid and iris even if they do not pass into the intra-ocular fluids. It is also possible that such occasional results as have been obtained may be secondary to the overcoming of an underlying general infection which is the cause of the intra-ocular inflammation.

The value of systemically administered penicillin in interstitial keratitis is still uncertain, as is its value in active choroiditis of syphilitic origin. It does not appear to influence syphilitic optic atrophy.

Other tentative methods

The failure of penicillin to penetrate into the interior of the eye when it is applied locally to the conjunctiva in the form of drops or ointments, has raised the question whether or not an adequate intra-ocular concentration could be obtained by the use of the corneal bath and of ionization. These methods present some difficulties in clinical application, and hitherto have not been fully investigated. It is possible that such readier penetration of penicillin into the interior of the eye as these methods allow is largely the result of damage of the corneal epithelium.

GENERAL OBSERVATIONS

Limitations of penicillin

To the oculist the outstanding limitation of penicillin is the fact that it does not readily penetrate into the interior of the eye. For this reason the use of penicillin in ophthalmology is largely confined to external infections. It is possible that the use of pure penicillin in intra-ocular infections may give more promising results than are obtained at present, and it is also likely that the use of pure penicillin injected subconjunctivally may increase the range of indications. For the moment penicillin has not established itself in intra-ocular infections.

Range of activity

Satisfactory results are obtained with penicillin in ophthalmia neonatorum of assumed virus origin. Promising results have also been obtained in trachoma. This would indicate that penicillin is effective against the large-size viruses of which the virus of trachoma and that of inclusion ophthalmia neonatorum are examples. As the tolerated dosages of penicillin applied locally are effective against the common causal organisms of ocular infection, penicillin may be regarded as specific in most infections of the outer eye. An exception must be made of epidemic kerato-conjunctivitis, and of some forms of nondescript keratitis which are probably caused by viruses of small size.

Comparison with the sulphonamides

In contrast to penicillin, the sulphonamides readily penetrate the interior of the eye, and have occasionally proved to be useful in low-grade intra-ocular infections of endogenous origin. The sulphonamides, however, are not effective locally, since they are inactivated by pus and by break-down products of the tissues; they have, therefore, proved to be ineffective as local applications in infections of the outer eye. It is in this field that penicillin finds its greatest use. Although the infections of the outer eye are readily amenable to the systemic use of the sulphonamides, the results obtained by local therapy of penicillin are distinctly better. This is well illustrated in ophthalmia neonatorum. Here the sulphonamides reduced the course of the affection from weeks to days; penicillin has reduced it from days to hours. In fact, penicillin is as superior to the sulphonamides as these in turn were to the classical methods of treating infections of the outer eye.

Penicillin in intra-ocular inflammation

A sharp distinction must be drawn between intra-ocular infection and inflammation. Characteristic examples of intra-ocular inflammation are iritis, iridocyclitis, and choroiditis. Their nature is obscure; it is only exceptionally that micro-organisms are found, and when these are present the condition is generally one of panophthalmitis. The sulphonamides, although occasionally they give striking results in cases of iritis and hypopyon keratitis, have on the whole influenced but little the course of the acute intra-ocular inflammations. It is unlikely that penicillin will be more effective, even if it should ultimately prove to be possible to achieve adequate concentrations in the interior of the eye. The underlying difficulty appears to be that most acutely inflamed eyes are not infective in nature, but are reactions to a whole series of unknown irritants of both bacterial and non-bacterial origin.

REFERENCES

[1] Struble, G. C., and Bellows, J. G. (1944) *J. Amer. med. Ass.*, **125**, 685.
[2] Leopold, I. H., and LaMotte, W. O., Jun. (1945) *Arch. Ophthal., N.Y.*, **33**, 43.
[3] Rycroft, B. W. (1945) *Brit. J. Ophthal.*, **29**, 501.
[4] Sorsby, A. (1945) *Brit. J. Ophthal.*, **29**, 511.
[5] Sorsby, A. (1945) *Ophthalmia Neonatorum.* Hamish Hamilton, Ltd., London.
[6] Juler, F., and Young, M. Y. (1945) *Brit. J. Ophthal.*, **29**, 312.
[7] von Sallman, L., Meyer, K., and Di Grandi, Jeanette (1944) *Arch. Ophthal.*, **32**, 179.
[8] Mann, Ida. (1946) *Brit. J. Ophthal.*, **30**, 134.

OTORHINOLARYNGOLOGY

By John F. Simpson, F.R.C.S.

Honorary Assistant, Ear, Nose and Throat Department, St. Mary's Hospital; Honorary Surgeon, Royal National Hospital for Ear, Nose and Throat, London

GENERAL CONSIDERATIONS

Infections of the ear, nose and throat constitute a large and important group of diseases, and range from a minor inconvenience to a case of the gravest severity. These infections are due to a variety of organisms, most of which are sensitive to penicillin, so that this non-toxic antibiotic becomes the most important form of therapy available at present in otorhinolaryngology.

The use of penicillin in this special field must be governed by the same cardinal principles as govern other fields of medicine and surgery. Since penicillin is specific in its action and success can be expected only when it is used to combat an infective process caused by organisms known to be sensitive to it, and since the substance must come in direct contact with the bacteria in the tissues in an adequate concentration and for a sufficient period of time if complete bactericidal and bacteriostatic effect is to be obtained, it follows that an accurate diagnosis must be made if treatment with penicillin is to be successful. The diagnosis must rest not only on the bacteriology but also on a sound understanding of the pathology so that any possible complication may be anticipated. These complications are especially liable to occur in those cases in which the fundamental principles of treatment have not been properly fulfilled. The outlook in the grave septic infections met with in this field has been transformed by the use of penicillin, as for example the complications of suppurative otitis media, frontal sinusitis, Ludwig's angina, and septic oedema of the larynx—to mention only a few. Nevertheless, unbridled enthusiasm leading to the indiscriminate use of penicillin will court disappointment, for even when the cardinal principles of therapy appear to have been fulfilled disappointment from time to time may occur. Such a calamity is illustrated by a case of cavernous sinus thrombosis seen by me in its earliest stage. It originated from a minute staphylococcal furuncle in the nasal vestibule. Contrary to all hopes and expectations, death occurred in 36 hours in spite of massive penicillin and heparin treatment. This fulminating staphylococcal infection, which included a meningitis and septicaemia, was apparently untouched by the penicillin, although the culture proved to be sensitive to it.

Used as a prophylactic, penicillin has proved to be most beneficial in the operations performed in otorhinolaryngology. Operations such as laryngectomy and pharyngectomy may be undertaken with greatly increased prospect of primary union if penicillin be given systemically before and after the operation and if it be applied locally to the operative field.

Shortage of supply of penicillin and of hospital accommodation has not allowed the treatment of minor infections to be carried out on a large scale. Further work remains to be done in regard to the catarrhal conditions of the upper respiratory tract and middle ear cleft which form so large a portion of hospital outpatient work. Perhaps new methods of administration which can be carried out by a patient in his own home—for example, inhalation—might be utilized.

Penicillin treatment and surgical intervention

The question how far penicillin therapy replaces surgery in otorhinolaryngology cannot be finally answered at present, and must be postponed until further experience has been obtained. As a general statement it may be said that the administration of penicillin does not mean that the fundamental principles of surgery may be neglected, although the routine surgical treatment advocated in the days before chemotherapy and penicillin will have to be substantially modified or even dispensed with in many instances. It must be emphasized that the surgeon must not be lulled into a sense of false security by the administration of penicillin and so dangerously delay having recourse to surgical intervention. When there is a collection of pus it should be evacuated, especially when it is imprisoned in a bony cavity which is in close proximity to the meninges. Penicillin therapy shows its most spectacular results in acute and spreading infections. Perhaps one of the most dramatic results of penicillin therapy is to be seen in the treatment of otogenic septic meningitis; its use in this condition has entirely replaced such surgical procedures as translabyrinthine drainage of the basal cistern. In chronic infections in which a high degree of tissue change has been produced, as for example in hypertrophic sinusitis, the results of penicillin therapy alone have not been favourable, and recurrence of symptoms is the rule. In cases of this kind surgery is required in order to remove the diseased and hypertrophied tissue and to promote adequate drainage before a radical cure can be effected. Similarly, penicillin cannot have any effect on cholesteatomatous formation, and this must be removed.

Methods of administration

The various methods, their techniques and dosage are dealt

with in detail elsewhere. In otorhinolaryngology penicillin is given both systemically and locally and in many respects these methods should be considered as being complementary. In severe and widespread infections heavy systemic treatment with little or no local treatment is required, whereas in the smaller and superficial ones local application often will suffice.

Systemic methods.—The intramuscular route is that most often adopted, as in general surgery, on account of its simplicity and the sustained concentration obtained of penicillin in the blood. A dose of 15,000 units every 3 hours is usual, although in some cases this may be increased. The period of administration must be governed by the response of the patient and a generous allowance must be made for "hibernating" organisms. A recent method of administration is the inhalation of a cloud of minute globules of penicillin solution produced by an atomizer. It has the advantage of being able to create a rate of concentration of penicillin in the blood high enough for therapeutic use; at the same time it allows the penicillin to settle like a dew on the mucosa of the respiratory tract and thus combines local with systemic effect. The advantage of this method in treating infections of the respiratory tract is obvious. By means of a small hand atomizer and mask a patient can keep up an adequate blood penicillin concentration without having to go into hospital, and this is of great importance in the treatment of non-urgent cases.

In cases in which penicillin is required to combat infections in the subarachnoid space of the brain and spinal cord it may be introduced either by lumbar or cisternal puncture or occasionally by direct injection into the ventricles.

Local methods.—These methods are very varied in order to meet the different needs in the treatment of ear, nose and throat infections. Penicillin in aqueous or isotonic saline solution in strengths varying from 1,000 to 2,000 units per millilitre is used for instilling directly into a cavity such as that made in the mastoid operation or into a nasal sinus; this solution is also used as a spray for the nose and throat. All solutions to be handled by patients in sprays and so forth should be protected from airborne contamination. Some of these contaminating organisms produce penicillinase which destroys the penicillin. Besides taking care to keep the spray clean by boiling it and by using fresh refills, as opposed to adding fresh solution to that remaining in the spray, it is suggested that, as a routine, a preservative such as Chlorocresol (*p*-chloro-*m*-cresol) be added to all solutions.

A gauze wick or pack saturated with the solution forms a most useful type of plugging. By using the method of replacement described by Proetz, a solution of $\frac{1}{2}$ per cent ephedrine sulphate in isotonic saline containing penicillin 1,000 units per millilitre, may be introduced into the sinuses. The additional advantage of the local effect on the respiratory tract obtained during the inhalation of the "atomized" solution has already been mentioned. It is not often that a solution of penicillin is used in otorhinolaryngology for infiltration in and around a septic process in the soft tissues. Penicillin is used as a cream for the dressing of surgical and accidental wounds or for such suitable skin affections as are met with in the practice of otorhinolaryngology. In a powder vehicle (sterile sulphathiazole) it can be blown through an insufflator so as to form a "frost" on any desired area, or it can be used for packing a small cavity such as the auditory canal. Finally, penicillin may be incorporated in lozenges, pastilles, or gum for dissolving slowly in the mouth.

Chemotherapeutic substances for attacking organisms insensitive to penicillin are sometimes added to the powder or solution. For example, a powder containing 2 per cent Flavazole in sterile sulphathiazole with penicillin (calcium salt) will eliminate the secondary invaders *B. proteus*, *B. pyocyaneus* (*Ps. aeruginosa*) and *Esch. coli.* Similarly, a solution of penicillin to which is added Phenoxetol (β-phenoxyethyl-alcohol), 2 per cent, or 5-amino-acridine hydrochloride, 1 in 1,000, will serve the same purpose. The strength of penicillin is usually 1,000 units per millilitre in both preparations.

Penicillin or sulphonamide ?

The answer to this question must be determined by both theoretical and practical considerations in the individual case. When a difference between the appropriate antibacterial activity of the two drugs exists, preference will naturally be given to the stronger; for example, penicillin is imperative in dangerous staphylococcal infections and is preferable when streptococci of the *viridans* type are to be dealt with.

The relative sensitivity of the various organisms met with in infections of the ear, nose and throat is indicated in the Table given below. In mixed infections each type of organism present must be assessed from this point of view. The sulphonamides possess the practical advantage of easy oral administration which so far is denied to penicillin. The importance of this advantage is obvious when such common conditions as acute sinusitis, uncomplicated acute otitis media and acute tonsillitis are being treated. Although the toxic reactions to the sulphonamides have been reduced by the introduction of the more recent preparations and the possibility of crystalluria has been minimized, such undesirable sequelae may still occur and, when compared with the non-toxicity of penicillin, must weigh against the choice of sulphonamides. For this reason, when a long period of administration is required penicillin will be chosen, and its use becomes essential in those patients who show a leucopenia or agranulocytosis after administration of sulphonamides. The above factors will usually determine the choice of therapeutic agent in clinical practice, but a combination of them in both systemic and local administration is often found to be a satisfactory procedure.

Organisms	Gram stain	Penicillin sensitivity	Sulphonamide sensitivity	Remarks
Haemolytic streptococcus (*Str. pyogenes*)	+	+++	+++	
Streptococcus, *viridans* type	+	Variable + to +++	Variable + to +++	
Pneumococcus, including type III, or *Str. mucosus*	+	+++	+++	− to sulphanilamide, but + to later preparations
Staph. aureus and *Staph. albus*	+	+++	+	− to sulphanilamide and sulphapyridine but + to later preparations
C. diphtheriae	+	++	++	Sulphonamides do not attack *C. diphtheriae* within the "membrane"
Meningococcus (*N. intracellularis*)	−	+++	+++	
N. catarrhalis	−	+++	+++	
B. fusiformis *Bor. vincentii*	−	++	−	
H. influenzae (Pfeiffer)	−	−	−	Some strains are sensitive to penicillin
K. pneumoniae	−	−	−	
B. pyocyaneus (*Ps. aeruginosa*)	−	−	−	These organisms are sensitive to Flavazole and Phenoxetol
B. proteus	−	−	−	
Esch. coli	−	−	++	

The above Table roughly indicates the susceptibility of some of the organisms met with in ear, nose and throat infections. It is true for most strains of the types shown, but some penicillin-insensitive and sulphonamide-resistant strains are sometimes found among them.

PENICILLIN IN VARIOUS INFECTIONS

Generalized infections of the upper respiratory tract

Many virus infections affecting the upper respiratory tract are complicated to a varying degree by secondary bacterial infections. The clinical effect is at first a catarrhal rhinosinusitis which may be followed by pharyngitis, tonsillitis and laryngitis. The rhino-sinusitis may progress in some instances to a suppurative sinusitis, or it may give rise to similar conditions in the tympanic cleft. Such a chain of events is not unusual in measles, influenza and the common cold, and because most of the secondary bacterial infections are due to organisms sensitive to penicillin, the drug must hold an important place in prophylaxis and treatment. Up to the present time, economic and other factors have prevented penicillin from being applied on a large scale. The possibility of new methods of administration being made available, however, raises the hope that the morbidity and man-hours lost to the nation may be reduced.

In scarlet fever the aural and other complications can be much reduced, as would be expected. Antitoxic serum is, however, sometimes required, since penicillin has no direct effect on toxins. Penicillin has a place in the management of laryngotracheo-bronchitis of infants, although this fortunately rare disease probably has a virus origin. Systemic therapy together with instillation through the tracheotomy tube combats the secondary infection; nevertheless, suitable antitoxic measures are also required.

In the acute forms of pharyngitis and laryngitis associated with generalized upper respiratory tract infection, the ordinary principles of treatment apply. Suitable sprays, paints and lozenges in which penicillin is incorporated are given for local use, but inhalation therapy will probably prove to be the method of choice, especially when a tracheitis and bronchitis are present. In the chronic forms treatment is often disappointing, particularly in those showing marked atrophic or hypertrophic changes.

Carriers of the haemolytic streptococcus are frequently cleared by the use of a penicillin spray or inhalation and sometimes by administration of lozenges alone. The clearance time shows wide variations in individual cases and reinfection is common.

The nose and nasal sinuses

Rhinitis.—Nasal catarrh (so called) is often the result of allergic rhinosinusitis. This primary cause tends to be hidden by secondary bacterial infections and is only too often unrecognized. Catarrhal rhinitis in the absence of allergy or of a definite infective focus, such as a chronic sinusitis, can often be relieved, however, by the local use of an isotonic solution of penicillin (1,000 units per millilitre) as a nasal spray to which $\frac{1}{2}$ per cent ephedrine hydrochloride may be added. A course of replacement therapy employing a similar solution often leads to good results when the spray by itself has failed. Unfortunately reinfection is very liable to occur in susceptible patients and treatment with a vaccine may be required in order to raise the immunity in these individuals. Atrophic rhinitis, both in the true and postoperative forms, is temporarily benefited by the spray mentioned above and by the regular removal of crusts. The condition tends to recur when the treatment is stopped, and recurrence happens also after systemic treatment.

Acute suppurative sinusitis.—Inhalations of penicillin—given so that it is inhaled through the nose and exhaled *via* the mouth and in sufficient quantity to produce adequate systemic therapy—would be ideal in the early stages of pansinusitis or single sinus infection. In the later stages when an empyema has occurred, introduction of penicillin solution into the affected sinus after evacuation and lavage is the proper course. This treatment should be accompanied by intramuscular injection of penicillin. It may be noted that penicillin has no deleterious effect upon the cilary action of the nasal or sinusal mucosa.

In maxillary sinusitis, daily lavage of the antrum followed by instillation of 4 or 5 millilitres of penicillin solution (1,000 units per millilitre) usually presents no difficulty. A Lanette wax SX cream containing a similar concentration of penicillin may be injected through the cannula instead of the solution and has the advantage that it will remain in the sinus for 3 or 4 days. An alternative method is to pass a ureteric catheter through a wide-bore cannula into the antrum. The catheter is retained *in situ* so that lavage and penicillin instillation may be carried out twice a day until disinfection is obtained.

More difficulty is experienced in introducing fluid into the frontal sinus. Penicillin solution may sometimes be introduced successfully by means of the method of replacement of Proetz, but the infundibulum of the infected sinus may be so tightly shut that this method fails. Catheterization *via* the ostium is difficult, but, under local anaesthesia, a small hole to take a ureteric catheter can be easily made into the frontal sinus. The hole is made with a dental burr which drills through the thin orbital plate which forms the floor of the sinus. The contents of the sinus may be aspirated for bacterial examination and penicillin solution may be instilled through the catheter. Ethmoiditis often accompanies infections of the other sinuses and is apt to be overshadowed by them. Evacuation and instillation into the ethmoidal cells is probably best achieved by replacement. In children an orbital oedema due to ethmoiditis is not uncommon and complete subsidence has been seen to follow systemic penicillin therapy. When a distinct orbital abscess has formed it should be surgically drained. In sphenoidal sinusitis lavage and instillation of penicillin solution through a catheter can be carried out when replacement fails.

Chronic suppurative sinusitis.—In chronic sinusitis there is a varying amount of tissue change which is irreversible and penicillin treatment is not as effective as it is in the acute form. Sometimes there is a temporary improvement in the symptoms but a relapse usually occurs. In chronic sinusitis surgical procedures are still required for the purpose of removing the thickened lining, polypoidal formations and the rare cholesteatomatous collections, which may be present.

Complications of sinusitis.—Osteomyelitis is the most feared complication, especially when it occurs in the frontal or sphenoid bones, for then spread of the infection to the meninges and brain threatens. The exact extent to which penicillin therapy replaces surgery of the frontal bone is still controversial. Cases of established frontal osteomyelitis are recorded as being completely cured by systemic therapy without a major operation. In such cases surgery was confined to opening a subperiosteal abscess and later perhaps picking out a sequestrum. Nevertheless, some patients so treated have suddenly presented signs of a cerebral abscess and have quickly died a few weeks after apparent cure. It may well be that if, in spite of apparent cure, medication be extended over a period of 3–4 weeks or even more, any "hibernating" organisms will be killed, and thus such disappointments will be less likely to happen.

Because of the evidence available a combination of radical surgery, immediate or delayed, together with prolonged systemic treatment, is probably the most reliable procedure. Furthermore, surgery may bring to light extradural collections unsuspected in these patients and in any case it will usually be required in order to deal with the sinus itself when this has been the seat of chronic disease.

The prophylactic use of penicillin in nasal operations.—Systemic penicillin therapy is of great value when it is given before and after such operations as radical antrostomy (Caldwell Luc), frontosphenoethmoidectomy (Ferris Smith), and extensive operations on the frontal sinus and excision of the upper jaw. The operative areas clean quickly, discharges cease and favourable conditions for postoperative irradiation are obtained. Nasal and postnasal plugging when used to arrest haemorrhage from the nose or nasopharynx, should be soaked in a solution of thrombin to which has been added penicillin 1,000 units per millilitre. Such tampons will remain sweet and clean for 2 or 3 days, and thereby the risks of aural infection associated with such procedures will be reduced.

The pharynx and larynx

The principles of penicillin therapy in the simple forms of pharyngitis and laryngitis have already been mentioned.

Tonsillitis and quinsy.—A commencing tonsillitis may sometimes be aborted when it is treated energetically with sprays and lozenges, but success cannot be counted upon. Severe acute tonsillitis will respond quickly to systemic treatment, often after administration of sulphonamides has failed. Local treatment alone is not sufficient. Peritonsillar abscess should be drained for the relief of pain, and on general surgical principles. Sometimes trismus is so great as to render stabbing of the quinsy impossible, in which case penicillin therapy must be relied on. Recurrence of tonsillitis after a course of systemic therapy is common, so that the need for tonsillectomy still remains.

Tonsillectomy.—Routine treatment with penicillin before the operation for removal of tonsils and adenoids has not been judged to be necessary but it can be employed if for any reason a heavy postoperative infection is feared. Penicillin may be given systemically at any time in the postoperative period should a marked degree of infection occur. Local administration by means of spray or in the form of lozenges as a postoperative routine has not been shown to produce a profound effect on the pain, the healing rate or the incidence of haemorrhage. If required a penicillin nasal spray must be used for the purpose of disinfecting the adenoidal area.

Diphtheritic infection.—Systemic penicillin therapy will dispose of *C. diphtheriae* but antitoxin will be required to relieve the toxaemia. In contrast to the sulphonamides, penicillin will attack the organism in the pseudomembrane. Carriers have been cleared by a systemic course of penicillin lasting a few days.

Vincent's angina.—Small ulcers are cured by repeated local application and by the giving of lozenges, but the more severe infections will require systemic therapy. When massive ulceration is present a tube to provide a constant drip into the mouth has been devised. This is used after the necrotic tissue has been cleared.

Dangerous septic infections of the neck.—These include retropharyngeal abscess, Ludwig's angina and the infections of the parapharyngeal fascial space. Ludwig's angina (submaxillary cellulitis) and parapharyngeal cellulitis may occur after infections of and operations upon, respectively, the lower molar teeth and tonsils. The organisms usually responsible for these forms of cellulitis are the haemolytic streptococci, but other organisms including *Esch. coli* are sometimes present. Systemic penicillin therapy provides a life-saving measure in these severe infections and frequently avoids the necessity of making incisions. Incisions are necessary when an abscess has formed, or for the purpose of relieving the considerable tension that may be present because of oedema. Large doses of penicillin—sometimes in the neighbourhood of 1,000,000 units in 72 hours—may be required.

Dangerous oedema of the larynx sometimes associated with severe laryngitis and tonsillar infections, or with the parapharyngeal infections, will subside rapidly with systemic penicillin treatment. This is important, since the necessity of tracheotomy may be avoided.

Septic perichondritis of the laryngeal cartilages is treated according to the usual principles of penicillin therapy and is helpful as a pre-operative measure when this condition is associated with cancer of the larynx.

Wounds of the oesophageal wall may be caused by sharp pieces of bone or other foreign bodies lodging there or during the removal of these through an oesophagoscope. Such cases are always an anxiety because of the possibility of an ensuing mediastinitis. When a tear is seen or suspected, systemic therapy may be given expectantly for 3 or 4 days. In cases in which mediastinitis has occurred from these or other causes, penicillin therapy offers the best chance of recovery.

The prophylactic use of penicillin in operations on the pharynx and larynx.—Pre-operative and postoperative penicillin therapy in connexion with extensive operations on the pharynx and larynx for malignant disease, is of the utmost value. These patients are often emaciated and toxic so that preference for non-toxic penicillin over the sulphonamides is obvious. After laryngectomy the incisions heal quickly with the aid of penicillin therapy and the chance of a pharyngostome forming as a result of sloughing is much reduced. Consequently, the plastic repairs required after such operations as lateral pharyngectomy and laryngopharyngectomy may be undertaken earlier. Pulmonary complications are rendered less likely, and advantage of this should always be taken into consideration when the operation of deliberate preliminary tracheotomy is performed. Cervical cellulitis and its possible spread to the mediastinum can be controlled or prevented.

The ear: the external ear

Infections of the pinna.—The pinna and neighbouring areas are commonly affected by eczematous and seborrhoeic conditions which become secondarily infected. Penicillin as a cream, in a jelly base, or as a powder, is used to eradicate the penicillin-sensitive invaders, but the underlying atopic conditions must be treated concurrently. In severe and longstanding cases systemic therapy may be required. Other infective conditions, such as erysipelas and impetigo, which are likely to be met with in this situation, are dealt with in the appropriate section. In haematoma of the auricle, penicillin in powder form may be spread in the cavity after the blood clot has been evacuated prior to placing the auricle in a moulded splint. When perichondritis has occurred drainage and systemic therapy is required.

Furunculosis and diffuse inflammation of the auditory canal.—These are usually due to staphylococcal infections, but streptococci and pneumococci may be found together with *Esch. coli* and the common secondary invaders. Systemic penicillin therapy is required in the severe or recurrent cases. Should there be definite pus formation in a furuncle, especially when there is great accompanying pain, incision is required. After incision or spontaneous rupture a gauze wick is placed in the canal; it should be moistened repeatedly with penicillin solution by means of a dropper. In the later stages penicillin powder may be insufflated. Local injection of penicillin solution into the furuncle has not proved to be convenient in this painful complaint.

It may be noted that the eruptions on the drum and adjoining skin of the canal seen in otitis externa haemorrhagica are unaffected by any form of penicillin administration. In the mycotic infections of the auditory canal treatment is essentially similar to that of the former conditions. Although the fungi themselves are not sensitive to penicillin they disappear when the commensals are eradicated. Careful toilet is essential for rapid cure. The gentle rubbing of the canal walls with a cottonwool swab moistened with silver nitrate solution 10 per cent and the allowing of the walls to dry prior to introduction of the wick or insufflation of the powder, is recommended.

The ear: the tympanic cleft

Acute otitis media.—The organisms usually met with in the acute infections of the tympanic cleft and its complications are streptococci, pneumococci, staphylococci and occasionally *H. influenzae*. As the majority of organisms here are penicillin-sensitive, the immediate institution of systemic treatment with penicillin would be ideal but for its intramuscular method of administration. The disadvantage of this, especially in children, is obvious. On this account the more convenient sulphonamide therapy is usually given in actual practice and is justified by the good results often obtained. At present, therefore, the tendency is to reserve penicillin for those cases which do not respond to a sulphonamide and for those cases in which otitis media complicates infections in the nose and throat such as quinsy or suppurative sinusitis. Systemic therapy must be instituted as soon as possible whether the tympanic membrane is intact or perforated and should be kept up until all the criteria of healing have been achieved. The question of performing myringotomy depends upon the response to treatment. Improvement should be distinct in 24 hours, otherwise the membrane should be incised; but pain and tenderness in the mastoid process demand incision, and it is always better to incise when there is doubt. The specimen for bacteriological examination must be taken with care in order to avoid contamination. Whenever possible the specimen should be taken directly from the tympanic cavity either by aspiration through the membrane or by means of a platinum loop applied at the perforation. A thick wool swab thrust into the meatus should never be employed.

It appears that resolution under sulphonamide therapy without incision may, on occasion, leave a residual hearing loss due to adhesive processes in the tympanic cavity. It is impossible to say, until further experience has been gained, whether or not such adhesions develop with penicillin administration. When the tympanic membrane is perforated, either spontaneously or by incision, the ensuing otorrhoea should be treated by local application of penicillin, in addition to systemic therapy.

The choice between the wet and dry methods of application rests with the personal preference of the surgeon, but no matter which method is chosen a precise and painstaking aural toilet remains an essential part of the treatment. A solution of 1,000 units of penicillin per millilitre of physiological saline with ephedrine ½ per cent may be used as a nasal spray in order to reduce the congestion and infection at the pharyngeal end of the pharyngotympanic tube. Tubal drainage is encouraged by this procedure. Concomitant infections in the throat or sinuses must be dealt with and local treatment must be maintained until the perforation is closed.

The dry method.—As a first step, as much discharge as possible is sucked through the tympanic perforation by means of a Siegel's pneumatic speculum, sometimes aided by gentle efforts at Valsalva's manoeuvre, and the canal is thoroughly cleansed and dried. Penicillin powder is then insufflated or poured into the canal through an aural speculum. The ear is covered with gauze on which penicillin cream has been spread in order to prevent possible secondary infection of the pinna and meatus. Change of dressing is regulated by the amount of the discharge; usually, 2 or 3 times a day is sufficient and the changes become less frequent as the discharge lessens.

The wet method.—After cleansing the ear as for the previous method, a wick saturated with penicillin solution is introduced into the canal right down to the tympanic membrane. The wick should be changed 2 or 3 times a day until the discharge diminishes. In the later stages the wick may be left in for a day if it is kept moist by having the solution poured on to it by means of a pipette. The ear should be covered as before.

Acute mastoiditis.—Before the advent of chemotherapy and penicillin there was a growing consensus of opinion against very early operation, other than myringotomy, in acute mastoiditis. To wait for a week or longer was not unusual in the presence of mastoid tenderness and pyrexia. During this period the disease is limited to the mucoperiosteum of the mastoid cells. At this stage systemic therapy will often lead to complete cure without operation. At the same time local therapy should be carried out; systemic therapy, however, remains the essential factor. Experience shows that penicillin alone is more efficacious than are the sulphonamides alone, although they are frequently used together. Cases with the clinical signs and symptoms of established mastoiditis such as tenderness, oedema, and loss of cell outline on X-ray examination, have responded satisfactorily after a few days' treatment with systemic penicillin; the average dose of 15,000 units, given intramuscularly, every 3 hours, is employed. A warning must be given, however, against the possibility of incomplete resolution. When this occurs the usual clinical features may be masked and the disease progresses insidiously in a manner reminiscent of a pneumococcus type III infection. Vigilant watch must be kept, and repeated radiological examinations made, for deterioration at any time or the absence of improvement after 5 or 6 days' treatment will probably call for operation. In these circumstances ripe judgment and experience is required; it is always safer to operate when there is doubt, especially when the disease is of more than 2 or 3 weeks' duration. In order to detect a relapse, observation for a week or more after the cessation of treatment is necessary in those cases which have escaped operation and are regarded as cured. The onset of meningitis in the early stages of acute otitis is due to the spread of infection through preformed channels and does not benefit by immediate mastoidectomy in the presence of adequate systemic therapy. Similarly, urgent operation on the mastoid process for a facial paralysis is not necessary in the early stages of acute mastoiditis. In the later stages when bone necrosis has probably occurred—making it likely that pus may be in contact with the dura mater or lateral sinus—operation must be undertaken despite penicillin therapy.

Chronic suppurative otitis media.—Chronic otitis media presents additional problems as it is a longstanding disease in which irreversible tissue change may have taken place and the presence of secondary invaders insensitive to penicillin may be a feature. Penicillin will not have any effect on chronic granulations and polypi so that these must be removed or suitably treated. Cholesteatoma is an indication for operation.

Provided that the above conditions have been complied with, good results will accrue from local treatment, especially when it is combined with appropriate measures for combating any penicillin-insensitive organisms that may be present. Unfortunately, recurrence of otorrhoea commonly accompanies the onset of catarrhal conditions in the nasopharynx in those cases which have been made dry.

The wet and dry methods of application accompanied by careful toilet are employed, as in acute otitis media. In chronic otitis media the tympanic perforation may be large enough to allow the introduction of the solution directly into the tympanic cavity when this is aided by displacement carried out with a Siegel's speculum. After this, the head should be kept in such a position as to retain the fluid for 20 minutes or more. Daily dressings, wet or dry, are usually sufficient. If cessation of the discharge has not been achieved in 3 weeks' time there is little prospect of success by these methods.

Complications of mastoiditis.—Meningitis and brain abscess are fully discussed in another chapter. When these conditions are otogenic the question of operation on the mastoid process will arise. The penicillin therapy primarily directed against the intracranial complication will usually cure the source of infection without operation, if this is a recent mastoiditis. When these complications follow an exacerbation in a chronic mastoiditis, especially in cases in which cholesteatoma is present, radical operation will be required. The timing of such an operation is important. The operation should be delayed until general improvement resulting from penicillin therapy permits it to be undertaken without undue risk. Extradural abscess, including the perisinus type, always requires drainage through the mastoid process. Petrositis without abscess in the petrotemporal bone, as may occur after a mastoidectomy, is usually successfully treated by systemic therapy. As soon as abscess formation is suspected, however, exploration should be carried out. With regard to labyrinthitis, it is conceivable that penicillin may reach the labyrinth through its blood supply, but up to the present time there is not any record in which the hearing has been preserved after labyrinthine suppuration. The improvement seen in serous labyrinthitis probably results from the removal of its cause.

Penicillin is a powerful weapon in the treatment of the dangerous complication of lateral sinus thrombosis. Cases are on record in which this condition has progressed to the formation of metastatic abscesses and yet the patient has recovered without operation, solely as a result of penicillin therapy. Such a line of treatment is permissible only when operation is refused or is impossible. The mastoid process must be opened and the clot must be removed whenever there is evidence of dissemination of infection in the blood stream as shown by the characteristic temperature chart, chills, and rigors. The operation is performed under an umbrella of pre-operative penicillin administration. At the same time the internal jugular vein and its common facial tributary may be tied or not according to the surgeon's preference. The plug used to compress the upper end of the sinus should be soaked in penicillin solution.

Postoperative therapy is always required so that bacteriaemia, septicaemia and metastatic infection, potential or established, may be controlled. When the thrombotic process has extended to the sinuses of the falx cerebri to produce otitic hydrocephalus, help cannot be expected from penicillin administration other than that it will deal with the source of infection should this still remain.

The use of penicillin in mastoid operations.—Complete closure of the postauricular incision, no matter how extensive the operation, is a safe routine procedure which almost always results in primary union when penicillin is instilled into the cavity of a cortical mastoidectomy. For this purpose a fine rubber tube is placed in the cavity and is secured in the upper end of the incision, which is covered with tulle gras. One millilitre of penicillin solution (1,000 units per millilitre) is syringed down the upper end of the tube, which should be accessible without removal of the bandages and should be closed by a spigot. This treatment is given 3 or 4 times daily for some 4–6 days, after which, in satisfactory cases, the tube can be withdrawn. Systemic therapy may be given at the same time, but good results are usually obtained without it when this method is employed and when it is accompanied by toilet of the meatus. By this procedure the stay in hospital is shortened, the necessity for repeated painful dressings is obviated and the prospects of complete restoration of hearing are further improved. These good results make it probable that the modified operation designed to conserve hearing in chronic otitis will tend to replace radical operation more often than is at present the case.

In the operation of radical mastoidectomy a gauze strip soaked in penicillin solution is used to pack the cavity. The packing may be moistened *in situ* by means of a pipette and need not be changed for 4 or 5 days. After 10 days or so powder insufflation and very light packing suffices.

In the fenestration operation for otosclerosis, penicillin can play an important part in preventing labyrinthitis, which renders the operation unsuccessful.

BIBLIOGRAPHY

Discussion on Penicillin (1944) *Proc. R. Soc. Med.*, **37**, 101.
Mothersill, M. H. (1945) *Ann. Otol., etc., St. Louis*, **54**, 166.
Kolmer, J. A. (1944) *Arch. Otolaryng., Chicago*, **40**, 17.
Stewart, J. P. (1945) "The Use of Penicillin in Certain Diseases of the Ear, Nose and Throat", *Penicillin Therapy and Control in* 21 *Army Group.*
Fowlkes, J. W. (1945) *Laryngoscope, St. Louis*, **55**, 155.
Greenfield, S. D., Kuritzky, I., and Jacobs, E. A. (1945) *Laryngoscope, St. Louis*, **55**, 20.
Baum, H. L. (1945) *Arch. Otolaryng., Chicago*, **41**, 175.
Discussion on Penicillin in Rhinology (1946) *Proc. R. Soc. Med.*, **39**, 279.
Hauser, I. J., and Work, W. P. (1945) *Arch. Otolaryng., Chicago*, **41**, 161.
Gaines, T. R., and Hatcher, M. B. (1945) *Arch. Otolaryng., Chicago*, **42**, 1.
Putney, F. J. (1945) *Arch. Otolaryng., Chicago*, **41**, 247.
Macbeth, R G. (1945) *J. Laryng.*, **60**, 16.

DERMATOLOGY

By A. C. Roxburgh, M.D., F.R.C.P.
Physician for Diseases of the Skin, St. Bartholomew's Hospital, London

PENICILLIN THERAPY

The types of skin disease in which penicillin is useful are, naturally, those due to infection with penicillin-sensitive organisms or those in which a secondary infection with penicillin-sensitive organisms complicates the original condition. The vast majority of skin diseases which yield to penicillin are those due to *Staph. aureus* and to *Str. pyogenes*, for example, impetigo, blepharitis, sycosis, pustular folliculitis, boils, carbuncles, erysipelas. Less common infections susceptible to penicillin are anthrax and erysipeloid (due to *Ery. rhusiopathiae*, the bacillus of swine erysipelas). *T. pallidum* and *Bor. vincenti* are also sensitive. Unfortunately, the fungi such as the ringworms and the monilias, the filter-passing viruses responsible for herpes labialis, herpes zoster, warts and molluscum contagiosum, the coliform group, *Str. faecalis*, *Proteus*, *Ps. aeruginosa* and the tubercle bacillus are quite insensitive. *A. bovis* is partly sensitive. Some penicillin-insensitive organisms may even destroy penicillin, so that in a mixed infection they indirectly protect penicillin-sensitive organisms. Even in cases in which the organism is at first sensitive to penicillin, when treatment has to be prolonged (for example, because the organisms are difficult of access, as in sycosis) the organism may eventually develop a resistance to penicillin.

In the majority of skin diseases in which it is helpful, penicillin can be used locally, applied to the lesion either in solution by spray, or as a cream. The advantages of local application are that a much higher concentration of the drug can be brought to the required site than is possible by systemic injection, there is an enormous economy in penicillin and the treatment can be applied by the patient himself in his home. Local application is useless, however, if the drug cannot reach the organisms, for example, because they are too deeply seated—as in boils, carbuncles, anthrax and erysipeloid; there is also the disadvantage that occasionally the skin of a patient is irritated by either the penicillin itself, or an impurity in it, or a constituent of the base in which it is applied, for instance, Lanette wax SX.

Media for local use

Solution.—A sterile solution of sodium or calcium penicillin of a strength of 500 or 1,000 units per millilitre is applied by means of a spray to the affected area 2 or 3 times daily. The solution for spraying should be prepared with distilled water, not saline, for if the latter is used an irritating deposit of common salt is left on the skin. The advantages of a solution for use in hospital are that it is cheaper than is a cream, it can be quickly applied to a large number of patients by means of a spray without risk of cross infection, and there is not any chance of irritation from the base, as there is with creams. The principal drawback is that spray apparatus is expensive and tends to become choked and broken. Solutions are not as convenient as are creams for individual use, and penicillin deteriorates more quickly in solution than it does in creams. Solutions of modern penicillin keep for from 2 to 3 months in a refrigerator but at room temperatures they lose activity after a week; therefore when possible they should be freshly made. When possible, all penicillin preparations should be kept in a refrigerator at 5° C. (41° F.).

Creams.—A commonly used cream consists of 30 per cent of Lanette wax SX in water. The objection to this formula is that on the skin the wax forms a film which later peels off and, moreover, is irritating to certain skins (Burrows and Russell[1]). If Lanette wax SX is sterilized at a temperature exceeding 110° C. it may become acid and so destroy the penicillin (Gough, Still and Wozencroft)[2].

The cream used by my colleagues and me in our original work on penicillin in skin diseases (Roxburgh, Christie and Roxburgh)[3], consisted of equal parts of Lanette wax SX, soft paraffin and water. The cream we are at present using at St. Bartholomew's Hospital consists of 27 per cent arachis oil in water with 13 per cent Lanette wax SX as an emulsifier. The formula for this was given by Jeffrey[4], as follows.

Arachis oil ...	125 millilitres
Lanette wax SX ...	60 grammes
Water	275 millilitres

Heat the sterilized oil to 70° C. Add the wax. Heat the water to 60–65° C. Add the water to the wax and oil with gentle stirring. Maintain at 65° C. for 2 hours in order to sterilize. Store in 100-gramme pots in a refrigerator until the cream is needed. Before use add 4 millilitres of penicillin solution of 10,000 units per millilitre to each 100-gramme pot of cream, mixing well under cover of a glass box. This gives a cream of 400 units per gramme.

A non-greasy tragacanth and glycerin jelly base has been recommended by Spencer, Bishop and Ricks[5]. There are several commercially prepared bases for penicillin creams.

Whatever base is used the penicillin solution should be added under sterile conditions immediately before it is issued to the patient or the ward. The solution is prepared by dissolving tablets of calcium or sodium penicillin in the appropriate amount of sterile distilled water to make a solution of 10,000 units per millilitre, and the necessary amount of this solution is then stirred into the penicillin cream. Sometimes phenoxetol (β-phenoxyethyl-alcohol) in a strength of 3 per cent is incorporated in the base in order to discourage the growth of organisms like *Ps. aeruginosa*, which may destroy the penicillin. At St. Bartholomew's Hospital we give to each patient, with his penicillin cream, the following printed instructions. (1) Keep the pot of cream in a cold place, preferably in a refrigerator. (2) Sterilize the blade of a table knife by holding it in boiling water for 3 minutes, and allow it to cool. (3) Take from the jar, on the knife blade, only sufficient cream for one application and immediately screw on the lid of the jar again. (4) Transfer the cream from the knife to the affected area with a clean finger, and smear it evenly over the surface. (5) The cream should be applied twice daily, preferably morning and evening. (6) Never put any cream back into the jar.

Diseases suitable for local application of penicillin in cream or spray

A strength of 400 units per gramme in the cream and 500 or 1,000 units per millilitre in the spray, is assumed. The cream is usually applied twice daily and the spray 3 times daily.

Impetigo.—Whether due to staphylococcal, streptococcal or mixed infections, this disease is usually cured in 5 or 6 days by the application twice daily of penicillin cream or 3 times daily of a penicillin spray. At the beginning of the treatment the crusts should be bathed off with physiological saline or removed by application of boric acid fomentations or starch poultices. The penicillin should be applied to the whole face each time in order to prevent the occurrence of new lesions. If improvement has not taken place in 5 days or if it has ceased before cure is complete, a change should be made to some other form of treatment (Roxburgh[6]).

In bullous impetigo of the newborn or of adults, the bullae should be cut away entirely with scissors and the cream or spray should be applied to the whole raw area and its surroundings; it should also be worked well in under the overhanging edges left by the blisters, since it is here that the staphylococci tend to lurk and to cause extension of the lesions.

Ecthyma.—The crusts must be removed by application of fomentations or starch poultices and the ulcers should be filled with penicillin cream twice daily or sprayed with solution 3 times daily. A waterproof dressing should be applied in order to keep the penicillin in place.

Intertrigo.—Cases of intertrigo which are of streptococcal origin respond to treatment with penicillin cream or spray. Those—more common—which are due to monilia infection are not improved.

Streptococcal fissures.—These, situated at the lower pole of the ear and at the angle of the nose or mouth, sometimes heal in a few days if penicillin cream is applied twice daily. In other cases they do not respond, no doubt because of the presence of insensitive organisms.

Otitis externa.—When streptococci or staphylococci play a considerable part in any given lesion there probably will be improvement with the use of penicillin cream or penicillin solution applied on a wick or sprayed into the ear, but many cases carry a heavy infection of insensitive organisms such as *Esch. coli*, and are little improved by penicillin treatment.

Blepharitis.—In many instances chronic blepharitis clears dramatically when it is treated with penicillin either in the form of a cream applied to the edges of the lids night and morning, or in the form of drops of the solution instilled between the eyelids 3 or 4 times a day. In some cases the cream irritates the conjunctiva and the use of drops is preferable.

Sycosis barbae.—Staphylococcal type. In most cases of chronic sycosis, penicillin applied either as a cream or a spray produces a dramatic apparent cure in about from 10 to 14 days, but should the treatment then be discontinued, the disease usually relapses sooner or later, especially if it has persisted for several years before penicillin treatment is begun. Probably the application of cream or spray should be continued once daily for weeks or even months after apparent cure, in the hope that the infection will eventually die out. In some cases, however, prolonged treatment leads only to the organisms becoming penicillin-resistant or to the patient becoming sensitized either to the penicillin or to one of its impurities, or to some constituent of the cream base, for example, Lanette wax SX. It is possible that combined systemic and local treatment with penicillin might be more effective than is local treatment alone, but so far I have had insufficient experience of this form of treatment to pronounce on it. Needless to say, all other possible foci of local staphylococcal infection in the teeth, sinuses, nostrils or external auditory meatus, as well as seborrhoea of the scalp, must be eliminated as far as possible; the patient should shave along the direction of the beard's growth and not against it. In the active stage of the disease he should not shave at all, but should clip the beard with scissors or clippers.

There is not any doubt that penicillin is a boon to most patients with chronic sycosis, as it does good far more rapidly than do most other treatments; but it does not by any means provide a cure for every case. For other treatments *vide* Roxburgh[6]. Penicillin is useless in ringworm of the beard.

Superficial pustular perifolliculitis (*Bockhart's impetigo*).—Staphylococcal perifolliculitis with small pustules at the orifices of the pilosebaceous glands, affecting especially the scalp, the thighs or other hairy areas. As this is an infection of the superficial parts of the follicle only, as opposed to the infection of the whole follicle which constitutes a boil, it often responds well to the application of penicillin cream or spray. One exceptionally severe example in a soldier of World War I, in whom all 4 limbs had been severely affected for 25 years, cleared in a few days with the use of penicillin cream only, but soon relapsed. After combined treatment with systemic penicillin for about one week and a cream for about 2 weeks the skin remained clear for a year except for two relapses of 3 and 4 weeks respectively.

Infective eczematoid dermatitis.—This sometimes arises around an infected wound or sinus. It improves rapidly with penicillin cream or spray when the sensitization of the skin happens to be to a penicillin-sensitive organism such as *Staph. aureus* or *Str. pyogenes*, but it does not improve when the sensitization is due to a penicillin-insensitive organism such as *Str. faecalis* or *Esch. coli.*

Skin lesions secondarily infected with penicillin-sensitive organisms.—It often happens that cases of eczema, seborrhoeic dermatitis, sulphonamide dermatitis, X-ray or radium dermatitis, scabies, lichen urticatus, varicose ulcer and other skin diseases not due in themselves to infection, become secondarily infected with penicillin-sensitive organisms such as *Staph. aureus* and *Str. pyogenes.* In such cases from 5 to 7 days' treatment with penicillin cream or spray clears the secondary infection, often with very beneficial results to the original condition, although it does not cure it. In many cases of secondary infection, however, insensitive organisms are present which are not only unaffected by penicillin but which may even destroy it, thus protecting indirectly any sensitive organisms which may be present.

Diseases which require systemic penicillin

Boils.—A course of 5 or 6 days of penicillin injections—15,000 or 20,000 units given intramuscularly 3-hourly—will usually clear a series of boils. In some cases the course has to be repeated as the boils recur. The local application of penicillin spray or cream to the surroundings of the boil helps to prevent others arising, especially in an area such as the axilla, but boils cannot be cured by local application alone since the staphylococci are too deeply seated in the follicles.

Carbuncles.—The same applies with even more force in the case of carbuncles. From 5 to 7 days of penicillin injections—20,000 units given intramuscularly 3-hourly—will often abort or cut short the course of a carbuncle. If the carbuncle has to be opened the cavity should be sprayed with penicillin solution 3-hourly or packed with gauze which is re-wetted with penicillin solution 3-hourly. Carbuncles sometimes relapse a week or so after penicillin treatment is stopped and, therefore, the penicillin must be resumed if necessary.

Erysipelas.—Since this is a streptococcal infection it usually responds so well to administration of sulphonamides that penicillin injections are hardly necessary, but if for any reason sulphonamides are contra-indicated, penicillin injections for 5 or 6 days usually cure erysipelas.

Recurrent cellulitis of the face.—Although this is supposed to be a streptococcal infection 3 of my patients treated with full courses of penicillin injections for from 5 to 7 days, have received hardly any benefit.

Erythema serpens (Morrant Baker), *Erysipeloid* (Rosenbach).—This infection of the skin with *Erysipelothrix rhusiopathiae* is usually seen in fishermen, butchers or cooks as a result of a prick or scratch with a meat bone or fish spine. The condition clears in from 2 to 4 days with penicillin injections of 15,000–20,000 units 3-hourly (Hodgson[7]; Barber, Nellen and Zoob[8]).

Actinomycosis.—Hamilton and Kirkpatrick[9] report on 2 patients who apparently were cured by between 5,000,000 and 6,000,000 units of penicillin given systemically.

Anthrax.—Penicillin injections are the treatment of choice in this severe infection. Fifteen thousand units administered 3-hourly for 4 or 5 days seems usually to be sufficient (Murphy, La Boccetta and Lockwood[10]; Abrahams[11]).

For records of results of penicillin treatment in diseases of the skin see Roxburgh, Christie and Roxburgh[3]; Taylor and Hughes[12]; Hellier and Hodgson[13]; Twiston Davies, Dixon and Stuart-Harris[14].

Side effects of penicillin

These are remarkably uncommon. I have encountered, I suppose, about a dozen in whom penicillin cream set up a dermatitis, and in some of these the spray was equally irritating; a patch test showed that it was the penicillin itself (or one of its impurities) which was responsible and not the cream base. In others the solution was tolerated, showing that it was the cream base which was causing irritation, and this was confirmed by patch test.

Contact dermatitis from penicillin has been recorded by Pyle and Rattner[15]; Barker[16]; Michie and Bailie[17]; Vickers[18].

The commonest reactions to intramuscular injections are urticaria, erythema, oedema and irritation of the skin sometimes accompanied by fever and abdominal colic (Lyons[19]; Cormia, Jacobsen and Smith[20]; Haswell and Wilkinson[21]). Cormia, Jacobsen and Smith mention a reaction like serum sickness, also acute syncope, transient miliaria-like eruptions, erythemato-vesicular eruptions, erythema nodosum and epididymitis. For an annotation on reactions to penicillin see the *Lancet* of 2nd March, 1946, p. 316, from which some of the above references are quoted.

REFERENCES

1 Burrows, A., and Russell, B. (1945), *Brit. med. J.*, **2**, 198.
2 Gough, J. B., Still, M., and Wozencroft, C. J. H. (1945), *Lancet*, **2**, 91.
3 Roxburgh, I. A., Christie, R. V., and Roxburgh, A. C. (1944), *Brit. med. J.*, **1**, 524.
4 Jeffrey, J. S. (1945), *Med. Annu.*, 222, Wright, Bristol.
5 Spencer, J., Bishop, E. J., and Ricks, A. (1946), *Lancet*, **1**, 127.
6 Roxburgh, A. C. (1946), *Common Skin Diseases*, 8th edition, H. K. Lewis, London.
7 Hodgson, G. A. (1945), *Brit. med. J.*, **1**, 483.
8 Barber, M., Nellen, M., and Zoob, M. (1946), *Lancet*, **1**, 125.
9 Hamilton, A. J. C., and Kirkpatrick, H. J. R. (1945), *Brit. med. J.*, **2**, 728.
10 Murphy, F. D., La Boccetta, A. C., and Lockwood, J. S. (1944), *J. Amer. med. Ass.*, **126**, 948.
11 Abrahams, A. M. (1945), *Brit. med. J.*, **1**, 771.
12 Taylor, P. H., and Hughes, K. E. A. (1944), *Lancet*, **2**, 780.
13 Hellier, F. F., and Hodgson, G. A. (1945), *Lancet*, **2**, 462.
14 Twiston Davies, J. H., Dixon, K., and Stuart-Harris, C. H. (1945) *Quart. J. med.* **14**, 183.
15 Pyle, H. D., and Rattner, H. (1944), *J. Amer. med. Ass.*, **125**, 903.
16 Barker, A. N. (1945), *Lancet*, **1**, 177.
17 Michie, W., and Bailie, H. W. C. (1945), *Brit. med. J.*, **1**, 554.
18 Vickers, H. R. (1946), *Lancet*, **1**, 307.
19 Lyons, C. (1943), *J. Amer. med. Ass.*, **123**, 1007.
20 Cormia, F. E., Jacobsen, L. Y., and Smith, E. L. (1945), *Bull. U.S. Army Med. Dept.*, **4**, 694.
21 Haswell, R. E., and Wilkinson, J. F. (1946), *Lancet*, **1**, 308.

DENTAL AND ORAL INFECTIONS

By E. Wilfred Fish, M.D., D.D.Sc., D.Sc.
Honorary Dental Surgeon, St. Mary's Hospital; Honorary Research Associate in Physiology, University College, London

INTRODUCTION

Since it is a fact that all the usual mouth organisms are more or less sensitive to penicillin, it is reasonable to expect considerable benefit from its use in oral and dental surgery; but an essential condition, if good results are to be obtained, is a complete knowledge of the habitat and distribution of the organisms in and about the oral tissues.

The vast majority of dental infections, apart from dental caries, are caused by streptococci and staphylococci to which may perhaps be added *B. fusiformis* and Vincent's spirochaete. All these organisms are markedly sensitive to penicillin, and because they are all serophytes, they cannot be killed by antibodies in the serum and can be eliminated only by the leucocytes or destroyed by chemotherapy.

When the inflammatory reactions produced by them are divided in the usual way into acute and chronic varieties, a very important difference in the distribution of the bacteria is observed. In the acute lesions the bacteria have actually invaded, or been thrust into, the normal tissues, and the acute reaction represents the effort of these tissues to destroy, expel or control them. In the chronic reaction the bacteria are already controlled and isolated in a necrotic nidus, from which, if they grow out, they will be destroyed, but in which they can flourish in an environment inimical to, or even beyond the reach of, the leucocytes.

A few examples will illustrate this important distinction. If a reamer be thrust through the apical foramen of a septic root canal it will carry with it the bacteria from the canal and implant them in the hitherto uninfected periapical tissues. An acute apical abscess will be the result. Conversely, as an example of a chronic lesion, an apical granuloma may be examined histologically *in situ* in serial sections, stained alternately with Gram's stain and haematoxylin-eosin. It will then be found that the bacteria are confined to the septic root canal, that a few polymorphonuclear leucocytes are lying round the opening of the canal, ready to engulf any organism that grows out, but unable to survive if they should enter the canal. Beyond these leucocytes is the granuloma, consisting largely of lymphocytes and plasma cells, but there are no bacteria amongst them. They are apparently attracted only by the presence of the soluble toxic matter which infiltrates the tissue round the opening of the infected canal. In such a lesion it is of no use to inject penicillin into the blood stream, for it is not possible for it to reach the organisms in the stagnant root canal in sufficient concentration to destroy them.

An even more convincing demonstration of the sterility of the tissue surrounding a chronic septic focus is possible in the case of pyorrhoea. This disease consists essentially of chronic septic ulceration of the epithelium lining the parodontal sulcus or pocket at the gum margin. If a tooth, thus affected but having a live pulp, be extracted, bacteria can almost always be cultivated from the apex of the extracted tooth; but it can be shown easily that these organisms were not on the apex of the tooth before extraction. They were confined to the surface debris on the ulcers in the parodontal sulcus; for if the sulcus be sterilized by a rapid sweep of the actual cautery all round the tooth, and the tooth be forthwith expeditiously extracted, both the pulp and the parodontal surface of the root will be found to be sterile[1].

It is possible that these bacteria on the surface of the gingival ulcer will be thrust into the deeper tissues by masticatory trauma or by injudicious use of a scaler, but in that event an acute lesion will supervene, and acute parodontal abscess, culminating in the isolated deep pocket of pyorrhoea profunda, is a frequently encountered complication of chronic marginal gingivitis[2].

The application of penicillin to oral lesions depends upon these basic findings. For instance, if a tooth is to be extracted, and it is not possible to sterilize the parodontal sulcus with the actual cautery—as is the case in a partially erupted and impacted lower third molar—an intramuscular injection of 50,000 units into the buttock 15 minutes before the operation will render the blood stream and the tissues surrounding the tooth, into which bacteria will very probably be thrust during the operation, inimical to the survival and growth of these organisms. It will, therefore, prevent, or at least limit, the widespread and extremely painful septic osteitis which hitherto has been so common a sequel. That does not excuse the surgeon from exercising the greatest care in limiting local trauma by every means in his power.

SOME CONDITIONS DESCRIBED

It will be practical to consider individually the various uses to which penicillin can be put in oral operations.

Vincent's acute necrotic stomatitis

Pathology.—In this condition the surface epithelium is ulcerated away, exposing the papillae of the corium. During mastication, or even speech, penicillin-sensitive bacteria (notably *B. fusiformis* and *Bor. vincenti*) are thrust into the subepithelial connective tissue, causing acute inflammation[2]. A photomicrograph has been published [2] showing *B. fusiformis* in considerable numbers in the tissues during the acute phase of the disease. No other Gram positive organisms were seen. When this happens at the bases of detached interdental papillae, as it often does, the accompanying congestion and stasis cause necrosis of the tip of the papilla. The necrotic apex of the papilla forms a yellowish green slough which is diagnostic of the disease; when the slough separates it leaves a crater in place of the pointed tip of the papilla, and this "scalloped" appearance of the gum margin is also distinctive of the later stages of Vincent's angina.

Indications.—These considerations indicate three modes of attack.

(1) The patient may be directed to suck penicillin lozenges, thereby destroying the penicillin-sensitive flora of the mouth.

(2) The surface of the ulcers may be tanned with chromic acid[2]. This limits the risk of further invasion of the tissues; and, with the same object, the patient is put on a soft diet for a few days and mouth washes are substituted for the toothbrush.

(3) Intramuscular injections of penicillin may be given for the purpose of destroying the bacteria which have already entered the tissues, or which may do so despite the precautions prescribed in (1) and (2) above.

Method of treatment.—The lozenge contains 500 units of penicillin and may be expected to remain effective for as long as 4 months if it is stored at a temperature below 10° C. and is kept in an airtight sterile container—although it will gradually lose strength. After 2 months at room temperature the penicillin content may drop to as low as 100 units but even if the potency of the lozenge has been reduced by one half it may still be sufficiently effective. Moisture causes rapid deterioration, therefore the bottle of lozenges should be kept tightly corked (see chapter on Pharmacology).

At the patient's first visit, any debris which can be removed from the necks of the teeth without injury to the ulcerated gum margin, should be cleared away. A section of the gum margin is painted with chromic acid (20 per cent solution in water) and this is followed at once by an application of hydrogen peroxide (Liquor Hydrogenii Peroxidi B.P., U.S.P. XI) before the lips are allowed to come in contact with it. The patient should rinse the mouth with warm hydrogen peroxide solution. Cotton rolls should not be used because they may hold the chromic acid in contact with the tissues and cause irritation, but there is no danger from traces of the solution spilling over the mucosa, provided that only a minim or so of the solution is used and that it is rapidly rendered inert. The other parts of the gum margin are treated in the same way, as also are any ulcers on the buccal mucosa.

When this treatment is completed, a penicillin lozenge is tucked into the buccal sulcus between the third upper molar and the cheek as high up in the buccal sulcus as it will go. The patient is told to avoid disturbing it or exploring it with his tongue, and to replace it when it has completely disintegrated—a process which should take 2 or 3 hours—at least in the daytime. One lozenge should last throughout the night. In a very severe case, or in one in which the lesions are widely distributed, it is advisable to place a lozenge on each side of the mouth at the same time.

The patient should avoid touching the gums with a tooth-brush, however soft, during the acute stage, in conformity with the principle of resting acutely inflamed tissues. A peroxide mouthwash (one part of 10 volume peroxide in 5 parts of warm water) is prescribed to remove gross debris, and a bland semi-fluid diet is ordered, together with a saline aperient and rest. The patient should even be discouraged from talking at first, and must not smoke.

The chromic acid treatment should be repeated once or twice daily and the acute phase will generally clear up in 2 or 3 days. It must not be thought, however, that the responsibility of the dental surgeon ceases at this point, for it is imperative that a complete toilet of the mouth should be carried out. Tartar must be completely removed, detached papillae and pockets of more than a millimetre in depth must be cut away, and the patient must be instructed how to keep the gum margins well keratinized by daily friction all round every tooth with brush and wood point. It is necessary to prescribe a soft brush and balsa wood points in the first place, but as the epithelium develops a more robust keratinous cuticle, a medium brush and whalebone points will be found to be more acceptable.

In an extremely severe case in which the necrotic ulceration has spread beyond the gum margins and has involved the buccal mucosa, tongue and palate, or even the tonsils and pharynx, it is advisable to confine the patient to bed and to institute systemic treatment with penicillin. An initial intramuscular dose of 50,000 units may be given, followed by 15,000 units every 3 hours or 100,000 units every 12 hours until the acute symptoms abate and, indeed, for one or two days longer (see chapter on Pharmacology).

Warning.—There is one note of warning. It is extremely inadvisable to use penicillin lozenges, either casually or often, for trivial reasons. It is possible to produce or select a resistant strain of streptococci by constant and incomplete use of the drug. It is then possible that these resistant bacteria will invade the lung or be transferred to some other person who may become gravely ill and be beyond the help which, in a normal case, penicillin could afford.

A second reason for the avoidance of indiscriminate use of the lozenges for trivial reasons is that they may cause a most painful stomatitis. The tissues of the lip, tongue and cheek become red and shiny and extremely sensitive to salt, acid, spices, tobacco and spirits. Salivation is very free and sleep is disturbed. The condition clears up on discontinuance of the lozenges. This stomatitis may be due to invasion of the oral cavity by insensitive bacteria following the destruction of the normal mouth flora, or it may have a chemical origin and be due to some constituent other than penicillin in the lozenge.

It is wise, therefore, to restrict the lozenges to those cases in which they are of specific value—for example, Vincent's acute ulcerative stomatitis, or even a simple streptococcal stomatitis brought on by excessive smoking—and to discontinue their use as soon as their primary function has been performed.

Cancrum oris

I have not had any experience of this rare condition since the advent of penicillin, but the pathology of the disease is similar to that of Vincent's stomatitis, although the necrosis of the soft tissues is more rapidly progressive and the bone may share the fate of the soft tissue. The treatment, therefore, may be similar to that described above. Penicillin should be administered intramuscularly as in a severe case of Vincent's infection, but the doses might be doubled and accompanied by the use of lozenges if the patient were well enough to tolerate them. The lesion should be dusted with penicillin and sulphathiazole powder by means of an insufflator. Severe caustics are contraindicated although the chromic acid and hydrogen peroxide sequence might be used with advantage to tan the surface of the lesion and to render it temporarily less permeable to bacteria. The sensitivity to penicillin of such organisms as could be cultivated should be tested as soon as possible.

SURGICAL INTERFERENCE IN SEPTIC AREAS

Pathology

Deliberate surgical interference for the purpose of securing drainage or for the elimination of a septic focus in bone is always liable—and indeed almost certain—to cause a transient bacterial shower into the blood stream[3] and to spread infection into the neighbouring tissue. A simple extraction in the presence of chronic marginal gingivitis falls in this category as would the passage of a cold root canal bristle or reamer into a pulp which had become exposed by caries. The former risk can often be combated, as we have seen, by cauterization of the gum margin, and the latter by the preliminary use of a pulp desiccator heated electrically to a temperature above 100° C[4].

In operations for the removal of impacted and partially erupted teeth it is not possible to cauterize the sulcus, and considerable trauma to the bone may be unavoidable in the course of operation. Premedication with penicillin is, therefore, of great advantage in order to render the surrounding tissues, as well as the blood, bactericidal to sensitive organisms.

There are cases in which a bacterial shower is a particular danger. Normally, the bacteria are rapidly killed by the reticulo-endothelial cells of the lymphoid tissue and of the spleen and liver; but in a patient with vegetations on the heart valves, there is always a danger of the organisms becoming implanted on the vegetations, causing an infective endocarditis to supervene. Whenever a dental operation likely to cause a bacterial shower is to be performed on any patient who has had rheumatic fever in earlier life it is wise, therefore, to take extra precautions; this is carried out by systemic premedication with penicillin. Another type of case is that in which it is particularly important to secure healing by first intention. The excision of small cysts followed by immediate suture, root resections, replantation of teeth and, indeed, any operation in the oral cavity in which it is intended to close up the wound at once, is an operation in which the chances of success are greatly enhanced by the use of penicillin either in the form of systemic premedication or by local application, or by both.

Method of treatment

Open wounds.—When the wound is to be left open, as in the case of removal of impacted teeth or ordinary extraction in patients who have a simple endocarditis or give a history of rheumatic fever, it is advisable not only to cauterize the gum margin (if that is possible) but also to give a preliminary dose of penicillin (50,000 units) intramuscularly, from 10 minutes to half an hour before operation. This dose may be doubled and supplemented with a further dose of 15,000 units 3-hourly for 24 hours after operation if it is thought that there is special risk.

Closed wounds.—When the wound is to be closed, as after total excision of a small cyst lining or a root resection, a 10,000 unit tablet, or a portion of such a tablet, may be left in the bone cavity. Impacted third molar wounds, even, may be treated in this way if systemic premedication with penicillin has been carried out and if all bone debris has been removed and bruising of the bone has been avoided. Intramuscular injection of penicillin should be continued for 4 days after operation.

Replantation of teeth.—Extraction of teeth with chronic granulomata and their subsequent replantation is being attempted with encouraging results in cases in which an apicectomy is impracticable. It cannot be said to have passed the experimental stage as yet, but there is good theoretical reason to suppose that a high percentage of successful results may be obtained. The procedure is contra-indicated when the apical lesion is acute, or of course if the tooth is already loose.

Hitherto failure has often followed attempts at replantation as a result of infection being implanted on the surface of the root or because, in an attempt to avoid this, strong antiseptics have been used, or the tooth has even been boiled. Strong disinfectants would kill the surrounding parodontal tissues, and in the latter event the boiling has so changed the nature of the dentine that it constitutes an irritant to the surrounding bone cells and becomes resorbed. Success, therefore, will depend upon excluding infection from the root surface as far as possible at the moment of extraction and upon using penicillin to kill such infection as may nevertheless gain access. It will be recalled that hyaline cementum is impermeable to bacteria or their products and that infection in the dentinal tubules cannot pass it and interfere with re-attachment.

The procedure is as follows. In the first place a splint is prepared which subsequently may be cemented in place. It must not interfere with the bite and should give stability by attachment to the adjoining teeth. The pulp chamber of the tooth is opened up, disinfected, cauterized and filled; the root canals, which may be inaccessible, may be left for the moment. As this interference with the pulp chamber might cause an acute alveolar abscess as a result of infection being inadvertently thrust through the apex, the extraction and replantation must be proceeded with immediately and must not on any account be postponed.

The sulcus should be cauterized before extraction and a 10,000 unit tablet of penicillin should be placed in the socket immediately afterwards and before it fills with blood. This is followed by a firm pack of sterile ribbon gauze. It will be obvious that if the extraction is a difficult one involving major damage to the tooth or its socket, the replantation may have to be abandoned. The extracted tooth is held in sterile gauze soaked in penicillin solution made by dissolving one 10,000 unit tablet in 2 millilitres of water. The root of the tooth is also painted with this solution. The apex or apices are amputated and the root canals are reamed out, cauterized and filled with cement and gutta-percha points from the amputated end. When the cement is set the surface of the amputated end is polished off flat with a sterile disc and is touched with a flat instrument heated just above boiling point. Its corners must not be rounded off as this would open up fresh tubules which might harbour infection. The gauze is removed from the socket and, after the root has been dipped in the penicillin solution, the tooth is replaced, being held in place by means of the previously prepared splint. The splint is cemented to both the replanted tooth and to the adjoining teeth; it should remain in place for 8 weeks.

The success of the operation depends upon certain minutae of technique which in turn depend upon the surgeon's being not unfamiliar with details of bacteriological method. For example, the tooth must be held so that when reaming out the canals the debris does not fall upon and infect the rest of the tooth. The tooth must not be shifted about in the gauze in which it is held in case organisms should be transferred from the crown to the root surfaces. Above all, the tooth should be x-rayed after 6 months, to ensure that bone has grown close up round the amputated end, which should have become surrounded by a continuous lamina dura, indicating that it was, and has remained, sterile. An added precaution would be to give an injection of 50,000 units of penicillin 15 minutes before operation and even, perhaps, a similar dose 3 hours afterwards.

When operating for the relief of acute suppuration in bone it is particularly important to give a preliminary dose of penicillin a quarter of an hour before operation. The common example of this is the acute alveolar abscess in which the danger of spreading the infection into the adjoining bone and soft tissues and throughout the blood stream in the course of extracting the tooth, is quite serious. In ordinary cases an intramuscular injection of 50,000 units would be sufficient but a case record may be instructive.

The patient, a girl of 19 years of age, had had a septic root canal treated in an upper lateral incisor. The next day it was causing pain and the dressing was removed. A few hours later the pain increased and that night the lip became swollen. Next morning, 48 hours after the first treatment, the patient had a rigor and the temperature was 105·6° F.; she was immediately admitted to hospital. She was given 100,000 units of penicillin, and 15 minutes later the tooth was extracted and the swelling incised in the labial sulcus; a large amount of streptococcal pus was evacuated. This was followed by 3-hourly injections of 15,000 units of penicillin intramuscularly for 4 days and the patient made an uneventful recovery. In contrast to this history, a case was reported to me, before the advent of penicillin for clinical use—in fact some 10 years ago—of a youth who died of septicaemia in similar circumstances.

Maxillo-facial injuries

Injuries of the soft tissues which do not involve bone may be heavily infected, and are often complicated by the presence of soiled fragments of non-viable tissue. The patient should be given an injection of 50,000 units of penicillin and, under general anaesthesia, the wound should be submitted to a thorough and delicately performed surgical toilet. Debris is removed and any hopelessly damaged tissue is cut away with sharp instruments—or, better still, a diathermy knife—in order to avoid spreading infection. The wound is dusted with penicillin and sulphathiazole powder. If it be possible to close the wound by suturing skin, or even skin to mucous membrane, this should be done in order to prevent deep scarring, even although it may be necessary to perform subsequent plastic repair. In severe cases a perforated drainage tube may be left in for 2–4 days; irrigation of the wound with penicillin solution is carried out 3 or 4 times each day. When the area is free from active inflammation the tube may be removed. Meanwhile, and perhaps for 2 or 3 more days, a 3-hourly injection of 15,000 units of penicillin may be given intramuscularly, depending upon the severity of the wound and the degree of infection.

When the wound involves fracture of the maxilla or mandible, fixation must be secured at the time of operation, which should not be postponed longer than necessary to combat shock; but in any case the systemic administration of penicillin should be inaugurated at once with an injection of 50,000 units followed by 3-hourly doses of 15,000 units for 5 days.

The use of penicillin does not supersede the necessity for efficient and thorough surgery—teeth in the line of fracture and detached bone fragments must be removed, together with any foreign body—but more latitude is permissible. Previously it might have been advisable to fix the fracture and to wait 2 or 3 days before removing the teeth in the line of fracture; these now may be extracted at the same time if the sepsis is being controlled by systemic penicillin treatment. Even greater risks may be accepted if there is adequate reason, as the following case will show.

A man, aged 25 years, was admitted to hospital with a compound fracture through the crypt of a deeply-placed horizontally-impacted lower third molar. Its removal would have caused the most severe disruption of the fracture, which was in good position and displayed little or no mobility. The wound into the mouth on the labial side of the fracture was small. The patient was given a full systemic course of penicillin commencing 48 hours after the injury, and the wound became clean in a further 48 hours. Union took place without the removal of the impacted tooth or further incident.

Osteomyelitis of the jaw

This condition occasionally occurs in an acute form as a sequel to tooth extraction. In its most simple form it results in "dry socket"; in its more extensive manifestation it may result in necrosis of the whole mandible.

Aetiology.—The cause of osteomyelitis of the jaw as a sequel to tooth extraction is reasonably clear. It has been shown already that when a tooth is extracted the blades of the forceps disturb the chronic ulcers which are extremely common in the parodontal sulcus, and carry infection some distance down into the parodontal membrane. The rocking of the tooth which follows alternately expands and compresses the vessels in the parodontal membrane, thereby pumping this infection into the blood stream.

If the bone trauma consequent upon the extraction is sufficiently severe, the vessels entering the bone may be crushed and damaged, and their contained blood will coagulate. Furthermore, this blood is known to be infected at this particular moment and there is a considerable risk that the bacteria in it will survive attack by the leucocytes and will multiply, forming multiple small bone abscesses. The abscesses will coalesce and cause necrosis of a larger or smaller area of bone. It may then happen that the thrombus in these small vessels will extend to the larger ones and, in the lower jaw, as pointed out by Mowlem[5], cause thrombosis of the inferior dental vessels. This so seriously reduces the blood supply to the medullary bone of the mandible on that side that the spread of infection from the thrombus into it is facilitated.

It appears, therefore, that any degree of bone infection and necrosis may develop as a sequel to tooth extraction when the alveolar bone forming the tooth socket is unduly crushed. When the infection remains localized to the crushed vessels and adjoining bone of the socket itself, only that part of the bone dies, and ultimately is separated off as a sequestrum. This is the typical "dry socket". When the infection from the thrombus spreads to the inferior dental vessels, widespread osteomyelitis of the mandible supervenes, with massive necrosis and sequestration. When the thrombosis spreads to the pterygoid plexus of veins a septic meningitis may supervene or a brain abscess develop; both of these conditions have been observed in isolated cases.

One more observation is necessary before the preventive and subsequent treatment of these unfortunate sequelae is described: bone which is infected by staphylococci and streptococci always dies and, becoming necrotic, sequestrates. It is not possible for any of the normal cells of bone—whether osteocytes, osteoblasts, osteoclasts or fibroblasts—to survive in the actual presence of infection. The demonstration of this fact is carried out by experimental infection of bone and subsequent histological examination of serial sections of the tissue which have been stained alternately with haematoxylin-eosin and Gram's stain[6].

Preventive treatment.—Preventive treatment consists in taking 3 precautions whenever a difficult extraction is to be performed. (1) An intramuscular injection of 50,000 units of penicillin should be given 15 minutes before extraction. (2) Cauterization of the sulcus should be carried out immediately before extraction, and after the induction of anaesthesia (preferably local or block anaesthesia if there is no acute inflammation; the trauma inflicted under nitrous oxide may be excessive). (3) Section of the root or roots should be made, if thought to be necessary after studying the skiagram, using a dental engine and appropriate burr. It is often possible in this way to minimize trauma to the bone.

Subsequent treatment.—When, however, osteomyelitis has supervened, systemic treatment with penicillin should be inaugurated at the earliest possible moment in order to render the bone surrounding the foci of infection—which is not as yet involved—inimical to the growth of the bacteria which may spread into it.

This is of decisive value only in the invasive phase of the disease and consists, as usual, of giving an initial intramuscular injection of 50,000 units of penicillin followed by 3-hourly injections of 15,000 units or 12-hourly injections of 100,000 units. Once the bone has become infected and necrotic, the value of the systemic treatment is much reduced since it cannot be expected to sterilize large sequestra. It does, however, have a most important value at a later stage when it becomes necessary to operate for the removal of the sequestrum; and with penicillin support it is possible to remove sequestra by opening up the bone and exposing the entire sequestrum, although in most cases it is better to wait until it can be removed by less heroic measures.

If radical removal through an external incision be decided upon, it is carried out after an initial intramuscular dose of 50,000 units. The bone is saucerized after all sequestra have been removed, and the wound is dusted with penicillin and sulphathiazole powder. A drainage tube is put in so as to permit irrigation with penicillin solution and the wound is closed[5].

When a "dry socket" has become fully established it is not very useful to insert a penicillin tablet covered with a pack of Vaseline gauze, though in the early stages this may be done. The difficulty is that the penicillin has to infiltrate and to diffuse through the necrotic tissue in order to reach the advancing edge of the infection, and success will depend upon the extent of this area. It is more satisfactory to approach the infection from the systemic side by intramuscular injection. This will limit the spread of necrosis but will not immediately relieve the pain.

PYORRHOEA

In conclusion, it may be pointed out that it is not a very hopeful procedure to use penicillin, either systemically or locally in the form of lozenges or penicillin wax, in cases of chronic parodontal disease. It may be possible to sterilize the pockets in this way, but as long as the pockets remain they are an ideal breeding ground for bacteria and are subject to the constant trauma of mastication so that a recurrence of the condition is inevitable. If there is no extensive deepening of the normal parodontal sulcus, that is, no "pocket" formation, a case of chronic marginal gingivitis will clear up, provided that the teeth are efficiently scaled and the patient is taught an effective system of oral hygiene. This consists in applying friction to the gum margin all round every tooth daily with the toothbrush and, when there are interdental spaces, with a wood point or with one made of whalebone or by some other effective method.

Pockets must be explored daily by the patient with wood points and very frequently by the dental surgeon with scalers and parodontal files. Otherwise they must be cut away—this will generally be found to be the only practical solution. In a severe case of pyorrhoea profunda in which the tissues are abnormally friable and are especially susceptible to the spread of infection, the operation of gingivectomy may be preceded by an intramuscular dose of penicillin (50,000 units). This is simply a particular case of the general axiom that penicillin treatment is seldom an alternative to sound surgery but, when it is intelligently used, is a means of raising sound surgery to a level of achievement far above any previous experience.

REFERENCES

[1] Fish, E. W., and Maclean, I. (1936) *Brit. dent. J.*, **61**, 336.
[2] Fish, E. W. (1944) *Parodontal Disease. A Manual of Treatment and Atlas of Pathology*. Eyre and Spottiswoode, London.
[3] Okell, C. C., and Elliott, S. D. (1935) *Lancet*, **2**, 869.
[4] Ross, W. S., and Rogers, K. (1943) *Brit. dent. J.*, **74**, 253.
[5] Mowlem, R. (1945) *Proc. R. Soc. Med.*, **38**, 452.
[6] Fish, E. W. (1939) *J Amer. dent. Ass.*, **26**, 691.

PENICILLIN IN ANIMAL DISEASES

By Reginald Lovell, M.Sc., Ph.D., M.R.C.V.S., D.V.S.M.
Deputy Director, Research Institute in Animal Pathology, Royal Veterinary College, London

INTRODUCTION

The treatment of animal diseases with penicillin has so far been curtailed by the limited amount of the drug available for this purpose. It was released in the United States of America in 1945 for use in veterinary medicine and trials concerning its application in the treatment of bovine mastitis were started. Supplies were released for similar work at 6 centres in Great Britain and as trials are still in progress information available is meagre. Its use in other animal diseases has been still further limited.

METHODS OF ADMINISTRATION

The determination of the best method of administration of penicillin for various diseases in different animals is of primary consideration, and as far as domestic animals are concerned, most of the treatment has been applied to cattle. The possibility of success in treating bovine mastitis by intravenous or intramuscular injection depends in part on the permeability of the lactating mammary gland. It appeared that absorption of penicillin from the blood stream by the mammary gland was unlikely after Bryan, Horwood and Huffman[1] had failed to treat bovine mastitis successfully by the intravenous administration of penicillin. Consequently Seeley and his colleagues[2] tested the milk of a healthy Jersey heifer for penicillin content after intravenous injections of 80,000 units and 500,000 units of the calcium salt. There was not any penicillin content in milk samples obtained during the 24 hours following administration and these authors consider that the lactating bovine mammary gland does not serve as a major systemic outlet for penicillin from the blood. Barker and Dussault[3] injected intramuscularly a total of 2,681,000 units of the calcium salt in a beeswax and peanut oil suspension into a Holstein cow at 8-hourly intervals for 4 days. The results of milk and urine assays indicated that the penicillin was excreted rapidly by the kidneys, but that it was not excreted by the mammary gland in a detectable amount or sufficiently to remove a mastitis infection due to *Str. agalactiae*. Beck, De Mott and Boucher[4] estimated the penicillin content of the urine and milk of 5 cows treated with 10,000,000 units of the sodium salt injected intramuscularly. The individual doses were

300,000 units every 4 hours for 5 days, or until 10,000,000 units had been administered. The assays of the urine indicated that there was ample concentration to affect *Cor. renale*—the causative organism of pyelonephritis in cattle. The milk assays showed negligible amounts of penicillin and in some cases the blood concentration was very low. Watts and McLeod[5] studied this problem and injected intramuscularly 100,000 units, 500,000 units and 1,000,000 units into groups of heifers and cows and did not find penicillin in the milk of any of the animals.

There is therefore sufficient evidence to show that the intramuscular and intravenous routes for the administration of penicillin are methods not to be advocated for treating bovine mastitis, but they may be used with advantage for treating bovine nephritis and possibly other diseases. The intramammary injection of penicillin for mastitis of cattle is the method most frequently used and as Murnane[6] points out an infected wound has certain disadvantages as compared with the udder which can be readily and frequently drained and the chemotherapeutic agent retained for any desired length of time between milkings. Penicillin concentration in the udder will, however, depend in part upon the extent and rate of absorption or loss and also upon dilution by the secretion of milk. There appears to be an inverse ratio between the concentration and the volume of milk and Murnane[6] has found that there is a considerable absorption of penicillin during the first few hours after an intramammary infusion. This loss was very much greater in the actively functioning gland than in one which was "drying off". In one case quoted there was a loss of 51 per cent during the first 4 hours, a 40 per cent loss during the second 4 hours, with a 4 per cent loss during the third period of 4 hours. Despite this loss in actively functioning glands Murnane has found that there is still an effective concentration in the milk 12 hours after the infusion of 15,000 units of penicillin. The intramammary injection of penicillin therefore seems to be the most effective and most economical method of administration when treating the infected udders of cows. Experience has shown, however, that in order to maintain an effective concentration more than one dose is desirable even though the initial one may be very large.

TREATMENT OF BOVINE MASTITIS

Mastitis of cattle is caused by a variety of bacterial species and in order to estimate the probability that a particular form of treatment is effective, bacteriological examination of the milk of infected cows is essential.

Some of the common forms of mastitis are caused by streptococci and these vary in incidence and importance. The most common form is a contagious one caused by *Str. agalactiae* (Lancefield's group B). The disease is usually chronic with little systemic disturbance, although acute cases may arise from the chronic ones causing the loss of function of one or more quarters of the mammary gland. The infected udder is the main reservoir of the causal organism but it has been found in other sites outside the animal body and may remain alive there for a considerable period (Watts[7]). At present the disease is widespread, and control is difficult. Consequently this form of mastitis has received the most attention especially regarding the value of penicillin therapy, and it is generally agreed that *Str. agalactiae* is penicillin-sensitive *in vitro*. Other streptococci which cause bovine mastitis include *Str. dysgalactiae*—an α-haemolytic streptococcus allied to Group C (Lancefield), *Str. uberis*—a non-haemolytic streptococcus—and *Str. pyogenes* (Lancefield's groups A and C). These latter infections are frequently sporadic and acute in nature and as yet there is little information concerning their treatment with penicillin.

Haemolytic staphylococci are responsible also for cases of bovine mastitis. A fulminating type may develop shortly after calving and is associated with severe systemic disturbance frequently followed by death. Similar organisms may cause a chronic catarrhal type of the disease and occasionally a granulomatous form. Bovine mastitis due to staphylococci, especially the catarrhal type, has been experimented with to decide the value of penicillin therapy and whether or not strains of haemolytic staphylococci *in vitro* are sensitive to penicillin.

Although many other bacterial species are sometimes involved in mastitis only one of these need be mentioned. *Cor. pyogenes* is a pus-producing organism and causes a suppurative mastitis more often in dry cows and maiden heifers. Because of its seasonal occurrence it is known as "summer mastitis" and acute and chronic cases are recognized; the former is associated with systemic disturbances.

One of the early accounts of penicillin therapy in streptococcal forms of mastitis is that of Kakavas[8], who used crude penicillin and found that infusion of this substance into the udder may induce a local tissue reaction, the degree and duration of the reaction depending upon the type of medium in which the penicillin was produced. It was, however, effective, as *Str. agalactiae* was eliminated from 21 of 23 quarters after 3 or 4 doses, each dose containing from 600 to 1,200 units. The sodium salt was also used by the author and it was well tolerated and effective in mastitis due to the same organism. Jensen and Jepsen[9] attempted treatment with a crude filtrate containing from 5,000 to 10,000 units per litre in herds in which the predominating organism was *Str. agalactiae*. A temporary rise in temperature and a transitory cessation of the milk secretion followed intramammary injections. The treatment was given to one herd in which the usual measures of isolation and disposal of incurable cases were adopted and the results are difficult to assess, but in 9 other herds 227 of 264 infected quarters were found to be free from streptococci when tested 1–2 months later. There were, however, relapses and recurrences in 20–25 per cent of certain cases in which the milk was examined regularly for periods of up to 15 months. Later authors have used the sodium or calcium salt of penicillin and attention has been paid to the amount injected, the number of doses necessary to effect a cure and the interval between doses; some authors regard the actual size of the inoculum as important. One dose only was given by Barker[10] and consisted of 100 millilitres of an aqueous solution containing 25,000 units; this was given into each infected quarter by means of a gravity infusion apparatus and was left in the udder for from 8 to 12 hours. Using a modified Hotis test for purposes of diagnosis he found that 16 of 32 quarters treated were free from infection when tested a month later. There were slight reactions in the treated cows which consisted of an occasional rise in temperature and udder disturbances with swelling and hardness of the gland but there were not any serious changes in its secretory capacity. Barker realized from the results of this trial that the optimal dosage and frequency of administration still required study. Murnane[6] used the calcium and the sodium salt in doses of 15,000 units and gave from one to 5 doses in acute and chronic cases of clinical infections due to *Str. agalactiae*. Two doses, given after successive milkings, gave a higher percentage of cures than one dose. One dose cured 9 of 24 quarters whereas 2 doses were successful with 41 of 57 quarters, giving a differential percentage of 37 and 72 respectively. After an initial treatment of one, 2, 4 or 5 doses infection still persisted in 32 of 86 quarters and these received up to 9 subsequent injections; eventually 28 of these were pronounced clear of infection and the success achieved by this treatment is shown by a total cure of 82 of 86 quarters treated, that is, 95 per cent. These were all clinical infections and similar results were obtained with both acute and chronic forms of the disease. Some treated at length were probably cases of reinfection but this is offset by the possibility that spontaneous recoveries may occur during the course of a trial. In a number of acute cases, however, despite the fact that infection was eliminated early, loss of function of the quarter became complete.

Whether or not such quarters will return to normal at the next lactation is a problem worthy of attention. There is a marked difference in the results obtained by Murphy and Pfau[11] according to the number of doses used. In one trial, 5 of 15 quarters were free from infection after one intramammary infusion of 5,000–200,000 units, whereas in a further trial in which they dealt with 32 quarters, 4 of which were not cured after a preliminary course of 5 doses of 10,000 units and one of which had become reinfected, treatment by the intramammary infusion of 5 doses of 20,000 units eliminated *Str. agalactiae* from them all. Slanetz and Allen[12] used larger doses of penicillin in their trials. They injected 100,000–200,000 units by the teat canal into quarters infected with this organism, and one administration cured 25 of 28 (89 per cent) and 2–4 doses eliminated the organism from 30 of 31 quarters (96 per cent). The criterion of cure accepted by these authors was the inability to find streptococci in the milk when tested at weekly intervals up to 4 or 5 weeks after treatment. They conclude that 100,000 units in 100 millilitres of sterile physiological saline or distilled water is sufficient to cure streptococcal mastitis, except in the more acute cases or in chronic cases of long standing when one or more injections of 200,000 units may be necessary. Byrne, Pullin and Konsk[13] made trials in 6 herds comprising 235 cattle and they paid attention not only to the number of doses and number of units injected but to the volume of the diluent used. The interval between the treatments was 4 days and this was adopted for the purpose of allowing sufficient time for the Hotis test to be completed and to determine from the result whether or not further treatments were necessary. A total of 179 quarters were found to be infected with *Str. agalactiae* and were treated with doses varying from 10,000 to 100,000 units in volumes of diluent which varied from 25 to 250 millilitres. If those cases treated with 40,000 units are considered, the following data are illuminating. One dose in 250 millilitres cured 28 of 73 quarters (38 per cent), one dose in 100 millilitres cured 26 of 52 quarters (50 per cent), whereas one dose in 25 millilitres cured 3 of 16 quarters (19 per cent). Two doses containing the same number of units in similar quantities of diluent increased the cures to 52 of 73 (71 per cent), 36 of 52 (69 per cent) and 6 of 16 (37 per cent) respectively. Three doses raised the cures to 80, 90 and 50 per cent respectively. The best results were therefore obtained when 40,000 units dissolved in 100 millilitres of diluent were employed; the results were slightly less favourable when the diluent was increased to 250 millilitres and were distinctly less advantageous when the diluent was decreased to 25 millilitres. Of 18 quarters treated with 100,000 units in 25 millilitres of physiological saline, 5 were cured after one dose, a further 5 after 2 doses, and 3 more after 3 doses, giving a total of 13 with a percentage cure of 72. The volume of the injection therefore appears to be important apart from the number of units it contains. Hardenbrook, Alberts and Bryan[14] confirm the value of penicillin therapy in the treatment of mastitis due to *Str. agalactiae*. They confined their attention largely to doses of 25,000 units in 10 or 20 millilitres of physiological saline and cured 27 of 44 quarters with one dose; 10 further quarters required more than one dose. The results obtained by workers at 6 centres who made trials under the general direction of the Mastitis Conference of the Agricultural Research Council are available in summary form only[15], and these also show that a high percentage of *Str. agalactiae* infections can be cured with a minimal amount of udder disturbance by injections of a solution of penicillin *via* the teat canal. One dose is usually insufficient, even though it is a large one. An injection of 100,000 units was effective in 81 of 140 quarters (57·9 per cent) whilst 2 injections 24-hourly of 20,000 units sterilized 123 of 154 quarters (79·9 per cent). There was little difference between the latter result and those obtained with 4 24-hourly doses of 20,000 units and with 4 doses of 10,000 units at successive milkings. It is concluded from these figures that on practical grounds 2 injections of 20,000 units at 24-hourly intervals is the method of choice. The Tables on pp. 343 and 345 give a selection of results obtained, showing the doses used and the intervals between successive treatments. It is not possible to make strict comparison as some authors waited for the results of the bacteriological examinations of milk samples after each treatment. An attempt, however, has been made to abstract comparable data and the Tables show the advantages of the use of more than one dose of penicillin.

There is less information concerning the effect of penicillin on mastitis due to other types of streptococci. Kakavas[8] achieved success with all of 6 quarters infected with *Str. dysgalactiae*, all of 3 quarters infected with *Str. uberis* and all of 4 quarters infected with other streptococci. Murnane[6] also records the successful treatment of 3 quarters infected with streptococci not belonging to Lancefield's group B. Byrne, Pullin and Konsk[13] used doses of 10,000–40,000 units in different quantities of diluent and 4 of 6 quarters infected with *Str. dysgalactiae*, 3 of 5 quarters infected with *Str. uberis* and 19 of 21 infected with unidentified streptococci were free from infection 1–2 months later.

The observations so far recorded on the treatment of staphylococcal mastitis are that these cases are more difficult to cure with penicillin than are streptococcal forms of the disease.

TREATMENT OF MASTITIS DUE TO *Str. agalactiae* BY THE INTRAMAMMARY INFUSION OF PENICILLIN

Number of doses	Units injected	Interval between doses	Number of quarters treated	Number of quarters cured	Percentage cure	Authors
3–8	600–1,200 (crude penicillin)	24 hours	23	21	91	Kakavas[8]
3–8	7,800–15,900	24 hours	15	10	66	
2	5,000–10,000 (crude penicillin)	1–3 days	264	227	86	Jensen and Jepsen[9]
1	25,000	—	32	16	50	Barker[10]
1	15,000	—	24	9	37	Murnane[6]
2	15,000	successive milkings	57	41	72	
1	5,000–200,000	—	15	5	33	Murphy and Pfau[11]
5	10,000	successive milkings	10	6	60	
1	100,000–200,000	—	28	25	89	Slanetz and Allen[12]
2–4	100,000 200,000	12 hours	31	30	96	
1	10,000–100,000	—	179	62	34	Byrne *et al.*[13]
1	25,000	—	44	27	61	Hardenbrook *et al.*[14]
1	100,000	—	140	81	57·9	Anon.[15]
2	20,000	24 hours	154	123	79·9	
4	20,000	24 hours	150	121	80·7	
4	10,000	successive milkings	150	125	88·3	

Kakavas[8] cured 16 of 27 quarters infected with *Staph. aureus* by means of crude penicillin and was also successful with 4 of 6 quarters when using an aqueous solution of the sodium salt. Two cases of acute mastitis were cured by giving 5,000 units daily for 4 days and the author noted the gradual disappearance of the swelling of the udder during treatment; staphylococci disappeared from the udder secretion. The results obtained by Klein, Crisman and Moor[16] were especially disappointing; they treated 5 cows of which 7 quarters were affected with the catarrhal type and there was an apparent temporary sterilization of the udders, which did not persist in 5 quarters even though several doses of 22,800 units of penicillin were given. Samples of milk were taken for examination immediately before the first injection, at intervals during the injection period and afterwards. Although staphylococci were not found in the samples taken up to 12 hours after the last injection they were present in samples from 5 quarters on the third or sixth day following; the 2 quarters which remained free had had 8 injections. Slanetz and Allen[12] also found staphylococcal mastitis more difficult to cure than the streptococcal forms although they had used large doses. Of 37 quarters with persistent subclinical infection treated by Murnane[6] only one was cured although *in vitro* tests showed the staphylococci to be penicillin-sensitive. Byrne, Pullin and Konsk[13] achieved better results than some; of 49 quarters infected 23 required 2 injections, 5 required 3 and a further 5 required from 4 to 6 injections. In all, 38 quarters were considered to have been successfully treated when examined 1–2 months later, giving a percentage of 77·5. An abstract of relevant data from the records of authors is given below.

There are not apparently any published records of the treatment with penicillin of mastitis due to *Cor. pyogenes*. The intramammary infusion of any therapeutic agent is likely to be difficult in many such cases because of the character of the lesion. The intramuscular or subcutaneous injection of alum precipitated toxoid (Lovell[17]) is often followed by a temporary improvement associated with an increase in the fluidity of the udder secretion. The suggestion is made therefore than an injection of toxoid might well precede penicillin therapy in mastitis due to *Cor. pyogenes*, an organism which is known to be penicillin-sensitive *in vitro*.

In bovine mastitis there is evidence that either the sodium or the calcium salt may be used and dissolved in sterile distilled water or sterile physiological saline for intramammary infusions *via* the teat canal. According to Little and others[18] suspensions of penicillin in mineral oil have been used experimentally and these are more stable than the aqueous solutions for they may be stored in a refrigerator for several weeks without appreciable loss in potency. The suspensions, however, must be adjusted to body temperature and shaken before use; irritation of the udder may be reduced if the volume does not exceed 50 millilitres. So far, most of the records available deal with physiological saline and aqueous solutions and there is general agreement that the penicillin must be retained in the gland for several hours. Although the activity of penicillin is not apparently inhibited by milk its efficiency may be reduced when the udder is secreting large

TREATMENT OF STAPHYLOCOCCAL MASTITIS BY THE INTRAMAMMARY INFUSION OF PENICILLIN

Number of doses	Units injected	Interval between doses	Number of quarters treated	Number of quarters cured	Percentage cure	Authors
3–4	600–2,300 (crude penicillin)	24 hours	27	16	59	Kakavas
3–7	1,200–9,000	24 hours	6	4	66	
4	22,800	12 hours	4	2	50	Klein *et al.*
8	22,800	6 hours	3	—	—	
1	100,000	—	8	5	62	Slanetz and
4	100,000–200,000	12 hours	6	6	100	Allen
1	15,000	—	3	1	33	Murnane
2	15,000	successive milkings	14	1	7	
4	15,000	successive milkings	25	1	4	
1	10,000	—	49	5	10	Byrne *et al.*

quantities and, furthermore, some absorption takes place. The amount of penicillin required to eliminate infection from the udder varies according to the type of infection and depends also on the stage of infection, the size of the udder and the volume of milk produced. There is thus a variation from cow to cow but mastitis is frequently treated on a herd basis and especially in the chronic form due to *Str. agalactiae*. On practical considerations it appears that 2 doses of about 20,000 units at an interval of 24 hours is the method most desirable for the treatment of this type of infection. Records of this treatment in Great Britain show a cure in about 80 per cent of cases whereas one larger dose is less efficient and 4 doses of 20,000 units each show little gain. Opinion in the United States of America is that 25,000–50,000 units once a day for 4 days is adequate in the majority of cases. That the size of the injection is important is shown by the work in Canada of Byrne, Pullin and Konsk[13], who recommended doses of 40,000 units dissolved in 100 millilitres of diluent. They preferred an interval of 4 days between treatments.

An extensive investigation into the modes of spread of *Str. agalactiae* infection in dairy herds was made by several workers and the opinion is given that the habitat of this organism is in or on the bovine udder and that it does not readily colonize in other sites[19]. If the infection which is present in or on the bovine udder could be eliminated it is considered that mastitis due to this organism might be effectively controlled. Penicillin apparently gives a high rate of bacteriological as well as clinical cure of this form of mastitis and should therefore tend to the effective control of this type of infection.

Mastitis due to staphylococci is not affected to the same degree. Murnane[6] suggests that the injection may not reach all foci of infection as treatment with penicillin usually lowers the bacterial count although this rises again when treatment ceases. It seems likely, therefore, that staphylococci will be more difficult to eliminate permanently from the udder than streptococci. Murnane mentions a further important point concerning the appearance of other bacteria including staphylococci in milk samples following the elimination of *Str. agalactiae* by penicillin. These staphylococci must be regarded as potential pathogens, the significance of which is at present difficult to assess.

TREATMENT OF STRANGLES IN HORSES

Strangles is an acute infective disease of horses characterized by inflammation of the nasal and pharyngeal mucosa with suppuration of the regional lymphatic glands. The causal organism is a haemolytic streptococcus—*Str. equi*—belonging to Lancefield's group C. Although the mortality is low, severe and fatal cases occur with involvement of the lungs and other tissues.

There are a few records of the successful treatment of this disease with penicillin. Semtner[20] treated 10 cases with the calcium salt and gave from 5 to 9 injections of 100,000 units intramuscularly at intervals of 3–4 hours. When distilled water was used as a diluent swellings appeared at the site of inoculation; these disappeared after from 18 to 24 hours, leaving no apparent ill effects. Such swellings did not occur when physiological saline was substituted for the distilled water. The diagnosis was confirmed by bacteriological examination and the infecting organisms were penicillin-sensitive *in vitro*. All the animals showed a fall in temperature and amelioration of symptoms. Six of them recovered completely but relapses occurred in 4 horses 24–48 hours after the cessation of penicillin therapy. These results were regarded as promising and the suggestion was made that fewer injections may be necessary when it is possible to retain the potency of the drug in animals for longer periods. Morcos[21] gave about 60,000 units intramuscularly thrice daily for 3 days in 3 cases and all the horses made a complete recovery. Roberts[22] records prompt recovery in one case which was diagnosed by clinical methods and treated with sulphamerazine and penicillin. The author emphasizes the rapidity of the recovery and the absence of a nasal discharge and cough within 7 days of beginning this treatment.

TREATMENT OF BOVINE PYELONEPHRITIS

A specific cystitis and pyelonephritis associated with *Cor. renale* occurs in cattle and the passage of turbid or sanguineous urine is a characteristic sign. The disease is chronic and some cases last for years, although exacerbations may periodically occur. As far as it is known natural recovery does not take place but there are marked periods of improvement during the course of the disease. *Cor. renale* may be found in large numbers in the urine of infected cattle and opinions differ whether these bacteria reach the kidneys and bladder *via* the blood stream or whether the infection is an ascending one *via* the urethra and ureters. *Cor. renale* is penicillin-sensitive *in vitro* and as penicillin is excreted rapidly in the urine it appears that this form of therapy would be profitable. Because of the nature of the condition with long periods of apparent good health, any assessment of the permanent value of penicillin therapy should be guarded. Morcos[21] records apparent recovery in one case after 2 days' treatment but gives few details as no laboratory examinations were made. Beck, De Mott and Boucher[4] treated 6 cows with a saline solution of the sodium salt. The intramuscular route was employed and doses of 300,000 units were given every 4 hours for 5 days or until 10,000,000 units had been given. Water was restricted and frequent assays were made of the penicillin content of the urine, blood and milk in 5 of the cases. The samples of urine contained from 75 to 100 units per millilitre 4 hours after the final injection whilst the blood did not contain any amount or contained only fractions of a unit, and the milk none or negligible amounts. After treatment all 6 cases showed clinical improvement with the disappearance of haematuria and other signs. Three of the cows appeared to have made a complete recovery as judged by clinical and bacteriological examinations made from 2 to 3 months later. Haematuria recurred in one case and *Cor. renale* was found in the urine of 2 others, in the urine of which, however, erythrocytes were not found. The authors consider that penicillin is of definite value in the treatment of cystitis and pyelonephritis of cattle but owing to the chronic nature of the disease and the tendency for cases to show clinical improvement without treatment, it is premature to presume actual cures. They hope to continue observations on these animals and to institute further trials.

SWINE ERYSIPELAS

Swine erysipelas is caused by *Ery. rhusiopathiae*, an organism which is also naturally pathogenic in sheep, mice and certain birds; in man it causes erysipeloid. There are not any published records of penicillin therapy in naturally occurring cases of swine erysipelas although Barber, Nellen and Zoob[23] record some success with the human disease. The data concerning the trials made in experimentally infected animals are confusing. Heilman and Herrell[24] claim to have cured mice experimentally infected with this organism, by using doses of 1,000 units in each mouse *per diem*, and Van Es, Olney and Blore[25] found that when given early and in adequate dosage penicillin would cure pigeons experimentally infected with *Ery. rhusiopathiae*. They suggest that penicillin may be of value if given in the early stages of swine erysipelas. Harvey, Libby and Waller[26] conclude from their experiments that the oral administration of penicillin is of value in protecting mice against experimental *Ery. rhusiopathiae* infection. They emphasize the necessity of instituting this form of therapy within 24 hours of exposure and the need for early administration is in accord with the opinion of previous authors. Under field conditions the institution of therapy at such an early stage of infection may be impossible and it appears therefore that penicillin may be of little value in treatment but possibly of some use in the control of an outbreak of this infection in domestic animals. Woodbine[27] is not optimistic and, basing his opinion on experiments with mice, concludes that infections of swine are unlikely to prove readily amenable to treatment with penicillin. Although the strains of this organism were penicillin-sensitive *in vitro* the degree of protection afforded *in vivo* was low. There is, however, some variation in dosage used by the different workers. Whereas Heilman and Herrell used doses of 1,000 units of penicillin *per diem* for each mouse the doses by the oral route used by Harvey, Libby and Waller were estimated to be of the order of 5,000 units; Woodbine gave 10–100 units daily. Trials on the natural disease of pigs is therefore awaited with interest but if swine erysipelas is amenable to penicillin therapy, the dosage will have to be large and it will have to be administered in the early stages.

MISCELLANEOUS DISEASES OF ANIMALS

On theoretical grounds, there are other animal diseases which should respond to penicillin therapy and this applies especially to those due to organisms of the clostridium group for several members of this genus are known to be susceptible *in vitro* to penicillin. There are not any records of adequately controlled trials in these natural diseases of animals but there are a few records of its use in one or two animals. Rydell[28] administered penicillin intravenously and intraperitoneally to calves ill with blackleg, presumably due to *Cl. chauvaei*; one of 3 calves treated survived.

Although given in large doses penicillin failed to save the life of a dog suffering from tetanus (Garlick[29]).

Penicillin was considered to be valuable in treating sheep suffering from pneumonia, associated with a diphtheroid (Morcos[21]), and this might be expected because of penicillin-sensitivity *in vitro* of some corynebacteria. Queen and Quortrup[30] claim that a particular strain of pasteurella recovered from wild ducks was unexpectedly found to be penicillin-sensitive *in vitro* and that the drug protected wild ducks infected experimentally with this strain.

REFERENCES

[1] Bryan ,C. S., Horwood, R. E., and Huffman, C. F. (1945) *Vet. Med.*, **40**, 87.
[2] Seeley, H. W., Jun., Anderson, E. O., Plastridge, W. N., and Pearson, Patricia (1945) *Science*, **102**, 44.
[3] Barker, G. A. V., and Dussault, H. P. (1945) *Canad. J. comp. Med.*, **9**, 332.
[4] Beck, J. D., De Mott, T., and Boucher, W. B. (1945) *Vet. Ext. Quart. Univ. Pa*, **100**, 10.
[5] Watts, P. S., and McLeod, D. H. (1946) *J. comp. Path.*, **56** (in press).
[6] Murnane, D. (1945) *Aust. vet. J.*, **21**, 82.
[7] Watts, P. S. (1941) *Vet. Rec.*, **53**, 61.
[8] Kakavas, J. C. (1944) *N. Amer. Vet.*, **25**, 408.
[9] Jensen, K. A., and Jepsen, A. (1945) *Skand. VetTidskr.*, **35**, 552.
[10] Barker, C. A. V. (1945) *Canad. J. comp. Med.*, **9**, 235.
[11] Murphy, J. M., and Pfau, K. O. (1945) *Cornell Vet.*, **35**, 88.
[12] Slanetz, L. W., and Allen, F. E. (1945) *J. Amer. vet. med. Ass.*, **107**, 18.
[13] Byrne, J. L., Pullin, J. W., and Konsk, H. (1946) *Canad. J. comp. Med.*, **10**, 16.
[14] Hardenbrook, H. J., Alberts, J. O., and Bryan, H. S. (1946) *J. Amer. vet. med. Ass.*, **108**, 140.
[15] Anon. (1946) *Vet. Rec.*, **58**, 138.
[16] Klein, L. A., Crisman, D. W., and Moor, J. W. (1945) *Amer. J. vet. Res.*, **6**, 3.
[17] Lovell, R. (1941) *J. Path. Bact.*, **52**, 295.
[18] Little, R. B., Bryan, C. S., Petersen, W. E., Plastridge, W. N., and Schalm, O. W. (1946) *J. Amer. vet. med. Ass.*, **108**, 127.
[19] Anon. (1944) *Imp. Bureau of Animal Health, Review Series* No. 2.
[20] Semtner, W. K. (1945) *Vet. Med.*, **40**, 226.
[21] Morcos, Z. (1945) *Vet. Rec.*, **57**, 425.
[22] Roberts, S. J. (1945) *Cornell Vet.*, **35**, 378.
[23] Barber, Mary, Nellen, M., and Zoob, M. (1946) *Lancet*, **1**, 125.
[24] Heilman, F. R., and Herrell, W. E. (1944) *Proc. Mayo Clin.*, **19**, 340.
[25] Van Es, L., Olney, J. F., and Blore, I. C. (1945) *Univ. of Nebraska Coll. of Agric. Exp. Sta. Research Bull.*, 141.
[26] Harvey, P. C., Libby, R. L., and Waller, B. B. (1945) *Proc. Soc. exp. Biol., N.Y.*, **60**, 307.
[27] Woodbine, M. (1946) *Vet. J.*, **102**, 88.
[28] Rydell, R. O. (1946) *J. Amer. vet. med. Ass.*, **108**, 37.
[29] Garlick, N. L. (1946) *J. Amer. vet. med. Ass.*, **108**, 83.
[30] Queen, F. B., and Quortrup, E. R. (1946) *J. Amer. vet. med. Ass.*, **108**, 101.

PENICILLIN AND THE GENERAL PRACTITIONER

By G. B. Mitchell-Heggs, O.B.E., M.D., F.R.C.P.
Physician in Charge, Skin Department, St. Mary's Hospital, London

GENERAL CONSIDERATIONS

Penicillin is not a panacea and this chapter is designed to indicate in general terms the types of case in which penicillin treatment may help and those in which it is unlikely to be of use.

It is important for the doctor in general practice to remember at all times that the essential principle in penicillin therapy is to bring the optimal concentration of penicillin into regular contact with organisms which are sensitive to it. Penicillin therapy does not replace the principles and practice of good treatment in medicine, surgery or the specialities.

Greatest success will be obtained in treating those cases where the predominant infection is penicillin-sensitive. It is obvious, therefore, that the organism responsible for the infection should undergo bacteriological examination. In practice this means that sterile specimens of blood, sputum or pus should be taken as soon as the practitioner realizes that a severe, acute, or chronic infection has occurred. This investigation need not necessarily be followed by penicillin therapy, because the patient's immunity, surgery, or less specific chemotherapy may be sufficient and correct.

It must always be borne in mind that systemic and local therapy demand a fair chance. This means a course of treatment lasting several days, entailing considerable extra nursing and medical attention. It will often be a trial rather than a pleasure to the patient and it is best for him to realize that it may cause pain. Brands of penicillin vary, however, in their tendency to produce pain. This is probably attributable to associated substances rather than to the penicillin. Immediately following the injection one experiences a sharp stinging pain which passes off in a few seconds. A dull ache may remain for half an hour and the site may be tender for 24 hours. Only those who have had penicillin injections every 3 hours for 7 or more days can realize how the loss of rest is followed by a dread of the next injection, however painless, however deftly given. Penicillin treatment, then, is a strain to patient, nurse and medical attendant.

Bacteriological diagnosis of an infection should be the practitioner's aim, but it is not obligatory. He must realize that this maxim is for his guidance, not bondage.

In cases where the invading infection is penicillin-sensitive, speedy adequate dosage will give the best result. In fact it can well be compared with intravenous quinine in malignant malaria, antitoxin in diphtheria, sulphaguanidine in bacillary dysentery or sulphapyridine in meningococcal meningitis. In these every hour of delay in treatment lowers the patient's resistance and may hasten his end. The sequelae and adverse effects of penicillin therapy are minimal in comparison with other methods of treatment.

Once bacteriological examination has shown that the organism is penicillin-sensitive or likely to be so, it is often better to stop other treatment and see how the patient fares with penicillin therapy. This applies particularly to local treatment. Soap and water and saline are the least detrimental to success, and antiseptics, especially solutions of the heavy metals and hydrogen peroxide, iodine and so forth, should not be used. Sulphathiazole, however, can be mixed with penicillin powder without detriment to the latter. Never forget that penicillin dusting powder for insufflation, mixed with sulphathiazole, is dangerous if applied to the skin for more than 5 days. Hypersensitivity to the sulphonamides has developed in many cases.

A busy practitioner may find it necessary under adverse conditions to paint the site of aspiration or penicillin injection with iodine or spirit. The danger of carrying much iodine into the skin is small in relation to the possible benefit of early treatment in such conditions.

Many of the early recipients of penicillin were Service personnel, and local anaesthesia was only occasionally used. This is necessary only if the needle is to be kept in for several hours, as in the continuous drip method. It is better, however, to give the painless injection of Novocain followed by penicillin from the same syringe, as indicated in the advice on intramuscular administration.

METHODS OF ADMINISTRATION

Penicillin can be administered by intravenous, intramuscular, or subcutaneous injections to obtain a systemic effect. In addition it can be injected into the cavities of joints, the theca spinalis, pleural cavities, pericardium, the centre of an abscess and an infected cyst. In the case of a peritoneal cavity, the bottom of a deep wound or the vagina intubation therapy is used.

In all the conditions enumerated in the last paragraph it is essential to ensure that there is adequate removal of pus or drainage of the potential space. Little good can be expected from injections of penicillin into a haemothorax or pyothorax which has been neither drained nor aspirated.

Penicillin must be given at once if it is considered that there is a thecal whitlow or infected joint. A spreading haemolytic streptococcus infection with the dangerous red streak of lymphangitis, severe pain at site of infection in the elbow and axilla accompanied by headache, sickness and high fever demands immediate treatment with penicillin to ward off death.

In all other such circumstances, the general practitioner should avoid penicillin therapy, especially in infections of the serous cavities, without specialized advice or reference to the relevant chapters in this book.

It is important to remember that penicillin helps to fight infection not only by killing the organism but by diminishing reproduction and the spread of sensitive organisms. The maxims of Hilton implying that painful and infected parts must be rested are most important if penicillin therapy is to give its best results. If these are not observed the penicillin effect will be diminished.

Equipment for a local injection

(1) a 5 millilitre and a 2 millilitre syringe
(2) a box of 5–8 cm. needles
(3) a box of ampoules of penicillin powder
(4) a bottle or ampoule of sterile water
(5) a box of files
(6) 2 dissection forceps
(7) soap and a bottle of surgical spirit
(8) cottonwool and lint
(9) a lint "purse-string" bag
(10) a saucepan to be used as a sterilizer
(11) 2 per cent Novocain in ampoule or bottle without adrenaline.

Method of sterilizing instruments

Take the syringe to pieces, wrap each part separately in a small piece of lint and place in the lint bag together with 2 needles and 2 dissection forceps. Place the bag in a saucepan half filled with cold water leaving the strings out of the water. Bring the water to the boil and allow to boil for a further 5 minutes. Lift the lint bag out of the water, allow it to drain and place on a clean plate. Take out the dissection forceps and proceed to prepare the syringe under aseptic conditions.

Selection of site for the injection

While the syringe is being sterilized, the selected site for the injection may be washed with soap and water. Surgical spirit may also be used should the skin need extra cleansing, but antiseptics generally should be avoided as they are contra-indicated in the use of penicillin. The usual area selected for this type of injection is the deltoid muscle or the gluteal muscles.

Method of injection

Penicillin is for the most part issued in rubber-capped bottles and the rubber is covered with a removable disc. The metal disc is removed and sufficient sterile physiological saline is introduced with the syringe. The penicillin rapidly dissolves and sufficient for one dose is withdrawn into the syringe (the amount of penicillin solution should be 1 millilitre for each injection), followed by $\frac{1}{2}$–1 millilitre of Novocain. Plunge the needle into the selected area and slowly inject without mixing anaesthetic and penicillin solution further. The local anaesthetic thus precedes the solution of penicillin.

Cleaning and storage

Wash instruments and all parts of the syringe under running water and dry thoroughly. Collect all the equipment and place on a tray in a safe place and ready for the next injection.

Complications in systemic administration

Complications in systemic penicillin therapy are rare. On the contrary the symptoms of headache, anorexia and lassitude are diminished with the first injections. Once penicillin therapy is commenced the pain tends to lessen. Patients who complain of pain at the site of injection more than 24 hours later should be examined for a tender red swelling since the possibility is that an organism which is insensitive to penicillin has been introduced with the injection. Appropriate conservative local measures such as a hot fomentation, kaolin poultice and radiant heat may be sufficient; even chemotherapy or surgery may be required. Urticaria and angioneurotic oedema may occur. There is no need to stop the injections as the eruption can frequently be controlled by ephedrine, a dose of $\frac{1}{2}$ grain thrice daily for several days being usually adequate for adults. Symptoms similar to serum sickness, malaise and joint pains with fever have been recorded but are extremely rare.

Site of injection

Thigh.—Over the greater trochanter where there is a lymph space or the vastus lateralis muscle which does not cover any vital structure.

Buttock.—Upper outer quadrant of the gluteal muscles, along a line joining the top of the natal cleft and top of the greater trochanter.

Shoulder.—The deltoid or triceps muscles.

It is a good plan to try to choose 6 sites, telling the patient their order of selection so that he can indicate the proper region for the next injection. In patients with multiple injuries or burns, or those who should not be moved, the choice will be much more limited. A good routine is: left shoulder, left hip, left buttock, right shoulder, right hip and right buttock. The patient will thus not have both sides simultaneously in a painful and tender state.

Frequency of injections and duration of the course

It is sometimes said by general practitioners that systemic penicillin treatment is too complicated for them in that it involves a multiplicity of injections. The common practice of giving 15,000 or 20,000 units every 3 hours day and night is hardly possible in general practice unless the patient has a special nurse, nor is the modification whereby the injections during the night are replaced by one large dose at bedtime. Fortunately, however, in most cases the infection responds to injections given at less frequent intervals and very satisfactory results have been obtained in ambulatory cases by a single dose of 300,000 units or twice daily doses of, say, 100,000 units. When the oil-wax or similar "depot" preparations are perfected this method of injections only once or twice a day may well become universal but even with watery solutions excellent results can be obtained in most infections. It is, however, less economical in penicillin and the doses indicated above are about the minimum. It is useless to give small doses such as 15,000 units once or twice daily. The duration of a course of systemic penicillin will depend upon the nature of the infection. It is far better to continue the administration for a few days too long than to cut the course short and risk a relapse.

PENICILLIN THERAPY COMBINED WITH SURGICAL MEASURES

When a doctor decides that incision of an abscess is necessary it is a good plan to aid the natural general immunities with the localizing effect of conservative measures such as rest and moist or dry heat. An additional aim is to establish a penicillin screen. Systemic penicillin should be administered for 24 hours before any other measures are undertaken which may result in spread of infection. Penicillin will thus diminish the risk of septicaemia or pyaemia.

In the event of an osteomyelitis or perinephric abscess being suspected, it is correct to start penicillin treatment at once, provided that arrangements also are made for early specialist surgery. Apparent early cure is so frequently followed by relapse. Chronic osteomyelitis is most resistant to massive doses of penicillin and always necessitates surgery. Perinephric abscess may remain discrete or loculated; the fever may decrease but not disappear. Blood count examination will show a fall in the polymorphonuclear leucocytes and a rise in the lymphocytes, but if the penicillin therapy is stopped for 24 hours all the symptoms and signs will recur.

LOCAL TREATMENT

The preparations of penicillin for local application are constantly increasing in variety, number and scope. Those available now are listed below.

It is desirable for preparations containing penicillin to include a substance which is bactericidal to Gram negative organisms, especially if the preparation is liable to be contaminated, as the majority of Gram negative organisms secrete a penicillinase which tends to inactivate penicillin.

In practice a physician can arrange for a spray or lotion to be prepared once daily or even once weekly if stored in a cool place. The penicillin may then be used at certain times in his surgery or during the course of a visiting round either by himself or a nurse. Penicillin cream will remain effective for as long as a month. The containers of spray lotions and creams should be sterilized by boiling before filling and when in use the cream may be removed from the pot by the use of a sterilized teaspoon.

Penicillin has been prepared for local use in the following preparations.

Lozenges
Suppositories
Snuff and powder
Solution for sprays and drops
Cream
Ointment

Full prescriptions are given elsewhere.

Administration of penicillin by inhalation

When a solution of penicillin in a very fine aerosol is inhaled the extremely small particles are carried far into the bronchial tree.

There are certain methods of producing a vapour of penicillin solution which can be used in infections of the respiratory tract.

The personal factor is so great in successful inhalation therapy that the patient must be taught correct breathing methods, and should be enjoined to keep at the vaporization. At St. Mary's Hospital, London, the routine in use is to instruct the patient to take a deep breath, breathe this air right out, hold the breath, squeeze the bulb four or five times while taking a deep breath.

The solutions used are 15,000–30,000 units per millilitre of penicillin. The inhaled penicillin is absorbed into the blood stream, thus combining local and systemic treatment. This method can be used in bronchitis and in bronchiectasis to obtain a therapeutic concentration in the affected areas. The effect on spasm is small, unless an antispasmodic such as ephedrine is combined with this treatment. Inhalations containing mixtures of penicillin solution and antispasmodics are beneficial.

Penicillin tent

This is used in the method of combining oxygen or oxygen and carbon dioxide with penicillin vapour in a tent. The oxygen is led from a cylinder into a hand type of inhaler and thence into a tent.

Conditions which are amenable to penicillin therapy are still being recorded. In general practice it is not wise to experiment with penicillin therapy and it is better to follow the special advice given in the appropriate chapters.

Infections by organisms which are penicillin-insensitive must be treated *secundum artem.* Penicillin, for example, is of little use in pyelitis or in cholecystitis where the infection is usually caused by *Esch. coli.*

COMMON DISEASES IN GENERAL PRACTICE

The following are conditions which are likely to be met with in general practice and which are amenable to penicillin therapy.

Acute rhinitis

Inhalation of snuff and spray shortens the duration and diminishes complications.

Chronic rhinitis

A considerable number of cases of chronic catarrh are relieved by penicillin inhalation.

Acute and chronic sinusitis

These conditions respond only when the spray can pass into the antra or sinuses.

Acute tonsillitis

This will be only slightly relieved by spray but greatly influenced by systemic penicillin therapy, especially when there is considerable cervical adenitis.

Chronic recurrent tonsillitis

Penicillin therapy may eliminate this septic focus but surgery will probably be essential.

Acute and chronic pharyngitis

These conditions are so often streptococcal that sprays are justified and severe cases necessitate systemic penicillin therapy.

Lozenges are of use in tonsillitis, pharyngitis and stomatitis but unfortunately cases of glossitis have been reported following their administration.

Quinsy

The lesion responds to systemic penicillin therapy if treated in the early stages, but after pus formation surgery is usually essential.

Acute recurrent bronchitis and chronic bronchitis

These conditions are benefited by inhalation therapy if the infecting organism is penicillin-sensitive.

Lobarpneumonia and bronchopneumonia

Lobarpneumonia and bronchopneumonia infections if penicillin-sensitive respond well to systemic penicillin therapy. A useful dosage is 15,000 units 3-hourly for an early adult case. Late cases should have an initial large dose of 60,000–100,000 units and then the 15,000 units 3-hourly.

The dosage for children depends upon their age and size. A good working guide is 1,000 units for each year of age given 3-hourly.

Where it is impracticable to give frequent injections the dose may be increased.

Bronchiectasis

It is particularly important to ensure good drainage of the cavities and the evacuation of the purulent sputum throughout the penicillin inhalation therapy.

Peribronchiectatic pneumonia responds to systemic penicillin therapy. Such cases should be placed under specialized observation as soon as possible.

Pleural effusion and empyemata

These conditions require very careful investigation before institution of any penicillin therapy.

Vincent's angina

This responds quickly to systemic and local therapy, but relapses are common. Penicillin lozenges are also used. Penicillin packs—made from dental wool and penicillin cream, packed round the teeth—have produced excellent results in St. Mary's Hospital, London. Skilled dental investigation and treatment are essential.

Stomatitis

When due to penicillin-sensitive organisms, this condition responds to the use of lozenges. Monilia infections (thrush) will not improve.

Genito-urinary infections

The conditions which respond to systemic therapy include acute pyelitis if the organism is penicillin-sensitive. After recovery radiological investigation will be necessary to exclude calculi. Usually the infection is due to *Esch. coli* and no response is obtainable.

Urethritis

Gonococcal infection responds in a dramatic manner. Such cases must be followed up and have a serological examination at the end of the second and fourth month. It is essential to read the chapter on venereal diseases before embarking on the treatment in general practice.

Otitis media

In early stages, with red tympanum, a large dose such as 100,000 units *statim* and 15,000 units 3-hourly is frequently successful. If the drum has perforated it is a good plan to add penicillin powder insufflation or drop instillation to the penicillin therapy.

If seen in the early stages a suspected mastoid infection should have penicillin, but must still be referred for surgical opinion.

Conjunctivitis

When due to the penicillin-sensitive organism, this condition responds well to penicillin drops.

Usually ophthalmia neonatorum responds quickly to instillations.

Other diseases

In general, cases of iritis, corneal ulcer and hypopyon should be referred to an oculist before treatment is instituted.

In abrasions following removal of a foreign body penicillin drops are a good prophylactic measure.

The uses in dermatology have been reviewed elsewhere. Penicillin spray and cream are extremely useful in impetigo, infected dermatitis, sycosis barbae and folliculitis.

Systemic therapy is useful in furunculosis, carbuncles, hidradenitis suppurativa axillaris, anthrax and erysipelas.

Indolent, static, varicose and traumatic ulcers become cleaner and healthier after the use of penicillin cream. Such treatment can be combined with a glycerin ichthyol gelatin dressing after a thorough cleansing and the bandage may be left on for 6 weeks to give good results.

Dramatic results follow the use of penicillin cream in pemphigus neonatorum but systemic therapy is indicated in severe cases.

The general practitioner must always realize that penicillin will not cure or improve many types of case and may even mask the pathological process, in particular, when gonorrhoea and syphilis are being treated, as the infection may be mixed. This limitation also applies to osteomyelitis, early lung abscess, pleurisy and infections of the uterine tubes. In cases such as these pus may form and surgery may become essential.

This chapter has been written to give general practitioners an idea of the conditions which will benefit from penicillin therapy. For further information the reader is advised to read the chapters on special subjects.

BIBLIOGRAPHY

ADMINISTRATION

ORAL

Little, C. J. H., and Lumb, G. (1945) *Lancet*, **1**, 203.

Leading Article (1945) *Lancet*, **1**, 215.

McDermott, W., Bunn, P. A., Benoit, Maria, DuBois, Rebeckah, and Haynes, Willetta (1945) *Science*, **101**, 228.

Libby, R. L. (1945) *Science*, **101**, 178.

György, P., Vandegrift, H. N., Elias, W., Colio, L. G., Barry, F. M., and Pilcher, J. D. (1945) *J. Amer. med. Ass.*, **127**, 639.

Heatley, N. G. (1945) *Lancet*, **1**, 590.

Annotation (1945) *Lancet*, **1**, 597.

Burke, F. G., Ross, S., and Strauss, C. (1945) *J. Amer. med. Ass.*, **128**, 83.

Perlstein, D., Kluener, R. G., Liebmann, A. J., and Dorrell, I. (1945) *Science*, **102**, 66.

Leading Article (1945) *Lancet*, **2**, 746.

Free, A. H., Parker, R. F., Biro, Barbara E. (1945) *Science*, **102**, 666.

Greey, P., and Macdonald, I. B. (1945) *Canad. med. Ass. J.*, **52**, 327.

ADMINISTRATION—*continued*

INHALATION

Mutch, N., and Rewell, R. E. (1945) *Lancet*, **1**, 650.

DERMATITIS CAUSED BY PENICILLIN

Bedford, P. D. (1946) *Brit. med. J.*, **1**, 51.
Vickers, H. R. (1946) *Lancet*, **1**, 307.
Park, R. G. (1945) *Brit. J. Derm.*, **57**, 151.

REACTIONS TO PENICILLIN

Barker, A. N. (1945) *Lancet*, **1**, 177.
Lumsden, R. B., and Weir, C. D. (1945) *Brit. med. J.*, **1**, 554.
Lamb, J. H. (1945) *Arch. Derm. Syph., N.Y.*, **52**, 93.
Jaslowitz, H. (1945) *Brit. med. J.*, **2**, 767.
Editorial (1945) *J. Allergy*, **16**, 302.
Annotation (1946) *Lancet*, **1**, 316.

DISEASES

DENTAL

Shaw, F. E., Sprawson, E., and May, H. B. (1945) *Brit. med. J.*, **1**, 551.
Fish, E. W. (1946) *S. Afr. med. J.*, **20**, 7.

DISEASES IN CHILDHOOD

Marks, M. B. (1945) *J. Pediat.*, **26**, 582.
Couper, E. C. R. (1945) *Arch. Dis. Childh.*, **20**, 117.
Aird, I. (1945) *Proc. R. Soc. Med.*, **38**, 569.
Gamble, T. O., Miller, L. C., and Tainter, M. L. (1945) *Amer. J. Obstet. Gynec.*, **50**, 514.

EAR, NOSE AND THROAT

Keith, J. D., Bynoe, E. T., Maclennan, J., Williamson, J., Carpenter, J. and Armstrong, C. (1945) *Canad. med. Ass. J.*, **53**, 471.
Cone, A. J. (1945) *Ann. Otol., etc., St. Louis*, **54**, 84.
Robinson, P. (1945) *Brit. med. J.*, **2**, 213.
Meadley, R. G. S., and Barnard, H. F. (1946) *Lancet*, **1**, 87.
Discussion (1946) *Proc. R. Soc. Med.*, **39**, 279.
Mothersill, M. H. (1945) *Ann. Otol., etc., St. Louis*, **54**, 166.
Berger, I. (1946) *Arch. Otolaryng., Chicago*, **43**, 19.

EYE

Bland, J. O. W., and Wilson, R. P. (1945) *Brit. J. Ophthal.*, **29**, 339.
Wright, R. E., and Stuart-Harris, C. H. (1945) *Brit. J. Ophthal.*, **29**, 428.

GONORRHOEA

Cutting, W. C., Halpern, R. M., Sultan, E. H., Armstrong, C. D., and Collins, C. L. (1945) *J. Amer. med. Ass.*, **129**, 425.

LUNG

Barach, A. L., Silberstein, F. H., Oppenheimer, Enid T., Hunter, T., and Soroka, M. (1945) *Ann. intern. Med.*, **22**, 485.
Leopold, S. S., and Cooke, R. A. (1945) *Amer. J. med. Sci.*, **209**, 784.
Kay, E. B., and Meade, R. H., Jun. (1945) *J. Amer. med. Ass.*, **129**, 200.

DISEASES—*continued*

Segal, M. S., and Ryder, Claire MacI. (1945) *New Engl. J. Med.*, **233**, 747.
Tillett, W. S., McCormack, J. E., and Cambier, Margaret J. (1945) *J. clin. Invest.*, **24**, 589.
Tillett, W. S., McCormack, J. E., and Cambier, Margaret J. (1945) *J. clin. Invest.*, **24**, 595.
Bunn, P. A., McDermott, W., Hadley, Susan J., and Carter, Anne C. (1945) *J. Amer. med. Ass.*, **129**, 320.
Poppe, J. K. (1945) *J. Amer. med. Ass.*, **129**, 435.
Leading Article (1945) *Lancet*, **2**, 819.
Smyth, C. J., and Billingslea, T. H. (1945) *J. Amer. med. Ass.*, **129**, 1005.
Anderson, T., Ferguson, Margaret S. (1945) *Lancet*, **2**, 805.
May, H. B., and Floyer, M. A. (1945) *Brit. med. J.*, **1**, 907.
Olsen, A. M. (1945) *Proc. Mayo Clin.*, **20**, 184.
Brobowitz, I. D., Edlin, J. S., Bassin, S., and Woolley, J. S. (1946) *New Engl. J. Med.*, **234**, 141.

MENINGITIS

CEREBROSPINAL

Forrest, A. R. (1945) *Brit. med. J.*, **2**, 805.

CHILDREN

Turner, E. K. (1946) *Med. J. Aust.*, **1**, 14.

EPIDEMIC

Lohrey, R. C., and Toomey, J. A. (1946) *J. Pediat.*, **28**, 86.

MENINGOCOCCAL

Tee, G. H. (1945) *Brit. med. J.*, **1**, 118.

PNEUMOCOCCAL

Genge, D. (1945) *Brit. med. J.*, **1**, 369.
Sweet, L. K., Dumoff-Stanley, Edith, Dowling, H. F., and Lepper, M. H. (1945) *J. Amer. med. Ass.*, **127**, 263.
Palley, A., and Shrand, H. (1945) *S. Afr. med. J.*, **19**, 73.
Hogg, P., and Bradley, C. D. (1945) *J. Pediat.*, **26**, 406.
White, W. L., Murphy, F. D., Lockwood, J. S., and Flippin, H. F. (1945) *Amer. J. med. Sci.*, **210**, 1.
Appelbaum, E., and Nelson, J. (1945) *J. Amer. med. Ass.*, **128**, 778.
Hutchins, Gretchen, and Davies, J. A. V. (1945) *J. Pediat.*, **27**, 505.
Milroy, W. H., and Hughes, B. L. (1945) *Med. J. Aust.*, **2**, 434.

STAPHYLOCOCCAL

White, W. L., Murphy, F. D., Lockwood, J. S., and Flippin, H. F. (1945) *Amer. J. med. Sci.*, **210**, 1.

STREPTOCOCCAL

White, W. L., Murphy, F. D., Lockwood, J. S., and Flippin, H. F. (1945) *Amer. J. med. Sci.*, **210**, 1.

SYPHILITIC

Annotation (1945) *Lancet*, **1**, 696.

MIXED INFECTIONS

Meleney, F. L., Johnson, B. A., Pulaski, E. J., and Colonna, F. (1946) *J. Amer. med. Ass.*, **130**, 121.

DISEASES—*continued*

ORAL INFECTIONS

Knott, F. A., and Blaikley, J. B. (1946) *Brit. med. J.*, **1**, 349.
Levitt, R. O., and Leathen, W. W. (1946) *Occup. Med.*, **1**, 81.

PYLEPHLEBITIS

Gamm, K. E. (1945) *J. Amer. med. Ass.*, **128**, 1159.

VINCENT'S ANGINA

Schwartz, B. M. (1945) *J. Amer. med. Ass.*, **128**, 704.
Shallenberger, P. L., Denny, E. R., and Pyle, H. D. (1945) *J. Amer. med. Ass.*, **128**, 706.
Pearce, W. F., and McDonald, J. B. (1945) *J. Amer. med. Ass.*, **128**, 342.

GENERAL

Spink, W. W., and Hall, W. H. (1945) *Ann. intern. Med.*, **22**, 510.
Price, D. E., McNairy, D. J., and White, E. L. (1945) *J. Amer. med. Ass.*, **128**. 183.
Goodman, H. (1945) *Urol. cutan. Rev.*, **49**, 492.
Woodward, F. D., and Holt, T. (1945) *J. Amer. med. Ass.*, **129**, 589.
Britton, C. J. C. (1946) *Practitioner*, **156**, 141.
Learmouth, J. R. (1946) *Edinb. med. J.*, **53**, 15.
Greey, P. (1945) *Canad. med. Ass. J.*, **52**, 550.

INDEX

INDEX

Abdominal infections, 229
appendix and ileocaecal angle in, 233
actinomyces, sensitivity of, 233
actinomycosis, 232
appendicitis, acute, in, 233
caecum, carcinoma of, 234
bacteriology, 229
B. proteus, 229
Esch. coli communis, 229
salmonella group, 229
Str. faecalis, 229
bladder, 238
cystitis, 238
Esch. coli, in, 238
B. proteus, in, 238
genito-urinary system, 237
urinary infections of, 237
B. proteus in, 238
Esch. coli in, 238
kidney, 238
abscess, perinephric, 238
carbuncle of, 238
pyelitis, 238
liver and gallbladder, 235
abscesses, multiple, 235
cholangitis, 235
cholecystitis, acute, 236
acute suppurative, 235
pylephlebitis, acute, 235
Weil's disease, 236
pancreas and spleen, 237
pancreatitis, acute, 237
sulphadiazine in treatment of, 237
peritoneal cavity, 230
abscess, local intraperitoneal, 231
cellulitis, 232
pelvic, 232
retroperitoneal, 232
diffusion into, 230
ileus, paralytic, 231
uraemia in, 231
peritonitis, 229
acute diffuse, 230
acute localized, 229, 230
general, 230
gonococcal, 231
pneumococcal, 231
streptococcal, 231
traumatic, 230
prostate and vesicles, 239
rectum and anal canal, 234
abscesses, ischiorectal, 234
buttocks and perineum, 234
injuries and infections of, 234
Cl. welchii in, 234
fissure of, 235
fistula in ano, 235
ulceration of, 234
gas gangrene, "autogenous" of, 234
small and large intestine, 232

Abdominal infections—*continued*
small and large intestine—*continued*
anthrax of, 233
colitis, 232
diverticulitis, 233
enteritis, 232
stomach and duodenum, 232
testis, 239
epididymitis, 239
chronic non-specific, 239
subacute, 239
epididymo-orchitis, acute, 239
therapeutics, general considerations 237
Abrasions, 359
Abscess, alveolar, acute, 331
bartholinitis, acute, 280
brain, 267
breast, 126, 247
intraperitoneal, local, 231
ischiorectal, 234
liver and gallbladder, of, 235
perinephric, 238
Actinomycosis, 126, 185, 232, 322
local application in, 186
Activity, 24
Adenocellulitis, 126, 128
Administration and dosage, methods of, 93
local, 102
creams, 103
dermatology, 103 (*see also* Dermatology)
infiltration, 103
anaesthetic combined with, 103
injection, in abscess cavity, 103
lamellae, 104 (*see also* Ophthalmology)
lozenges, 104
ointments, 103 (*see also* Dermatology)
sprays, 103
oil and wax suspensions in, 93
oral, 102
capsules, 102
duodenal tube, 102
pills, 102
rectal, 102
systemic, 93
continuous, 93
drip transfusion, 95
clock-drip (Last), 96
Eudrip apparatus, 95
thrombosis, liability to, 93
inhalation, 100
asthmatics, 100
B.L.B. type mask, 100
Collinson atomizer, 100, 101
vapours, 100
injection, by, 103
abscess cavity, into, 103
intermittent, 97, 98

Administration and dosage, methods of—*continued*
systemic—*continued*
injection—*continued*
intermittent—*continued*
anaesthetic in, use of, 97
oil and beeswax suspension in, 98
intramuscular, 97
intravenous, 97
site of, 97
Anaerobic myositis, 171
Animal diseases, 337
administration, methods of, 337
intramammary, 338, 343
intramuscular, 337
suspension, beeswax and peanut oil, in, 337
intravenous, 337
permeability of mammary gland, 337
consideration of, 337
milk test to assess, 337
blackleg, 349
Cl. chauvaei causing, 349
cystitis, 347
mastitis, bovine, 337, 338
bacteriology of, 337
Cor. pyogenes, 339
Staph. aureus., 343
Str. agalactiae, 337
Str. dysgaclatiae, 339
Str. pyogenes, 339
Str. uberis, 339
criterion of cure of, 341
Hotis test, diagnosis in, of, 340
"summer mastitis", 339, 341
treatment of, 344
alum precipitated toxoid in, 344
injection, by, 344
infusion *via* teat canal, 344
intramuscular, 344
subcutaneous, 344
pneumonia, 349
Pasturella causing, 349
wild ducks, in, 349
pyelonephritis, bovine, 338, 347
Cor. renale causing, 338, 347
treatment of, 347
strangles, horses, in, 346
signs of, 346
Str. equi causing, 346
treatment of, 346
swine erysipelas, 348
Erysipelothrix rhusiopathiae causing, 348
erysipeloid in man, causing, 348
Anthrax, 233, 322
Apicolysis, 160 (*see also* Chest surgery)
Appendicitis, acute, 233
Arthritis, 196
gonococcal, acute and chronic, 280
septic, 257
Ascites
syphilis, latent, in, 287
Atrophy
primary optic, 287

B. fusiformis, 305
Bacteriological control, 76
estimation, methods, 80
agar diffusion, 84
blood serum, 80
capillary tube, 83
test organism, 83
haemolytic streptococcus, 83
staphylococcus, 83
cerebrospinal fluid, 84
Fleming's, 80
Heatley and Garrod's, 81
pus, 85
Rammelkamp's, 83
sensitivity of organism, methods, 87
agar diffusion, 87
Morley's, 87
serial dilution, 87
slide cell, 80
sputum, 85
urine, 84
penicillinase, 87
B. subtilis, 88
culture material, precautions, 91
M. lysodiekticus, 88
neutralization, 90
methods, 90
agar diffusion, 90
titration, 90
organisms producing, test of, 89
potency, 76
assay, methods, 77
agar cup, 79
agar diffusion, 77
cylinders, 79
filter paper discs, 79
Heatley's, 78
rapid, 79
test organisms, 79
titrations, 80
turbidemetric, 80
serial dilution, 79
creams and ointments, 80
measurement, 76
International Standard, 77
standard solution, 77
test organisms, 76
B. subtilis, 76
B. welchii, 80
National Collection of Type Cultures, 77
pneumococcus, 76
staphylococcus, 76
streptococcus, 76
Therapeutic Substances Act, 76
powders, snuffs and lozenges, 80
Blepharitis, 296, 320
Boils, 321
Bone and joint infections, 223
Bone grafts, 184

Brain and meningeal infections, 265
abscess, 267
brain, of, 267
complications causing, 269
Dandy method in, 267
dissection *en coque* of, 271
sulphadiazine following, 271
Vincent's technique in, 271
encephalitis in, 270
intrathecal therapy in, 271
mixed infections causing, 268
oedema in, 270
otogenic, 269
postoperative sepsis, 272
Ps. aeruginosa in, 270
sulphonamides in, 268
systemic therapy in, 271
Thorotrast in, 267
ventriculography in, 267
cerebellar, 269
cerebral, 277
in meningitis, 277
extradural, 266
complications causing, 266
treatment of, 266
Carrel tubes in, 266
intracranial, 265
temperosphenoidal, 269
needling in, 269
fracture of base, 265
treatment of, 265
meningitis, 273
abscess, cerebral, in, 277
diagnosis by ventriculography of, 277
cisternal puncture in, 276
complications of, 277
arachnoiditis, 277
complications of, 277
obliterative, 277
paraplegia, causing, 277
atrophy, convolutions, of, in, 277
Magendie's foramen, obstruction of, 277
hydrocephalus, causing, 277
H. influenzae, due to, 273
loculations, 276
catheter, use of, 276
mastoid disease causing, 276
lumbar puncture in, 276
meningococcus in, 273
middle ear disease causing, 265
nasal sinus, infections from, in, 265
pneumococcal, 273
pneumococcus in, 276
Ps. aeruginosa in, 277
spray, prophylactic use of, in, 265
staphylococcal, 273
streptococcal, 273
subarachnoid space, in, 276, 277
fibrin formation in, 276
sulphonamides in, 273, 276
operations, intracranial, 277
Brain and meningeal infections—*contd.*
osteomyelitis, 265
skull, of, 265
staphylococcus causing, 265
systemic therapy in, 266
scalp wounds, causing, 265
sulphadiazine, 265
fracture of base, in, 265
penicillin drops, with, 265
thrombosis, 272
cavernous sinus, of, 272
signs of, 272
intracranial, septic, 272
carbuncles causing, 272
furuncles causing, 265
middle ear infection causing, 265
lateral sinus, of, 273
Bronchiectasis, 70, 147, 158, 357
prophylactic use in, 158
Bronchitis, 148, 306, 357
acute recurrent and chronic, 357
Bronchopneumonia, 357
Burns and plastic surgery, 180
actinomycosis, 185
local application, 186
bone grafts, 184
burns, 187
Lanette wax SX, 187
penicillin-insensitive organisms, 187
intra-oral operations, 185
pastilles, 185
osteomyelitis, 186
skin, 182
grafts and losses, 182
flaps, full thickness, 184
granulating areas, treatment, 183
Eusol, 183
trypsin, 183
therapeutic methods, 180
local application, 181
preparation for, 181
systemic administration, 180
wounds, 181
cream, 182

Cancrum oris, 328
Carcinoma of lung, 159 (*see also* Chest Surgery)
Carbuncles, 126, 127, 321, 359
kidney, of, 238
Cellulitis, 126, 212, 309, 310
face, recurrent, of, 322
fingers, of, 212
pulp infections, 212
pelvic, 232, 249
retroperitoneal, 232
Chancroid, 289
Chemistry and manufacture, 24
chemistry, 27
enzymatic breakdown, 30
formula, constitutional, 27
penicillamine, 28
penillic acid, 29
sodium penicilloate, 29

Chemistry and manufacture—*continued*
history, 24
activity, 24
different strains of *P. notatum*, 32
inactivation, 25
various metals, in the presence of, 25
purification, 26
chromatography, by, 26
partition, 26
stability, 25
*p*H in, 25
studies of, 25
various solvents, in, 25
manufacture, 30
processes, 30
concentration, 38
deep (tank) fermentation, 32, 38
agitation, 33
aeration with sterile air, 33
asepsis, 33
drying, 39
freeze, 41
spray, 41
harvesting, 38
incubation, 37
medium, 34
preparation of, 34
Czapek-Dox solution, 34
"corn steep liquor," 34
spore suspensions and inoculation, 36
sterilization and cooling, 35
surface culture, 33
Chest infections, 141
bacteriology, 141
D. catarrhalis, 141
H. influenzae, 141
K. pneumoniae, 141
staphylococci, 141
streptococci, 141
bronchiectasis, 147
inhalation method in, 148
bronchitis, 148
inhalation method in, 149
empyema, 145
systemic administration in, 145
lung abscess, 146
acute single, 147
bronchiectatic, 147
chronic single, 147
mixed infection, 147
multiple staphylococci, 147
pneumonia, 143
sulphadiazine in, 144
Sulphamezathine in, 144
sulphonamides in, 142
traumatic haemothorax, 146
tubercle bacillus in, 142
tuberculous pyothorax, 146
Chest surgery, 150
administration, methods of, 150
inhalation, 151
Collinson inhaler, 151
Chest surgery—*continued*
administration, methods of—*contd.*
inhalation—*continued*
Rybar inhaler, 151
instillation, 151
local, 150
systemic, 150
clinical applications, 151
bronchiectasis, prophylaxis in, 158
empyema, 151
aspiration, 154
bacteriology, 153
chemotherapy, 153
children, 155
chronic type, 156
secondary infection in, 156
treatment of, 156
drainage of, 154
postural, bronchiectasis, in, 158
fistula formation in, 159
sulphathiazole powder in, 159
general considerations in, 151
haemothorax, in penetrating wounds in, 157
Lipiodol in diagnosis of, 154
lobectomy, 158
Phenoxetol cream in, 155
rib resection in, 155
secondary infection in, 153
treatment, principles of, 152
tuberculous type, 157
lung, 158
abscess, 158
drainage of, 159
result of obstruction, 158
suppurative conditions of, 159
major, 159
apicolysis in, 160
carcinoma, 159
bronchial in, 159
heart, 160
endocarditis, acute and infective, 160
pericarditis, suppurative, 160
pneumonectomy in, 159
mediastinitis, 161
causes of, 161
treatment of, 161
pneumonectomy, 159
thoracoplasty, 160
Cholangitis, 235
Choroiditis, 299
Clostridial myositis, 173
Colitis, 232
Conjunctiva, 320
cream, irritation by, 320
Conjunctivitis, 295, 358
Corneal ulcer, 359
C. diphtheriae, 305
Cystitis, 238

Dacrocystitis, 297

Dental and oral infections, 324
  cancrum oris, 328
    insufflation, 328
      sulphathiazole powder in, 328
    intramuscular administration in, 328
  gingivectomy, 335
    intramuscular injection in, 335
  infections, in, 324
    B. fusiformis, 324
    staphylococcal, 324
    streptococcal, 324
    Vincent's spirochaete, 324
  lesions, 325
  maxillo-facial injuries, 332
    intramuscular injection in, 332
    sulphathiazole powder in, 332
  osteomyelitis of jaw, 333
    aetiology, 333
    treatment, 334
      preventive, 334
        intramuscular injection in, 334
        root, section of, 334
        sulcus, cauterization of, 334
      subsequent, 334
        sulphathiazole powder in, 334
        systemic administration in, 334
  pyorrhoea, 325, 335
  surgical interference in septic areas, 329
    pathology, 329
    treatment, method of, 330
      teeth, replantation of, 330
        abscess, acute alveolar, 331
        bone, acute suppuration in, 331
        intramuscular injection for, 331
        method of, 330
      wounds, 329, 330
  Vincent's acute necrotic stomatitis, 326
    indications for, 326
    pathology of, 326
    treatment, methods of, 326
      chromic acid in, 327
      lozenges in, 326
      systemic, 327
        buccal mucosa, ulceration involving the, 327
      warning note in, 328
Dermatitis, 73, 321
  infected, 359
  infective eczematoid, 321
  radium, 321
  seborrhoeic, 321
Dermatology, 317
  Actinomycosis bovis, 317
  administration, 318
    local, 318
      creams, 318, 319
        Phenoxetol, 319
      spray, 318, 319
Dermatology—*continued*
  administration—*continued*
    systemic, 321
  boils, 321
  carbuncles, 321
  diseases, 317
    actinomycosis, 322
    anthrax, 322
    blepharitis, 320
    cellulitis of face, recurrent, 322
    dermatitis, 321
      infective eczematoid, 321
      radium, 321
      seborrhoeic, 321
    ecthyma, 319
    eczema, 321
    erysipelas, 321
      swine erysipelas, 317
    erysipeloid, 317
    erythema serpens, 322
      Rosenbach's, 322
    herpes labialis, 317
    herpes zoster, 317
    impetigo, 319
      Bockhart's, 321
      bullous type, 319
    intertrigo, 320
    lichen urticus, 321
    molluscum contagiosum, 317
    otitis externa, 320
    ringworm, 317
    scabies, 321
    seborrhoea of scalp, 320
    sycosis barbae, 320
  fissures, streptococcal, 320
  penicillin-sensitive organisms, 317
    inhibiting penicillin, 317
    secondary lesions caused by, 317
  reactions, 323
  side effects, 322
  staphylococcal foci, 320
  Treponema pallidum, 317
  tubercle bacillus, 317
  ulcer, varicose, 321
  warts, 317
Diphtheria, 309
Diverticulitis, 233
Dorsal hand infections, 216

Ecthyma, 319
Eczema, 311, 321
Empyema, 127, 130, 133, 145, 151
  fistula formation in, 159
  sulphathiozole powder, 159
Encephalitis, 270
Endocarditis, bacterial, 134
  acute, 140
    septicaemia, complication of, in, 140
  subacute, 134
    administration methods and general care, 137
      America, United States of, 138
        intravenous drip in, 138

Endocarditis, bacterial—*continued*
subacute—*continued*
administration methods and general care—*continued*
continuous intramuscular infusion, 137
intermittent intramuscular injections, 137
dose, daily, 135
in vitro sensitivity tests, significance of, 137
Medical Research Council, 135
Penicillin Clinical Trials Committee, 135
penicillin and heparin in, 134, 139
subcutaneous deposition, by, 134
prognosis, 139
aortic regurgitation, severe, 139
infecting organism, sensitivity of, 140
prophylaxis, 139
congenital heart disease, in, 139
rheumatic endocarditis, in, 139
relapses, 138
response to, 138
dangers, 138
embolic phenomena, 138
infarcation, 138
erythrocyte sedimentation rate in, 138
treatment, 135
death rate during, 137
heart failure, due to, 137
major emboli, due to, 137
uraemia, due to, 137
duration of, 135
importance of early and adequate, 137
Enteritis, 232
Epididymitis, 239
acute, 280
chronic non-specific, 239
subacute, 239
Epididymo-orchitis, acute, 239
Erysipelas, 126, 311, 321
swine erysipelas, 317
Erysipeloid, 317
Erythema serpens, 322
Rosenbach's, 322
syphilis, in treatment of, 285
Ethmoiditis, 307

Fever, reaction to therapy, 72
Fissures, streptococcal, 320
Folliculitis, 359
Forearm infections, 227
Furunculosis, 359

Gas gangrene "autogenous", 234
General practice, 350
administration, methods of, 351
injections, 352
equipment for local, 352
frequency of, and duration of course, 354

General practice—*continued*
administration, methods of—*contd.*
injections—*continued*
intramuscular, 351
novocain with, 351
intravenous, 351
methods of, 353
site of, 353
buttock, 354
selection of, 352
shoulder, 354
thigh, 353
subcutaneous, 351
systemic, 353
complications in, 353
local, 355
cream, 355
inhalation, 355
methods of producing, 355
tent, 356
lozenges, 355
ointment, 355
snuff and powder, 355
sprays and drops, solution for, 355
suppositories, 355
bacteriological examination in, 350
penicillin-sensitive organism, 351
diseases in, 356
abrasions, 359
bronchiectasis, 357
bronchitis, 357
acute recurrent and chronic, 357
bronchopneumonia, 357
carbuncles, 359
conjunctivitis, 358
corneal ulcer, 359
dermatitis, infected, 359
folliculitis, 359
furunculosis, 359
genito-urinary infections, 358
hidradenitis suppurativa axillaris, 359
hypopyon, 359
impetigo, 359
iritis, 359
otitis media, 358
pemphigus neonatorum, 359
pharyngitis, 357
acute and chronic, 357
pleural effusion and empyemata, 358
pneumonia, lobar, 357
quinsy, 357
rhinitis, 356
acute, 356
chronic, 356
sinusitis, 356
acute, 356
chronic, 356
stomatitis, 358
sycosis barbae, 359
tonsillitis, 357
acute, 357

General practice—*continued*
diseases in—*continued*
tonsillitis—*continued*
chronic recurrent, 357
ulcers, 359
idolent, 359
static, 359
traumatic, 359
varicose, 359
urethritis, 358
Vincent's angina, 358
haemolytic streptococcus infection, 352
instruments, 352
cleaning and storage, 353
methods of sterilizing, 352
sulphonamides, 351
hypersensitivity to, 351
sulphathiazole, 351
surgical measures, 354
osteomyelitis, in, 355
perinephric abscess, in, 355
Genito-urinary infections, 358
Gonorrhoea, 69, 126
prenatal, 241
Granuloma venereum, 289

Haemolytic streptococcus infection, 352
H. influenzae, 273, 305
Haemothorax, traumatic, 146
Hand infections, 211
administration, methods of, 211
cream, 211
local, 211
solution, 211
systemic, 211, 212
arthritis, infective, of wrist and carpus, 227
ankylosis, end result, 227
bacteriology, 211
anaerobic streptococci, 211
fusiform bacilli, 211
haemolytic streptococci, 211
Staph. aureus, 211
cellulitis of the fingers, 212
pulp infections, 212
cream in, 213
osteomyelitis from, 212
foreign bodies in, 226
infections, 214
anaerobic, 226
fusiform bacilli, 226
anterior subaponeurotic, 216
administration, 216
local, 216
systemic, 216
bone and joint, 223
systemic administration, 225
dorsal, 216
forearm, 227
primary tendon sheath, 217
haemolytic streptococcus, 218
local administration, 219

Hand infections—*continued*
infections—*continued*
primary tendon sheath—*continued*
Staph. aureus, 218
space, 215
mid-palmar, 217
thenar, 217
web, 215
subcutaneous, of proximal and middle phalanges, 214
butchers, in, 214
cream in, 214
erysipeloid, 214
Erysipelothrix rhusiopathiae, 214
intramuscular injection, 215
systemic administration, 214
tenosynovitis, 220
acute pyogenic, 223
suppurative, 220
paronychia, 212
flap operation, 212
cream in, 212
Heart, 160
endocarditis, acute and infective, 160
pericarditis, suppurative, 160
Herpes labialis, 317
Herpes zoster, 317
Herxheimer reaction, 72, 285, 287
Hidradenitis suppurativa axillaris, 359
History and development, 1
administration, 20
bacteria, morphological changes, 17
B. brevis, 14
Cor. acnes, 9
culture, 5, 16
method, 5, 16
Czapex-Dox medium, 13
diffusibility, 4
dosage, 21
experiments, preliminary, 4
H. influenzae, 8
H. pertussis, 8
insensitivity (*see* Table, p. 19)
instability, 9
Lysozyme, 6
meningitis, first case, 17
mould, 3
isolation, 3
nature, 3, 16
Oxford workers, 15
miniature factory, 15
Penicillin Committee, 17
Penicillium, 1
P. chrysogenum, 16
P. notatum, 16
purity, 18
sensitivity (*see* Table, p. 19)
stability, 14
staphylococci inhibited, 8
sulphonamides, 14
combination with, 14, 22
toxicity, 10
treatment, 17
extension of use in, 17

History and development—*continued*
treatment—*continued*
general rules for, 18
infection, nature of, conditioning, 20
limitations of, 22
inconvenience, 22
instability, 22
penicillinase, 22
sequestered infections, 22
unit, 18
International, 18
"Oxford unit", 18
United States visit, 15
Hypopyon, 295, 359

Ileus, paralytic, 231
uraemia in, 231
Impetigo, 126, 311, 359
Bockhart's, 321
bullous type, 319
Inactivation, 25
various metals, in the presence of, 25
Infections, generalized, 116
abscess, breast, of, 126
actinomycosis, 126
adenocellulitis, 126, 128
aspiration, 133
bacteriology, 121
causative organism, 121
Staph. aureus, 127, 128, 129, 130
staphylococcus, 127
Streptococcus, 128
haemolytic, 129, 130
non-haemolytic, 128
pyogenes, 128
viridans, 129
breast, inflammation of, 128
carbuncles, 126, 127
cellulitis, 126
complications, 128
endothelium in, 128
epithelium in, 128
constitution, 132
convalescence, 124
diagnosis, 119
pus, 119
presence of, 119
toxaemia, evacuation of, in, 120, 123
underlying organic lesion, 120
carcinoma, 120
leukaemia, 120
skin disease, chronic, 120
tuberculous, 120
X-ray examination, 119
dosage, summary of, 125
drainage, 123
effusions, 133
empyema, 127, 130, 133
endocarditis, 126
bacterial, subacute, 129
erysipelas, 126

Infections, generalized—*continued*
eye, diseases of, 126 (*see also* Ophthalmology)
infection, intra-ocular, 126
gonorrhoea, 126
impetigo, 126
jaundice, 130
Ludwig's angina, 128
lymphangitis, 130
mastoiditis, 126, 129
meningitis, 126, 133
osteomyelitis, 126, 128, 129, 130
otitis media, 126, 129
puerperal sepsis, 130
pulmonary lesions, 126, 129
matastatic, from carbuncle, 127
empyema, 127, 130, 133
rat-bite fever, 124
Spirillum minus, 124
Streptobacillus moniliformis, 124
Weil's disease, 125
Leptospira icterohaemorrhagiae, 125
septicaemia, 126, 129, 130
sinusitis, 126
therapy, 121
adjuvant measures, 123
aim, 121
institution of, 121
localization of lesion, 121
organism, 121
avascular tissue, in, 121
identification of, 121
phases of, 122
first, 122
control, initial, 122
erythema, 123
oedema, 123
pulse rate, 122
pyrexia, 122
vasomotor dilation, 123
second, 122, 123
control, continued, 122
pus, 123
absorption of, 123
aspiration, 123
drainage, 132
intravenous, 132
meninges, in, 123
pleura, in, 123
theca, in, 123
sterilizing the lesion, 121
trauma, influence of, 127, 128
venous channels, 131
influence of, 131
periphlebitis, 131
thrombosis, infective, 131
Vincent's angina, 126
Injections, 352
equipment for local, 352
frequency of, and duration of course, 354
intramuscular, 351
novocain with, 351

Injections—*continued*
intravenous, 351
methods of, 353
site of, 353
buttock, 354
selection of, 352
shoulder, 354
thigh, 353
subcutaneous, 351
systemic, 353
complications in, 353
Instruments, 352
cleaning and storage, 353
methods of sterilizing, 352
Intertrigo, 320
Intra-oral operations, 185
pastilles, in, 185
Iridocyclitis, 299
Iritis, 299, 359
gonococcal, 280

K. pneumoniae, 305
Keratitis, interstitial, 288, 297
syphilis, congenital, in, 288

Larynx, 287
syphilis of, 287
Lichen urticus, 321
Lobectomy, 158
intrapleural therapy, following, 158
Ludwig's angina, 128, 309
Lung (*see also* Chest Surgery, Chest Infections)
abscess, 146, 158
infections, 255
suppurative conditions, 159
Lymphangitis, 130
Lymphogranuloma inguinale, 289

Manufacture, 30
deep (tank) fermentation, 32, 38
Mastoiditis, 126, 129, 313
Measles, 306
Mediastinitis, 161
causes of, 161
treatment of, 161
Meningitis, 66, 126, 133, 261, 273
septic otogenic, 302
Meningococcus, 273
Middle ear disease, 265
molluscum contagiosum, 317

N. intracellularis, 305
Naspharyngitis, 254
Nephritis, 67
Nuflav, 169

Obstetrics and gynaecology, 241
intranatal use, 243
caesarean section, in, 243
pelvic cellulitis, 249
pelvic peritonitis, 249
postoperative sepsis, 248

Obstetrics and gynaecology—*continued*
postpartum use, 246
breast abscess, in, 247
nipples, cracked, in, 247
ophthalmia neonatorum, prophylaxis, 246
puerperal sepsis, prophylaxis, 246
prenatal use, 241
gonorrhoea, in, 241
syphilis, in, 242
prophylactic value in, 245
puerperal sepsis, prevention of, 245
salpingitis, 249
salpingo-oophoritis, 249
vulva, infections of, 251
Oedema, 270
Ophthalmia neonatorum, 246, 254, 294
Ophthalmology, 291
administration, 292
injections, 292
intra-ocular, 297
anterior chamber, into, 297
vitreous body, into, 297
subconjunctival, 292, 297
interstitial keratitis, in, 297
methods, other tentative, 298
systemic, 298
choroiditis, in, 298
endophthalmitis, septic abortion, after, 298
optic atrophy, syphilitic, 298
applications, clinical, 292
local therapy, 292
clinical conditions amenable, 294
blepharitis, 296
conjunctivitis, 295
acute purulent, 295
mucopurulent, 295
cornea, infections of, 296
dacrocystitis, 297
ophthalmia neonatorum, 294
corneal complications of, 295
atropine sulphate in, 295
drops in, 294
socket, infected, 296
trachoma, 296
ulcer, 295
corneal, infected, 296
dendritic, 296
hypopyon, 295
atropine drops in, 295
concentration, 292
frequency, 293
lamellae, 293
mode, 294
ointments, 293
Eucerin, 293
Oculentum B.P., 293
paraffin, soft, 293
penicillin, 298
activity, range of, 299
ophthalmia neonatorum, 299
trachoma, 299

Ophthalmology—*continued*
penicillin—*continued*
intra-ocular inflammation, in, 299
choroiditis, 299
iridocyclitis, 299
iritis, 299
panophthalmitis, 299
limitations of, 298
sulphonamides, comparison with, 299
theoretical considerations, 291
adnexa oculi, 292
infections of outer eye, 292
therapy, local, 292
Orthopaedic surgery and fractures, 189
arthritis, 196
bacteriology, 197
diagnosis, 197
aspiration, 197
gonococcal, 196 (*see also* Venereal Diseases)
primary, 196
pyogenic, 196
secondary, 196
suppurative, 196
acute, ankylosis following, 198
scarlet fever, following, 197
treatment, 198
fractures, 189
compound, 190
haemolytic streptococcus in, 190
staphylococci in, 190
treatment, 190
delayed primary suture, 190
local, instillation, by, 190
parenteral, 190
penicillin - sulphanilamide powder, 190
infected, 191
treatment, 191
grafts, 191
cancellous bone, 191, 192
cortical bone, 191
haematoma following, 192
skin, 191
insufflation, 192
intramuscular, 191
infection, cause of, in, 189
treatment, 190
joints, wounds of, 192
direct, 193
treatment of, 193
fracture, compound, involving, 193
after-treatment, 194
treatment, 193
immobilization, 193
injection, 193
contamination of, 193
systemic, 193
haemarthrosis, 192
osteomyelitis, 194
acute, 194
bacteriology, 194
Orthopaedic surgery and fractures–*con.*
osteomyelitis—*continued*
chronic, 195
Brodie's abscess, 195
haematogenous, 194
pyogenic, 194
treatment, 194
dangers of, 195
abscesses, large, in, 195
pyaemia, 196
tendons, 189
flexor, of hand, 189
grafts, 189
sheath, suppuration of, 189
sutures, 189
tuberculosis, surgical, 198
sinuses, prevention of, 199
wounds, 193
treatment, 193
Osteomyelitis, 126, 128, 129, 130, 186, 194, 200, 257, 265
acute haematogenous, 200
administration, methods of, 201
local, 201
systemic, 201
arthritis, associated, 204
suppurative staphylococcal, of infants, 204
treatment of, 204
compound fracture, complicating, 208
dosage, 201
flat bones, of, 208
immobilization, 203
local response of the bone lesion, 206
long bones, 200
metastatic lesions, management of, 205
pericarditis, in, 205
operative intervention, scope of, 202
subperiosteal abscess, evacuation of, 203
preliminary investigation, 200
radiological appearances, 206
short bones, 208
streptococcal, 208
systemic response of septicaemia in, 205
treatment, 201
commencement of, 201
duration of, 202
chronic, 208
Brodie's circumscribed abscess of bone, 208
jaw, of, 333
penicillin-resistant organisms, due to, 209
bacteriological examination, importance of, 209
Otitis, 311, 314
externa, 320
media, 126, 129, 255, 358

Otorhinolaryngology, 301
abscess, 309
extradural, 314
metastatic, 315
peritonsillar, 309
retropharyngeal, 309
subperiosteal, 308
administration, methods of, 302
local, 303
instillation, 303
bronchitis, infantile, 306
mastoidectomy, following, 303
nasal sinus, into, 303
powder, 304
Flavazole in, 304
sulphathiazole in, 304
solutions, 303
ephedrine sulphate in, 303
Phenoxetol in, 304
sprays, 303
chlorocresol, addition of, 303
pharyngotympanic tube, in, 312
systemic, 303
inhalation, atomizer, by, 303
injection, ventricles, into, 303
intramuscular, 303
puncture, 303
cisternal, 303
lumbar, 303
subarachnoid space, into, 303
B. fusiformis, 305
B. proteus albus, 304, 305
Bor. vincenti, 305
bronchitis, 306
C. diphtheriae, 305
cellulitis, 310
cholesteatoma, 314
diphtheria, 309
ear, 311
eczema of, 311
external, 311
auricle, 311
haematoma of, 311
perichondritis of, 311
canal, auditory, 311
furunculosis of, 311
infections, mycotic, 311
otitis externa haemorrhagica of, 311
pinna, infections of, 311
erysipelas of, 311
impetigo of, 311
mastoid operations, 315
postoperative therapy in, 315
mastoiditis, 313
acute, 313
complications of, 314
abscess, 314
matastatic, 315
extradural, 314
labrynthitis, 315
lateral sinus thrombosis, 315
otitic hydrocephalus, 315
Otorhinolaryngology—*continued*
ear—*continued*
mastoiditis—*continued*
acute—*continued*
complications of—*continued*
petrositis, 314
venous ligation in, 315
signs and symptoms of, 313
otosclerosis, 316
fenestration in, 316
labrynthitis, prevention of, 316
treatment, 302
catarrhal conditions, 302
drainage, translabrynthine, 302
meningitis, septic otogenic, 302
method, 312
dry, 312
Siegal's pneumatic speculum in, 312
wet, 313
pus, evacuation of, 302
sulphonamides in, 304
tympanic cleft, 311
otitis media, 311
acute, 311
complicating other infections, 312
meningitis, causing, 312
perforation in, 312
chronic suppuration, 314
cholesteatoma in, 314
otorrhoea in, 314
treatment, 312
dry, 312
wet, 313
tympanic membrane, 312
perforation of, 312
otorrhoea following, 312
treatment of, 312
erysipelas, 311
Esch. coli, 304, 305, 310
ethmoiditis, 307
furuncle, staphylococcal, 311
furunculosis, 311
H. influenzae, 305
impetigo, 311
infection, 306
respiratory tract, 306
staphylococcal, 301
meningitis with, 301
septicaemia with, 301
streptococcal, 311
mycotic, 311
K. pneumoniae, 305
labrynthitis, 316
laryngectomy, postoperative therapy, 310
laryngitis, 306
larynx, 310
cancer of, 310
oedema of, 310
Ludwig's angina, 309
measles, 306

Otorhinolaryngology—*continued*
meningitis, 302
otogenic, septic, acute, 302
myringotomy, 312
N. catarrhalis, 305
N. intracellularis, 305
neck, 309
cancer of, 310
cellulitis of, 309
larynx, oedema of, 310
Ludwig's angina, 309
retropharyngeal abscess of, 309
septic infections of, 309
septic perichondritis of, 310
nose, 306
rhinitis, catarrhal, 306
rhinosinusitis, 306
sinuses, nasal, 306
catarrh of, 306
sinusitis, 306
acute suppurative, 307
chronic suppurative, 308
osteomyelitis complicating, 308
subperiosteal abscess in, 308
maxillary, 307
osteomyelitis, frontal, 308
otitic hydrocephalus, 315
otitis, 311
externa haemorrhagica, 311
media, 311
acute, 311
chronic, 314
suppurative, 314
otorrhoea, 312
otosclerosis, 316
perichondritis, 310
petrositis, 314
pharyngectomy, 310
pharyngitis, 306
pharynx, 309
prophylaxis, 308
antrostomy, radical, 308
frontosphenoethmoidectomy, 308
jaw, upper, excision of, 308
larynx, operations on, 309, 310
pharynx, operations on, 309, 310
systemic, 309
Ps. aeruginosa, 304, 305
quinsy, 309
respiratory tract, infections of, 306
carriers, haemolytic streptococci, of, 306
rhinitis, 306
rhinosinusitis, 306
scarlet fever, 306
seborrhoea, 311
sinus, 301
cavernous, 301
thrombosis of, 301
furuncle causing, 301
lateral, thrombosis of, 315
sinusitis, 301
frontal, 301

Otorhinolaryngology—*continued*
sinusitis—*continued*
hypertrophic, 302
suppurative, 307, 308
Staphylococcus, 305
albus, 305
aureus, 305
Streptococcus, 305
haemolyticus, 305
mucosus, 305
pyogenes, 305
viridans, 305
tonsillectomy, 309
tonsillitis, 306, 309
tracheitis, 306
Vincent's angina, 309

Pancreatitis, acute, 237
sulphadiazine in treatment of, 237
Panophthalmitis, 299
Paronychia, 212
Parotitis, septic, 257
Pemphigus neonatorum, 359
P. notatum, different strains of, 32
Periphlebitis, 131
Peritonitis, 229
acute diffuse, 230
acute localized, 229, 230
general, 230
gonococcal, 231
pelvic, 249
pneumococcal, 231
streptococcal, 231
traumatic, 230
Pharmacology, 59
administration, 59
infusion, continuous, 60, 63
intramuscular, 59, 64
intravenous, 64
injection, 60
continuous intramuscular, 60
intermittent, 60
blood bacteriostatic, 61
dosage, 61, 62
intramuscular, 59, 60
neurosyphilis, 66
intravenous, 59, 60
thrombosis following, 50
subcutaneous, 60
pain following, 72
oral, 68
achlorhydria, 69
gastric acid, 69
substances neutralizing, 69
gonorrhoea, 69
indications, 69
methods, 69
pneumonia, 69
other routes, 69
cavities, infected, 70
abscess, 70
joints, 70
theca 70

Pharmacology—*continued*
administration—*continued*
other routes—*continued*
intestine, 70
intubation, duodenal, 70
lumbar injection, 66
lungs, 70
bronchiectasis, 70
intratracheal, 70
intubation, 70
inhalation, 70
rectum, 70
suppository, 70
blood level, therapeutic, 59
distribution, 65
bile, 65
cerebrospinal fluid, 65
meningitis, 66
intrathecal injection, 66
lateral ventricle, 66
eye, 65
foetal, 65
lacrimal secretion, 65
placenta, 65
red cells, 65
saliva, 65
serous sacs, 65
urine, 65
excretion, renal, 59, 66
retardation, 67
nephritis, 67
blood bacteriostatic, assay, 67
oliguria, 67
p-aminohippuric acid, 67
urinary antiseptic, 66
Proteus vulgaris, 66
Str. faecalis, 66
instability, acid solution, in, 59
Staph. aureus, standard H strain, 61
therapeutic effect, prolongation of, 67
absorption, delayed, 68
methods of effecting, 68
adrenaline, 68
glucose, 68
Neo-synephrine hydrochloride, 68
oily suspension, 68
subcutaneous injection, 68
excretion, delayed, 67
benzoic acid, 68
diodrast, 67
p-aminohippuric acid, 67
toxic effects, 70
animals, 71
man, 71
central nervous system, 72
brain, 72
cauda equina, 72
convulsions, 72
lateral ventricle, 72
meningeal irritation, 72
fever, 72
Herxheimer reaction, 72
pain, 72
procaine hydrochloride, 72

Pharmacology—*continued*
toxic effects—*continued*
man—*continued*
sensitization, 73
chance inhalation, 73
dermatitis, 73
urticaria, 73
site, inflammation at, 72
chemical change, 72
effusion, 72
thrombophlebitis, 72
Pharmacy, 46
dispensing, 50
regulations governing, 47
general considerations, 46
Therapeutic Substances Act, 46
injections, 50, 51
aseptic precautions, 52
bacteriostatic level, 50
inactivation, 52
Injection of Penicillin B.P., 51
intrathecal, 52
Oily Injection of Penicillin B.P., 52
parenteral, 50, 51
properties, 47
activity, 47
bactericidal, 47
compatibility, 49
alcohols, 50
antiseptics, 49
cysteine, 50
drugs, 50
emulsifying waxes, 50
glycerin, 50
heavy metal ions, 48, 50
sulphonamides, 49
decomposition, 48
acids, 48
alkalis, 48
inactivation, 48
metallic ions, 48
*p*H, 48
resistance, 48
excretion, 47
stability, 48
factors influencing, 48
autoclaving, 49
buffers, 49
hygroscopicity, 49
moisture, 48
penicillinase, 48
*p*H, 48, 49
purity, 48
rancidity, 49
solutions, 49
suspensions, 49
temperature, 48
storage, 48
thermolability, 47
topical use, 52
cream, penicillin and Phenoxetol, 55
eye drops, 56
inhalations, 57

Pharmacy—*continued*
  topical use—*continued*
    lamellae, 56
    Lozenge of Penicillin B.P., 56
    Oculentum Penicillini B.P., 56
    Ointment of Penicillin B.P., 55
    Penicillin Cream B.P., 54
    powder, insufflation, 57
    spray solutions, 57
    Sterilized Penicillin Cream B.P., 53
    snuff, 57
    tablets, 56
Pharyngitis, 357
  acute and chronic, 357
Pleural effusion and empyemata, 358
Pneumococcus, 276
Pneumonia, 69, 143
  lobar, 357
Prophylactic use, 105
  bacteriology, 108
  carriers, 105
    hospitals, in, 105
      maternity, in, 105
      pastilles in, 105
      sprays in, 105
  civil practice, 113
    application to, 113
    treatment, 114
      dosage, 114
      Eudrip III apparatus, 114
      methods, 114
      parenteral, 106, 114
    wounds in, 113
      anaerobic organisms causing, 113
      minor, 113
      potentially infected, 113
      powder in, 113
        sulphonamides as diluents in, 114
  diphtheria, 105
  hospitals, 106
    maternity, in, 106
      labour following, in, 106
    wards, 106
      operations, following, in, 106
  infections, 105
    airborne, 105
      lozenges in, 105
      pastilles in, 105
    categories of, 112
    epidemic, 105
  proflavine, 113
  Sulphamezathine, 112
  sulphathiozole, 112, 113
  sulphonamides, 105
  venereal diseases, 105
    resistant strains in, 105
  wounds (*see also* civil practice), 106
    war, 106
      infection, materials harbouring, 109
      methods, 107
      sulphanilamide, 111
      sulphonamides, 111
Prophylactic use—*continued*
  wounds—*continued*
    war—*continued*
      surgery, primary, 107
      treatment, 107
        dosage, 107
        methods, 107
        time-distance factor, 109, 110
Puerperal sepsis, 130, 246
Purification, 26
  chromatography by, 26
  partition by, 26
Pyaemia, 256
Pyelitis, 262
Pylephlebitis, acute, 235
Pyorrhoea, 325
Pyothorax, tuberculous, 146

Quinsy, 309, 357

Reactions, 323
Rhinitis, 356
  acute, 356
  chronic, 356
Ringworm, 317

Salpingitis, 249
  gonococcal, acute, 280
  gonococcal, chronic, 280
Salpingo-oopharitis, 249
Scabies, 321
Scarlet fever, 306
Seborrhoea of scalp, 320
Sensitization, 73
Sepsis neonatorum, 252
  general considerations, 252
    bacteriology, 252
      coliform organisms, 252
      Staph. aureus, 252
      streptococci, 253
    clinical manifestations, 253
      diarrhoea and vomiting, 253
      eye infections, 253
      meningitis, 253
      nasopharyngitis, 253
      otitis media, 253
      pericarditis, 253
      pneumonia, 253
      pyelitis, 253
      septicaemia, 253
      skin sepsis, 253
      tetanus, 253
      thrush, 253
      umbilical infection, 253
    infections, incidence of, 252
      portal of entry of, 253
        alimentary tract, 253
        skin, 253
        umbilicus, 253
        upper respiratory tract, 253
  specific diseases, 254
    congenital syphilis, 259
    lung infections, 255
    meningitis, 261
    nasopharyngitis, 254
    ophthalmia neonatorum, 254
    otitis media, 255

Sepsis neonatorum—*continued*
specific diseases—*continued*
pyelitis, 262
septicaemia and pyaemia, 256
septic arthritis and osteomyelitis, 257
septic parotitis, 257
skin sepsis, 256
stomatitis, 262
tetanus, 258
umbilical sepsis, 255
treatment, general principles, 262
administration, methods of, 263
cream, 264
eye drops, 264
local, 263
systemic, 263
vapour, 264
dosage, 262
Sepsis, postoperative, 248
Septicaemia, 256
Sinusitis, 126, 356
acute, 356
chronic, 356
Skin, 182
grafts and skin losses, 182
flaps, full thickness, 184
granulating areas, treatment of, 183
Eusol in, 183
trypsin in, 183
sepsis, 256
Stability, 25
*p*H in, 25
studies of, 25
various solvents in, 25
Stomatitis, 262, 358
necrotic, acute, Vincent's, 326
Sulphadiazine, 144
Sulphamezathine, 144
Sulphathiazole, 351
Sulphonamides, 142, 351
hypersensitivity to, 351
sulphathiazole, 351
Sycosis barbae, 320, 359
Syphilis (*see* Venereal Diseases)
congenital, 259
prenatal, 242

Tabes dorsalis, 287
Tendons, 189
Tetanus, 258
Thoracic surgery, major, 159
bronchial carcinoma, in, 159
pneumonectomy in, 159
Thrombophlebitis, 72
Thrombosis, 272
intracranial, 272
sinus, 272
cavernous, 272
lateral, 273
Tonsillitis, 306, 309, 357
acute, 357
chronic recurrent, 357
Trachoma, 296
Tubercle bacillus, 142, 317
Tuberculosis, surgical, 198

Ulceration, 326, 327
buccal mucosa, of, 327
Ulcers, 359
idolent, 359
static, 359
traumatic, 359
varicose, 321, 359
Umbilical sepsis, 255
Urethritis, 358
non-gonococcal, 282
Urticaria, generalized, 73
syphilis, in treatment, 285

Venereal diseases, 278
chancroid, 289
gonorrhoea, 278
chancre, primary, in, 279
complications of, 279
endocarditis, 281
local, 280
females, in, 280
abscess, 280
bartholinitis, acute, 280
salpingitis, 280
acute, 280
chronic, 280
blood sedimentation rate in, 280
vulvovaginitis, 280
non-gonococcal, 280
males, in, 279
epididymitis, acute, 280
prostatitis, 279
acute, coliform organisms in, 279
chronic, vesical irrigations in, 279
metastatic, 280
arthritis, acute and chronic, 280
iritis, 280
"rheumatism", 281
Ps. aeruginosa in, 281
concurrent with syphilis, 279
injection, subcutaneous, in, 279
magnesium sulphate in, 279
oil-wax suspension in, 278
ethyl oleate in, 278
proof of cure of, 281
granuloma venereum, 289
lymphogranuloma inguinale, 289
syphilis, 282
cardiovascular, 287
Herxheimer reaction in, 287
chancre, 279
intra-urethral, 282
primary, with gonorrhoea, 279
congenital, 288
infantile, 288
Herxheimer reaction in, 288
marasmic children with, 288
late, 288
combined treatment of, 289
interstitial keratitis in, 288, 297
oil-wax suspension in, 289
dosage of penicillin in, 283

Venereal diseases—*continued*
  syphilis—*continued*
    late, 286
      Herxheimer reaction in, 286
      cerebrospinal fluid, examination of, 286
    latent, 286
      bismuth in treatment of, 286
      cerebrospinal fluid in, 286
      cutaneous conditions in, 287
      diagnosis of, 286
      larynx, 287
      liver, 287
        ascites, resulting in, 287
      mucocutaneous conditions, 287
      osseous conditions, 287
    neoarsphenamine in, 283
    neurosyphilis, 285, 287
      asymptomatic, 285, 288
        exclusion of, 285
      cerebrospinal fluid in, 284, 287
      general paralysis of insane, 288
      injections, intrathecal in, 288
      lightning pains, 287
      meningovascular, acute, 287
        Herxheimer reaction in, 287
      optic atrophy, primary, 287
      tabes dorsalis in, 287
    treatment, 284
      cerebrospinal fluid during, 284
      combined, schedules of, 283, 284
        synergistic action of, 283, 284
      follow-up of, 284
      oil-wax suspension in, 284
      primary syphilis, 284
      reactions to, 285
        adenitis, 285
        erythema, generalized, 285
        Herxheimer, 285
        pyrexia, 285
        toxicodermal, 285
        urticaria, generalized, 285
      secondary, 284
        combined schedules of, 284
  urethritis, non-gonococcal, 282
    staphylococci present in, 282
Vincent's angina, 126, 309, 358
Vulva, infections of, 251
Vulvovaginitis, non-gonococcal, 280

Warts, 317
Weil's disease, 125, 236
Wounds and gas gangrene, 162
  anaerobic myositis, 171
    bacteriology, 177
      Cl. oedematiens, 177
      Cl. perfringens, 177
    causes, predisposing, 176
    incidence, 177
      factors influencing, 178, 179
    mortality, 177
    surgery, 173
      clostridial myositis, 173
        treatment, 173

Wounds and gas gangrene—*continued*
  anaerobic myositis—*continued*
    surgery—*continued*
      devitalized tissue, 173
      drainage, 173
      nutrition, state of, 174
      primary, 173, 174
      prophylaxis, 173
        drugs, 174
        gas gangrene antitoxin, 174
        serum, 174
        sulphonamides, 174
      tension, 173
      time factor, 174
    therapy, 174
      civil practice, 179
      drugs, 174
      gas gangrene antitoxin, 175
        dosage, 175
      serum, 174
      sulphonamides, 175
    wounds, 176
      parts affected, 176
      types, 176
  wounds, 162
    classification, 164
    summary, 170
      civil practice, 170
        administration methods, 171
        contamination, 171
        dosage, 171
        laceration, 171
          dosage, 171
        minor wounds, 171
        powder, 171
    therapeutic applications, 162
      closure, 163
        methods, 163
          grafting, 163, 171
          partial, 163
          plastic, 163, 171
          time-distance factor, 168, 171
        sutures, 163
          definition, 163
          delayed primary, 163
          primary, 163, 171
          secondary, 163
      convalescence, 163
      cosmetic results, 163
      prophylaxis, 162, 171
    treatment, 164
      dosage, 165
      injection, local, 165
      insufflation, 165
      Nuflav, 169
      parenteral, 165
      research investigation, 166
      results, 166 (*see* Tables I and II)
        failure, causes, 170
      sulphonamides, 165
      surgical methods, 164
Wrist and carpus, 227
  arthritis, infective, of, 227